Modification of Radiosensitivity in Cancer Treatment

Modification of Radiosensitivity in Cancer Treatment

EDITED BY

Tsutomu Sugahara

Kyoto National Hospital
Kyoto, Japan

1984

ACADEMIC PRESS, INC.

(Harcourt Brace Jovanovich, Publishers)

Tokyo   Orlando   San Diego   San Francisco   New York
London   Toronto   Montreal   Sydney   São Paulo

ACADEMIC PRESS JAPAN, INC.
Hokoku Bldg. 3-11-13, Iidabashi, Chiyoda-ku, Tokyo 102

United States Edition published by ACADEMIC PRESS, INC.
Orlando, Florida 32887

United Kingdom Edition published by ACADEMIC PRESS, INC. (LONDON) LTD.
24/28 Oval Road, London NW1   7DX

Library of Congress Cataloging in Publication Data

Main entry under title:

Modification of radiosensitivity in cancer treatment.

    Includes index.
    1. Cancer--radiotherapy. 2. Radiation-sensitizing
agents. I. Sugahara, Tsutomu. Date. [DNLM: 1. Radiation
protection--Methods. 2. Neoplasms--Radiotherapy.
3. Radiation tolerance. 4. Radiation-sensitizing agents.
WN 650 M692]
RC271.R3M594 1983   616.99'40642   83-11858
ISBN 0-12-676020-9

PRINTED IN THE UNITED STATES OF AMERICA

84 85 86 87   9 8 7 6 5 4 3 2 1

Contents

PART THREE   Hypoxic Cell Sensitizers

7. A New Hypoxic-Cell Radiosensitizer Containing the Oxidized Sulfur Group instead of the Nitro Group: 2-Mercaptoimidazole Derivatives
Seiichi Inayama and Tomoyuki Mori

8. Design, Synthesis, and Activity of New Hypoxic-Cell Sensitizers: Spermine and Spermidine Amides Having Nitro Groups
Eiichi Fujita and Tomoyuki Mori

9. Anoxic Cell Radiosensitization Induced by Heterocyclic Compounds
Eiichi Kano, Susumu Tsubouchi, Takashi Kondo, Michi Inui, Shinji Yoshikawa,
and Masayo Furukawa

PART FOUR   *Biological Sensitization*

14. Repair of DNA Damage Induced by Ionizing Radiation in Ataxia Telangiectasia Cells and Potentially Lethal Damage Repair Inhibitors

Tsuneo Kada, Tadashi Inoue, Akiko Yokoiyama, Hajime Mochizuki, Shigekazu Nakatsugawa, and Tsutomu Sugahara

15. Radiation Sensitivity and Intracellular cAMP

Takashi Aoyama, Hiroshi Kimura, and Toshiko Yamada

Contents

PART SIX   Cellular Radiosensitivity and Its Mechanisms

24.   Radiosensitivity, DNA Repair, and DNA Replication in Cells Derived from Patients with Ataxia Telangiectasia

Osamu Nikaido, Masami Watanabe, and Tsutomu Sugahara

25.   Physical Modification of Thermal Neutron-Induced Biological Effects

Yowri Ujeno

26.   Radiosensitivities in Acute and Late Effects on Human Cells

Sadayuki Ban

Contributors

Numbers in parentheses indicate the pages on which the authors' contributions begin.

Mitsuyuki Abe (177, 365), Department of Radiology, Faculty of Medicine, Kyoto University, Kyoto 606, Japan

Takashi Aoyama (265), Department of Experimental Radiology, Shiga University of Medical Science, Otsu 520-21, Japan

Sadayuki Ban[1] (487), Department of Pathology and Clinical Laboratories, Radiation Effects Research Foundation, Hiroshima 730, Japan

J. Martin Brown (139), Division of Radiobiology Research, Department of Radiology, Stanford University School of Medicine, Stanford, California 94305

M. Edgren (13), Department of Tumor Biology II, Karolinska Institute Medical School, 104 01 Stockholm, Sweden

Eiichi Fujita (121), Institute for Clinical Research, Kyoto University, Kyoto 611, Japan

Masayo Furukawa (129, 439), Department of Anatomy, School of Medicine, Osaka City University, Osaka 545, Japan

Shin-ichiro Heki (335), Department of Radiation Biology, Kyoto College of Pharmacy, Kyoto 607, Japan

Masahiro Hiraoka (365), Department of Radiology, Faculty of Medicine, Kyoto University, Kyoto 606, Japan

Seiichi Inayama (109), School of Medicine, Keio University, Tokyo 160, Japan

Tadashi Inoue (251), Department of Induced Mutation, National Institute of Genetics, Mishima, 411, Japan

Michi Inui (129, 439), Department of Experimental Radiology and Health Physics, Fukui Medical University, School of Medicine, Fukui 910-11, Japan

Tsuneo Kada (251), Department of Induced Mutation, National Institute of Genetics, Mishima 411, Japan

Tsutomu Kagiya (85), Department of Hydrocarbon Chemistry, Faculty of Engineering, Kyoto University, Kyoto 606, Japan

Eiichi Kano (129, 335, 439), Department of Experimental Radiology and Health Physics, Fukui Medical University School of Medicine, Fukui 910-11, Japan

[1]Present address: Biology Department, Brookhaven National Laboratory, Upton, Long Island, New York 11973.

Hirokazu Kato (315), Department of Radiology, Shimane Medical University, Izumo 693, Japan

Hiroshi Kimura (265), Department of Experimental Radiology, Shiga University of Medical Science, Otsu 520-21, Japan

Takashi Kondo (129, 439), Department of Experimental Radiology and Health Physics, Fukui Medical University, School of Medicine, Fukui 910-11, Japan

Ashok Kumar (45), Bio-Science Department, H. P. University Summer-Hill, Simla 171005, India

Clara Yukie Mitsutani (291), Laboratory of Radiation Biology, Department of Zoology, Faculty of Science, Kyoto University, Kyoto 606, Japan

Junji Miyakoshi (335, 439), Department of Radiation Biology, Kyoto College of Pharmacy, Kyoto 607, Japan

Hajime Mochizuki (251), Department of Induced Mutation, National Institute of Genetics, Mishima 411, Japan

Tomoyuki Mori (109, 121), Department of Radiation Oncology, School of Medicine, Tokai University, Kanagawa 259-11, Japan

Hiroji Nagata (31), Kyoto National Hospital, Kyoto 612, Japan

Toshifumi Nakajima (381), Department of Radiology, Osaka City University Medical School, Osaka 545, Japan

Shigekazu Nakatsugawa[2] (221, 251), Department of Experimental Radiology, Faculty of Medicine, Kyoto University, Kyoto 606, Japan

Osamu Nikaido (351, 463), Division of Radiation Biology, Faculty of Pharmaceutical Sciences, Kanazawa University, Kanazawa 920, Japan

T. Nishidai[3] (13), Department of Tumor Biology II, Karolinska Institute Medical School, 104 01 Stockholm, Sweden

Sei-ichi Nishimoto (85), Department of Hydrocarbon Chemistry, Faculty of Engineering, Kyoto University, Kyoto 606, Japan

Ohtsura Niwa (291, 523), Department of Experimental Radiology, Faculty of Medicine, Kyoto University, Kyoto 606, Japan

Koji Ono (177), Department of Radiology, Faculty of Medicine, Kyoto University, Kyoto 606, Japan

Yasuto Onoyama (195, 381), Department of Radiology, Osaka City University Medical School, Osaka 545, Japan

L. Révész (13), Department of Tumor Biology II, Karolinska Institute University Medical School, 104 01 Stockholm, Sweden

Tsutomu Sugahara (3, 31, 251, 351, 463), Kyoto National Hospital, Kyoto 612, Japan

[2]Present address: Radiation Oncology Research Laboratory, CED-200, UCSF, San Francisco, California 94143.

[3]Present address: Department of Radiology, Faculty of Medicine, Kyoto University, Kyoto 606, Japan.

Yoshimasa Tanaka (61), Department of Radiology, Kansai Medical University, Moriguchi 750, Japan

Takeshi Todo (291), Laboratory of Radiation Biology, Department of Zoology, Faculty of Science, Kyoto University, Kyoto 606, Japan

Susumu Tsubouchi (129, 439), Department of Experimental Radiology and Health Physics, Fukui Medical University, School of Medicine, Fukui 910-11, Japan

Masashi Tsumura (381), Department of Radiology, Osaka City University Medical School, Osaka 545, Japan

Raymond U (415), Department of Radiology, Duke University and V.A. Medical Centers, Durham, North Carolina 27710

Yowri Ujeno (477), Department of Experimental Radiology, Faculty of Medicine, Kyoto University, Kyoto 606, Japan

Takeshi Wada[4] (85), Department of Hydrocarbon Chemistry, Faculty of Engineering, Kyoto University, Kyoto 606, Japan

Masami Watanabe (351, 463), Division of Radiation Biology, Faculty of Pharmaceutical Sciences, Kanazawa University, Kanazawa 920, Japan

Li-Hui Wei (523), Department of Gynecology and Obstetrics, People's Hospital of Peking Medical College, Peking, China

Boyd T. Worde (415), Department of Radiology, Duke University and V.A. Medical Centers, Durham, North Carolina 27710

Toshiko Yamada (265), Department of Experimental Radiology, Shiga University of Medical Science, Otsu 520-21, Japan

Akiko Yokoiyama (251), Department of Induced Mutation, National Institute of Genetics, Mishima 411, Japan

Shuji Yonei (291), Laboratory of Radiation Biology, Department of Zoology, Faculty of Science, Kyoto University, Kyoto 606, Japan

Shinji Yoshikawa (129, 439), Department of Experimental Radiology and Health Physics, Fukui Medical University, School of Medicine, Fukui 910-11, Japan

---

[4]Present address: Osaka University of Economics and Law, Osaka 581, Japan.

Preface

Radiosensitivity and its modification have been studied both *in vitro* and in animal systems for the past 30 years. However, for modification of sensitivity to be of use in cancer therapy, there must be a differential effect on malignant and normal tissues. In this volume, attention is directed to physical, chemical, and biological means of achieving such a differential effect. Particular attention is paid to some of the more recent advances that have potential for application in cancer treatment, such as the use of radiosensitizers to enhance the cytotoxicity of various anticancer drugs to tumors, the use of inhibitors of potentially lethal damage, and the development of hyperthermia. These and other new approaches to cancer treatment are being vigorously pursued in various laboratories throughout the world.

This volume deals with molecular, cellular, and animal aspects of the modification of radiosensitivity as well as with some of the many clinical trials being conducted. The studies clearly demonstrate the close cooperation between radiobiologists and radiotherapists in the search for effective, life-preserving treatments for cancer; they should provide the researcher with much important current and background material.

I extend my sincere thanks to all the contributors who provided the chapters for this volume and to my colleagues who have honored me by making the publication of this book possible. Special gratitude is extended to Drs. Y. Ujeno and O. Niwa and to M. Ohara for compilation and preliminary editing of the manuscripts.

T. Sugahara

PART ONE

General Review

1 History and Perspectives

Tsutomu Sugahara

Kyoto National Hospital
Kyoto 612, Japan

I. Introduction

A hypothesis on cellular radiosensitivity was formulated by Bergonié and Tribondeau (1906) from the response of seminiferous tubules in rats to radiation: that X rays are more effective on cells with a greater reproductive capacity, an extended dividing life span, and the least fixed morphology and function. Thus, it was assumed that cancer cells have a greater radiosensitivity than normal cells.

The success achieved in treating superficial tumors with X-ray therapy led to its use in treating deep-seated tumors. Early radiobiological studies emphasized protection of the skin, which was exposed to a higher radiation dose than the tumor. Protraction and fractionation were rationalized by Regaud (1922) and Strandqvist (1944) to improve the selective effects of radiation in destroying proliferating tumor cells while protecting the skin. Conventional radiotherapy techniques are based on these proposals with some modifications for practical working conditions.

Since the description by Howard and Pelc (1953) of the principal phases of the intermitotic cycle, cell cycle analyses using radioactive labeling have been adapted to normal and malignant cells. Work such as that of Steel (1977) made it clear that reproductive activity of tumor tissue is not always higher than that in normal tissue such as intestinal mucosa and bone marrow. Furthermore, the colony formation method in cultured mammalian cells developed by Puck and Marcus (1955, 1956) demonstrated that cancer cells are no more radiosensitive than normal cells.

Modification of Radiosensitivity in Cancer Treatment

These results clearly indicated that the hypothesis of Bergonié and Tribondeau could not be applied to all tumors. Furthermore, the introduction of *in vivo* colony assay revealed that some tumor cells *in situ* were more radioresistant than normal clonogenic cells. Since the mid-1950s, radiobiologists have been attempting to improve tumor radiotherapy by radiosensitizing cells, possibly tumor cells selectively.

The use of hyperbaric oxygen or bromodeoxyuridine for radiosensitization of tumors has failed to obtain full support by radiotherapists; therefore considerable attention has been directed to high-LET radiations such as fast neutrons and π mesons. The high-LET radiations introduced for their low oer (oxygen enhancement ratio) have other beneficial features for tumor therapy, that is, low repair and low age dependencies. Encouraged by success with high-LET radiations, scientists have extensively studied the modification of cellular radiosensitivity by chemical (sensitizers) as well as physical (hyperthermia) means. These new modalities are experimentally effective for sensitizing tumor cells, not only in case of ionizing radiation but also with some antitumor drugs. The development of and prospects for these new aspects of cancer treatment are discussed in this book by the relevant specialists.

II. Radiosensitization in the Past

Radiosensitization using Synkavit was first reported by Mitchell (1953); however, this drug was not introduced for radiotherapy because it sensitized various types of cells *in vivo*. The first drug used for cancer therapy was 5-bromodeoxyuridine (BrdU), first reported in 1960 by Djordjevic and Szybalski. This compound sensitizes cells to ionizing radiation, probably by the distortion of the molecular structure, under conditions of which Br replaces methyl in the thymidine bases. BrdU sensitizes tissue with a high cell proliferation rate, that is, some tumors and the normal mucosa of the G.I. tract. Brain tumors have been selectively sensitized, because the normal tissues are protected by the blood–brain barrier. Head and neck tumors have also been treated by intraarterial infusion of BrdU, but its clinical use has been limited by both radiosensitization of the surrounding normal tissue and carcinogenicity.

Since the first trial by Churchill-Davidson and Foster (1966), hyperbaric oxygen has been used extensively to evaluate the effectiveness of improved oxygen tension in a tumor exposed to radiotherapy. Although improved effectiveness has been reported, hyperbaric oxygen treatment is generally not recommended because improvement has not been adequate, despite expensive, troublesome, and sometimes risky procedures.

Even hyperbaric treatment does not increase oxygen tension of tumor tissue sufficiently to cause a radiosensitivity that results from a large consumption of oxygen by the hypoxic tissue.

Unlike radiosensitization, chemical radioprotection has a long history, since Patt *et al.* (1949) demonstrated that mice were protected against ionizing radiation by cysteine. Clinical applications of this phenomenon to radiotherapy have only recently been actively studied. Only in Japan (Sugahara, 1973) has protection against leukopenia of patients on radio- therapy by 2-mercaptopropionylglycine been investigated. In work by Yuhas and Storer (1969), differential protection of normal tissue versus tumors was noted with application of WR-2721.

Radiosensitization in hypoxic cells by membrane-binding drugs has also been reported. Shenoy and Singh (1980) found that chlorpromazine hy- drochloride radiosensitized sarcoma 180A in Swiss mice. Yau and Kim (1980) demonstrated that local anesthetics such as procaine and lidocaine are hypoxic radiosensitizers, oxic radioprotectors, and potentiators of hyperthermic killing in murine L-5178Y cells. In the field of cancer che- motherapy, Medoff *et al.* (1974, 1981) and Akiyama *et al.* (1980) reported that various polyenes such as amphotericin B and vitamin A enhanced the cytotoxicity of various antitumor drugs. Tsuruo *et al.* (1981) demon- strated that verapamil (an antiarrhythmic) increased the effect of vincris- tine in p338 leukemia cells. In case of membrane-binding drugs, their effect may differ depending on cell type, as demonstrated in the report by Yonei *et al.* (Chapter 16, this volume). For example, when applied to L- 5178Y cells, lidocaine had a radiosensitizing effect in hypoxic cells and radioprotective effects in oxic cells but no effect in HeLa cells and only intermediate effects in L-1210 cells.

III. High-LET Radiation in Radiotherapy

In development of modern radiotherapy of refractory tumors, the con- tribution of high-LET radiations, from fast neutrons to π mesons, has been invaluable. Clinical trials of fast-neutron radiotherapy have been carried out in Europe, North America, and Japan. Improved dose distri- bution in deep-seated tumors, not only physically but also in the sense of biologically effective doses, is one of the main benefits of high-LET radia- tions such as heavy ions and π mesons. Although fast neutrons widely used for high-LET radiations have no greater dose distribution than do conventional X rays, biologically, these neutrons do have beneficial fea- tures in common with heavy ions or π mesons, that is, low oer, low repair, and low age response. In the beginning, high-LET radiations were introduced to radiotherapy to attack hypoxic cells in a tumor, on the assumption that these cells were the cause of radioresistance and recurrence because of their low oer. Later biological studies revealed other features of high-LET radiations assumed to be beneficial for radiotherapy. The influence on oxygen effects, the extent of repair, and the age response seem to differ with various high-LET radiations. Although most radiation oncologists still insist on the importance of low oer in high-LET radiotherapy, the role of repair and age response remains to be determined.

As outlined in the present book, there are now other methods of modifying the oxygen effect, repair, and age response. Hypoxic cell sensitizers, repair inhibitors, and hyperthermia are being applied. These new modalities should contribute not only to the improvement of radiotherapy of refractory tumors but also to analyses of radioresistance and recurrence of these tumors. Furthermore, their greater availability the world over should greatly enhance cancer treatments.

IV. Specificities of Cancer Cells

Radio-, chemo-, hormone, and immunotherapies depend on biological characteristics unique to cancer cells as opposed to normal cells. These biological features include the following: hypoxia, low pH, cell kinetics, high repair capacity, membrane structure, antigenicity, and other genetic and/or epigenetic and unknown features. These characteristics are arranged roughly in the order of (1) circumstantial to intrinsic, (2) verified to speculative, and (3) general and specialized. Often scientists in chemotherapy are more interested in looking for something unknown than in screening for chemicals that modify cells with more established and general characteristics. Immunotherapy based on still unproven specific antigenicity of cancer cells has attracted the attention of many oncologists. Recent studies on biological characteristics of cancer cells have indicated that their inter- as well as intratumor variability may relate to the therapeutic results. Individualization may become a prerequisite for this type of cancer therapy.

Radiobiologists prefer generalized methods, and efforts have been made to screen agents that are generally effective. Stimulated by the results of chemical modification of radiosensitivity related to oxygen tension, repair, or age response, analysis of antitumor chemicals on these cellular conditions has also been carried out. Effects of most cytotoxic chemicals depend on cell kinetics, because the cytotoxicity is based on either particular molecular damage or disturbance in the metabolism. For low-LET radiations, radioresistance of hypoxic cells has been considered the most important factor in radiotherapy. The cytotoxicity of some chemicals depends on oxygenation of cells; however, no clear relationship between chemicals and hypoxia in tumor treatment has been established. The repair of potentially lethal damage (PLD) after chemical treatment was seen in case of antitumor drugs such as bleomycin, adriamycin, ACNU, and Ara-C. Using PLD repair inhibitors, the differential cytotoxicity of tumor cells by anticancer drugs can be attained without modifying the chemical structure.

V. Concluding Remarks

In an attempt to bring about a closer cooperation among radiobiologists and clinical oncologists, I edited a book in collaboration with L. Révész and Sir Oliver Scott: *Fraction Size in Radiobiology and Radiotherapy* (1973). The main topic at that time was how to cope with hypoxia. There were numerous clinical trials on hyperbaric oxygen radiation therapy and fast-neutron therapy. Development of hypoxic cell sensitizers produced considerable interest.

Since that study was published, clinical trials of high-LET radiation therapy have been extended. In particular, experience using fast-neutron therapy has accumulated, and data on π-meson clinical trials have attracted the attention of oncologists and physicists. In 1975, I organized a research group supported by Research-in-Aid from the Ministry of Education, Science and Culture, Japan, on the modification of radiosensitivity for cancer treatment, mainly on hyperthermia and the drugs misonidazole and WR-2721. This group has expanded rapidly, and syntheses and *in vitro* screening of new hypoxic cell sensitizers have been carried out. The two inhibitors of PLD (potentially lethal damage) repair, Ara-A (β-arabinofuranosyladenine) and cordycepin (3'-deoxy-adenosine), were reported almost simultaneously by Iliakis (1980) and Nakatsugawa and Sugahara (1980). Iliakis (1981) extended the study on Ara-A to the analyses of PLD repair, while Nakatsugawa and Sugahara extended the study on cordycepin to the development of more stable and less toxic inhibitors and their application to cancer therapy (Sugahara and Nakatsugawa, 1981; Nakatsugawa and Sugahara, 1980; Nakatsugawa *et al.*, 1982).

Recent research and development of these physical and chemical means to modify radio- and chemosensitivity of tumor cells are ushering in a new era in cancer radio- and chemotherapy. This book should serve as a preliminary introduction to these new modalities.

References

Akiyama, S., Kuwano, M., Komiyama, S., and Saneyoshi, M. (1980). Antitumor effect of a combination of 6-methylthioinosine and amphetericin B on mouse leukemia L1210. *Cancer Lett.* **9**, 305–311.

Bergonié, J., and Tribondeau, L. (1959). Interpretation of some results of radiotherapy and an attempt at determining a logical technique of treatment. *Radiat. Res.* **11**, 587–588. (Originally published in 1906, *C. R. Hebd. Seances Acad. Sci.* **143**, 983–985).

Churchill-Davidson, C. A., and Foster, G. W. (1966). The place of oxygen in radiotherapy. *Br. J. Radiol.* **34**, 321–331.

Djordjevic, B., and Szybalski, W. (1960). Genetics of human cell lines. III. Incorporation of 5-brome- and 5-iodo-deoxyuridine into the deoxyribonucleic acid of human cells and its effect on radiation sensitivity. *J. Exp. Med.* **112**, 509–531.

Howard, A., and Pelc, S. R. (1953). Synthesis of deoxyribonucleic acid in normal and irradiated cells and its relation to chromosome breakage. *Heredity* (Suppl. 6), 261–273.

Iliakis, G. (1980). Effects of β-arabinofuranosyladenine on the growth and repair of potentially lethal damage in Ehrlich ascites tumor cells. *Radiat. Res.* **83**, 537–552.

Iliakis, G. (1981). Characterization and properties of repair of potentially lethal damage as measured with the help of β-arabinofuranosyladenine in plateau-phase EAT cells. *Radiat. Res.* **86**, 77–90.

Medoff, G., Valeriote, F., Lynch, R. G., Schlessinger, D., and Kobayashi, G. S. (1974). Synergistic effect of amphetericin B and 1.3-bis (2-chloroethyl)-1-nitrosourea against a transplantable AKR leukemia. *Cancer Res.* **34**, 974–978.

Medoff, G., Valeriote, F., and Dleckman, J. (1981). Potentiation of anticancer agents by amphetericine B. *J. Natl. Cancer Inst. (US)* **67**, 131–135.

Mitchell, J. S. (1953). Assessment of tetra-sodium-2-methyl-1 : 4-naphthohydroquinone diphosphate as a radiosensitizer in the radiotherapy of malignant tumors. *Br. J. Cancer* **7**, 313–328.

Nakatsugawa, S., and Sugahara, T. (1980). Inhibition X-ray-induced potentially lethal damage (PLD) repair by cordycepin (3'-deoxy-adenosine) and enhancement of its action by 2'-deoxycoformycin in Chinese hamster *hai* cells in the stationary phase *in vitro*. *Radiat. Res.* **84**, 265–278.

Nakatsugawa, S., Sugahara, T., and Kumar, A. (1982). Purine nucleoside analogues inhibit the repair or radiation-induced potentially lethal damage in mammalian cells in culture. *Int. J. Radiat. Biol.* **41**, 343–346.

Patt, H. M., Tyree, E. B., Straube, R. L., and Smith, D. E. (1949). Cysteine protection against X-irradiation. *Science (Washington, D.C.)* **110**, 213–214.

Puck, T. T., and Marcus, P. (1955). A rapid method of viable cell titration and clone production with HeLa cells in tissue culture: the use of X-irradiated cells to supply conditioning factors. *Proc. Natl. Acad. Sci. USA* **41**, 432–437.

Puck, T. T., and Marcus, P. (1956). Action of X-rays on mammalian cells. *J. Exp. Med.* **103**, 653–666.

Regaud, C. (1922). Influence de la durée d'irradiation sur les effets détérmines dans le testicule par le radium. *C. R. Seances Soc. Biol. Ses Fil.* **86**, 787–790.

Shenoy, M. A., and Singh, B. B. (1980). Cytotoxic and radiosensitizing effects of chlorpromazine hydrochloride in sarcome 180A. *Indian J. Exp. Biol.* **18**, 791–795.

Steel, G. G. (1977). "Growth Kinetics of Tumors." Oxford Univ. Press (Clarendon), Oxford.

Strandqvist, M. (1944). Studien über die kumulative Wirkung der Röntgenstrablen bei Fraktionierung. *Acta Radiol.* **55** (Suppl.), 1–293.

Sugahara, T. (1973). Possible application of chemical radioprotectors to radiotherapy. *In* "Fraction Size in Radiobiology and Radiotherapy" (T. Sugahara, L. Révész, and O. Scott), pp. 84–93. Igaku-Shoin, Tokyo.

Sugahara, T., and Nakatsugawa, S. (1981). Radiation sensitization studies in Japan. *Cancer Treat. Rep.* **8,** 51–61.

Tsuruo, T., Iida, H., Tsukagoshi, S., and Sakurai, Y. (1981). Overcoming of vincristine resistance in p388 leukemia *in vivo* and *in vitro* through enhanced cytotoxicity of vincristine and vinblastine by verapamil. *Cancer Res.* **41,** 1967–1972.

Yau, T. M., and Kim, C. C. (1980). Local anaesthetics as hypoxic radiosensitizers, oxic radioprotectors and potentiators of hyperthermic killing in mammalian cells. *Br. J. Radiol.* **53,** 687–692.

Yuhas, J. M., and Storer, J. B. (1969). Differential chemoprotection of normal and malignant tissues. *J. Natl. Cancer Inst. (US)* **42,** 331–335.

PART TWO

Chemical Protection

2 Mechanisms of Inherent Radioprotection in Mammalian Cells

L. Révész
M. Edgren
T. Nishidai

Department of Tumor Biology II
Karolinska Institute Medical School
Stockholm, Sweden

I. Introduction[1]

Much of the radiobiological research conducted in our department over the past two decades has been devoted to investigations of factors that determine the inherent radiosensitivity of cells. Our interest was focused on intrinsic cellular substances that possess radioprotective properties and may play a role in defining the overall radiosensitivity of cells. Our

---

[1] *Abbreviations:* AET, S-(2-aminoethyl)isothiouronium; DTT, dithiothreitol; GSH, glutathione; GSH$^-$, glutathione-deficient; GSH$^+$, glutathione-proficient; MEA, cysteamine; MISO, misonidazole; MN, micronucleus; MPG, mercaptopropionylglycine; NPSH, nonprotein-bound sulfhydryls; NPSS, non-protein-bound disulfides; ER, oxygen enhancement ratio; PSH, protein-bound sulfhydryls; PSSG, mixed disulfides of glutathione and protein; ssb, single-strand DNA breaks.

Modification of Radiosensitivity in Cancer Treatment

work was greatly influenced by investigations conducted by Dr. Sugahara, whose scientific interests are similar to ours in many respects. Many of our approaches were initiated by his considerations and experimental results, and his suggestions and comments aided greatly in developing many of our ideas and formulating our concepts. We feel that it is most appropriate to review the experimental studies done following the stimulus provided us by Dr. Sugahara. Besides summing up and discussing our investigations conducted over a 20-year period on different aspects of the inherent radioprotection in mammalian cells, observations recently obtained will also be included.

II. Chemical Radioprotection: Historical Remarks

One of the first reports that sulfur-containing chemicals can protect against radiation damage appeared in 1942 (Dale). Colloidal sulfur and thiourea were found to protect some enzymes against inactivation by X rays. In 1948 Latarjet and Ephrati reported that bacteriophages were effectively protected against radiation damage by thioglycolic acid, GSH, cysteine, and cystine. In 1949 Barron *et al.* provided evidence that radiation-induced inactivation of some SH-containing enzymes could be inhibited by GSH. The observation that cysteine treatment aided survival of irradiated rats was described in the same year (Patt *et al.*, 1949). In 1950 Chapman and Cronkite found that GSH protected mice from lethal radiation injury, and in 1951 (Bacq *et al.*) the protective effect of MEA on radiation survival of mice was demonstrated. Aminoalkylisothioureas were found to be effective radioprotective compounds in 1955 (Doherty and Burnett). Considerable efforts were made to develop potent chemical radioprotectors in the 1950s, but due to their low efficiency and/or toxicity, none of the compounds could be practically applied. Only two types of compounds have emerged with potential, practical usefulness. Thiola (2-mercaptopropionylglycine, MPG) was introduced in Japan as a chelating drug for the treatment of liver disease and mercury and lead poisoning, and has radioprotective properties with little or no side effects (Tanaka and Sugahara, 1970). Thiophosphate derivatives developed in the United States also appear promising and are now at the stage of clinical trials (Yuhas *et al.,* 1980).

III. Cellular Glutathione

Glutathione (γ-glutamylcysteinylglycine, GSH) is almost universally present in animal cells. In mammalian cells, it constitutes the dominant low molecular weight thiol-containing substance. Its synthesis is accomplished in two main steps: A peptide bond is first formed between glutamic acid and cysteine by the action of glutamylcysteine synthetase, and the product is then bound to glycine by the action of glutathione synthetase. Details of this synthesis through the γ-glutamyl cycle are being studied (Meister, 1973, 1981b). In mammalian tissues, GSH has a rapid metabolic turnover (Griffith and Meister, 1979a); for example, it has a half-life of 2 to 4 h in the liver (Douglas and Mortensen, 1956) and 50 to 90 h in erythrocytes (Edler and Mortensen, 1956). In most cases, about 5% of GSH is present in the oxidized form (GSSG) (Kosower and Kosower, 1974). The balance between the reduced and oxidized forms is maintained mainly by the action of two enzymatic systems involving glutathione peroxidase and glutathione reductase, but protein-bound GSH also probably plays an important role (Tietze, 1970; Eriksson, 1974).

Glutathione participates in many metabolic functions in mammalian cells (Kosower and Kosower, 1978; Meister, 1981a). It regulates the activity of several enzymes and is known to be the prosthetic group and cofactor in a number of enzymatic pathways. It plays an important role in cell growth and replication (Mazia, 1961) and functions as a detoxifying agent (Boyland and Chasseaud, 1969; Boyd et al., 1982). Diseases linked to a disturbed GSH metabolism include leukemias and anemias (Sabine, 1964; Macdougall, 1968), cataract of the lens (Beutler and Srivastava, 1974), and 5-oxoprolinuria (Larsson, 1981). In view of the numerous complex functions of GSH, the biological role of this compound is still a matter of intensive research.

IV. Cellular Radiosensitivity and Glutathione

Glutathione protects against radiation only moderately *in vivo* (Alexander et al., 1955) or in cellular experiments *in vitro* (Vergroesen et al., 1964). However, (Barron, 1952) it is equally efficient in protecting enzymes in solution against X-ray damage, as are compounds that have a protective effect in biological systems. This difference in the radioprotective capacity can be explained by the slow and difficult penetration of GSH through the cell membranes. We have shown (Modig and Révész, 1967) that ascites cells incorporate 10 times more MEA than GSH when treated with the compounds at equimolar concentrations.

In early work in which a number of cellular sublines with differing radiosensitivity derived from a serially irradiated Ehrlich ascites tumor were studied, chemical (Révész et al., 1963) and cytochemical (Caspersson and Révész, 1963) measurements indicated that the decreased sensitivity of some sublines was associated with a comparable increase of the level of non-protein-bound sulfhydryls (NPSH). No increase in the level of non-protein-bound disulfides (NPSS) or protein-bound SH groups (PSH) was observed in the radioresistant lines. It was also noted that the increased radioresistance of some sublines is evident only when the tissue is irradiated under anaerobic conditions, and only statistically insignificant variations of sensitivity between the different lines were noted when X-ray exposure took place in the presence of oxygen. The reduced sensitivities in the presence of oxygen are in fairly good agreement with observations (Dewey, 1963) that radiation protection by thiols is decreased or even disappears in an oxygenated medium. Under such conditions, oxygen is clearly present in an excess to cellular NPSH and, in line with the "competition hypothesis" (Alexander and Charlesby, 1955), the radiation damage in target molecules may be permanent. However, in the absence of oxygen or where oxygen is present only in a reduced concentration, cellular NPSH may, to an extent proportional to its concentration, repair radiation-induced target radicals by hydrogen donation. The validity of this consideration can be supported by such observations (Howard-Flanders, 1960) as that T2 bacteriophages were better protected by MEA from radiation inactivation when exposed under anoxic conditions.

Our observations of an association of radioresistance with increased cellular thiol levels were subsequently confirmed in studies using various biological materials. Thus, in a radioresistant mouse lymphoma cell line, the level of NPSH was increased in comparison to a related, radiosensitive line (Alexander *et al.*, 1965). The radiosensitivity of three bacterial strains was directly related to their total SH content (Bruce and Malcham, 1965). Similar observations were obtained using yeast cells (Brunborg, 1977). Radiosensitivity changes noted during the progression of mammalian cells through the cycle were also directly related to changes in NPSH levels, the radioresistant phases being associated with an increased NPSH content (Sinclair, 1969, Ohara and Terashima, 1970).

V. Intracellular Release of Glutathione

Whereas the free GSH content and its variation have been determined in different cell lines and with great accuracy, little quantitative information is available on the GSH bound to cellular proteins. We determined the cellular concentration of such mixed disulfides in Ehrlich ascites tumor cells after isolating the cellular proteins and reducing the disulfide bonds by treatment with sodium borohydride. Protein-bound GSH amounted to 60% of the cellular free GSH content and 35% of the total cellular GSH (Modig, 1968). Protein–GSH mixed disulfides (PSSG) have been subsequently found to occur in about the same proportion in the liver (Harisch and Schole, 1974) and other rat tissues (Harrap et al., 1973), and the lens (Harding, 1969; Beutler and Srivastava, 1974).

Little is known of the spatial distribution of the free or protein-bound GSH, although related information can be of particular importance for understanding the radiobiological role of the compound. Our studies indicated that histones obtained from Ehrlich ascites tumor cell nuclei were rich in thiol and disulfide groups. Evidence was obtained that at least two peptides, one being GSH, were bound to the nucleoproteins, as mixed disulfides (Modig, 1973).

Several enzymatic systems may regulate the interchange between free and protein-bound GSH, but the mechanisms of regulation are poorly understood (Tietze, 1970; Eriksson, 1974). We found that a considerable amount of GSH can be released intracellularly by treatment of cells with different thiols. Because our attention was directed to effects of radioprotectors, we used MEA, AET, MPG, and 5-mercaptopyridoxine, all known to have radioprotective properties, in these experiments (Modig and Révész, 1968; Modig et al., 1971; Révész et al., 1974). Treatment of the cells with these compounds resulted without exception in an increase of the cellular free GSH content. The increase varied specifically with the concentration of the particular compound used for treatment. Release of GSH from mixed disulfides with proteins in an exchange reaction with the particular radioprotective compound was put forward as an explanation for the GSH increase. Such thiol–disulfide interchange reactions apparently occur in biological systems (Gorin, 1965).

Support for this explanation has been obtained in different experimental tests. When ascites cells were labeled with [^{35}S]cysteine in vivo and subsequently exposed to unlabeled MEA in vitro, an intracellular increase of the ^{35}S-labeled GSH concentration occurred (Modig et al., 1971). This finding provides evidence that the MEA-mediated rise of the intracellular GSH concentration is of an intrinsic origin. In other experiments, ^{35}S-labeled MEA was used (Modig et al., 1971) to treat the ascites cells. After a lapse of time, about 40% of the incorporated MEA was bound to the cellular proteins. In comparing the amount of released GSH, the amount of protein-bound cysteamine was always in excess. The amount of protein-bound GSH was also present in quantities large enough to explain the observed GSH increase in the cells following MEA treatment.

In view of the radioprotective properties of GSH, and the increased concentration of the compound after treatment of cells with different radioprotectors (probably by the thiol–disulfide interchange reaction just proposed), it was suggested (Révész and Modig, 1965; Modig et al., 1971) that the action of various protectors is, at least in part, attributable to the capacity of these substances to raise the cellular GSH content. According to this concept, artificial radiation protection would act by enhancing the physiological protection afforded by endogenous GSH. This hypothesis finds particular support in observations made in experiments with two homologous compounds: 4-mercaptopyridoxine and 5-mercaptopyridoxine (Modig and Révész, 1968). The former compound lacks radioprotective action, whereas the latter increases the mean lethal radiation dose for mice by a factor of about 1.4. In testing the effect of the compounds on Ehrlich ascites cells in an *in vitro* system, we found that the protective substance raised the GSH level to a significantly greater degree (by >20%) than its homologue, even though the latter was incorporated into the cells in larger concentrations. The differential radioprotection afforded by these compounds is thus clearly associated with the difference in their capacity to induce an intracellular increase in concentrations of GSH.

VI. Mechanisms of Chemical Radioprotection

Various hypotheses have been put forward to explain the radioprotection afforded by some aminothiols. Thus, among other processes, the induction of anoxic conditions, the formation of mixed disulfides, radical scavenging, repair by hydrogen atom donation, change of membrane properties, modification of enzyme activities and different metabolic processes, and specific binding to DNA have all been considered, alone or in combination. Access to bacteria (Fuchs and Warner, 1975; Apontoweil and Berends, 1978) and human cell lines (Larsson, 1981) that are either almost totally deficient in GSH or have a reduced content of the compound provides new approaches to experimental tests of many of the hypotheses. Earlier studies in which the cellular content of GSH was reduced by treatment with different sulfhydryl-reactive agents, have proved useful in this type of test (Bridges, 1969; Harris and Power, 1973). However, because of irrelevant side effects of these agents (Harris and Biaglow, 1972), many of the observations have to be carefully considered. The GSH deficiency in the types of cells now used is due to a specific genetic defect in the activity of a particular enzyme, glutathione synthetase (Larsson, 1981). Our experiments were performed with different cell strains, homozygous or heterozygous, with regard to this defect. The cells were derived from blood samples or subcutaneous biopsies from patients with 5-oxoprolinuria, or from their close relatives with no clinical symptoms of the disease. In most of our work, untransformed fibroblast cultures derived from the biopsies were used. The homozygous cells had a

GSH level of about 6% of the level in GSH-proficient controls, whereas the level in the heterozygous cells was about 50%. In addition to GSH, a considerable amount of other non-protein-bound thiols were present in both the homozygous and heterozygous cell types, consisting of cysteine, γ-glutamylcysteine, and probably also some as yet unidentified thiols. In comparison to the controls, the total NPSH concentration was, however, decreased in both cases (about 50 and 70%, respectively) (Edgren *et al.*, 1981).

VII. Glutathione and the Oxygen Effect

As indicated in Section IV, the enhancement of radiosensitivity by oxygen (oxygen effect) is probably determined by competition between oxygen and cellular thiols for radiation-induced radicals in key targets. Glutathione-deficient (GSH⁻) cells are a particularly useful biological material for experimental tests of the competition hypothesis. A large series of such tests have been performed using the yield of single-strand DNA breaks (ssb), micronucleus (MN) frequency, and clonogenic survival as end points (Edgren *et al.*, 1980; Deschavanne *et al.*, 1981; Midander, 1983). Figure 1 illustrates the relationship between the cellular GSH content and the oxygen enhancement ratio (oer) for the induction of ssb. A clear correlation appears to exist between oer and GSH content, the enhancement of sensitivity being critically dependent on the GSH available. Because GSH⁻ cells have a considerable concentration of aminothiols other than GSH (cf. Section VI), the data in Fig. 1 suggest that GSH is specific for determining the enhancement of radiosensitivity by oxygen, and the role of other cellular aminothiols may be insignificant. The observations illustrated in Fig. 1 are thus in agreement with the competition hypothesis, with the reservation that GSH is a competing species of a particular significance, at least for the radiation damage expressed by ssb.

When MN frequency (Midander, 1983) or clonogenic survival (Deschavanne *et al.*, 1981) were the criteria chosen for the radiation effect, the relationship between oer and cellular GSH concentration was in a general agreement with that seen with ssb as end point. However, the oer calculated for the survival of GSH⁻ cells was, although close to unity, still significantly different with a value about 1.5. Because survival, in contrast to MN frequency and ssb, is determined several days after radiation exposure, it is conceivable that oer, in this case, will also reflect the influence of different postirradiation processes that may modify the result of the competition reactions occurring immediately after irradiation.

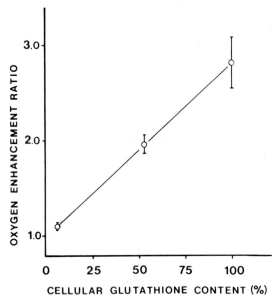

Fig. 1. Dependence of the oxygen enhancement ratio (oer) on the relative cellular glutathione content. Fibroblast cultures, homozygous or heterozygous with respect to glutathione synthetase deficiency, were used with a genetically related control cell strain that had normal enzyme activity. The oer was determined from the yield of ssb of the cells irradiated with different X-ray doses in the presence of oxygen or in oxygen-free argon. Means ±SE are presented, calculated from the data in Edgren *et al.* (1980, 1981); M. Edgren (unpublished).

VIII. Radioprotection of Glutathione-Deficient Cells by Exogenous Thiols

In a particular series of investigations, changes in the sensitivity of GSH⁻ cells were determined after treatment with some thiols known for their radioprotective effect. The tests made use of MEA, MPG, GSH, and DTT (dithiothreitol) (Edgren *et al.,* in press). Using ssb yield as the end point, dose-modifying factors were calculated that were always greater with exposure under anoxic conditions than when oxic conditions prevailed during irradiation. As a consequence, the oer for GSH⁻ cells, which was close to unity in the untreated cells (cf. Section VII), increased and had values varying from 2.8 (treatment with 20 mM GSH) up to 3.4 (treatment with 10 mM DTT). The comparable values for GSH⁺ controls were 5.1 and 5.6, respectively (M. Edgren, unpublished).

The observation that the protective effect was in all cases considerably greater under hypoxic exposure conditions—that is, the finding of an increased oer in the cells in which exogenous thiols substitute the missing

GSH—agrees with the expectation based on the competition model discussed earlier, although part of the effect may be due to a scavenging process. However, the finding that oer for the thiol-substituted GSH⁻ cells do not reach the values calculated for GSH⁺ cells treated in a similar manner suggests that none of the added exogenous thiols can fully replace endogenous GSH in the competition process. This conclusion also concerns exogenous GSH in considering the significantly lower oer = 2.8 calculated for GSH⁻ cells treated with 20 mM GSH in comparison to oer = 5.1 calculated for GSH⁺ cells treated with GSH in the same concentration. The more advantageous spatial distribution of the endogenous GSH, possibly in close contact with the critical radiation target (cf. Section V), as compared to the possibly less convenient localization of the incorporated GSH, may be one explanation.

Preliminary observations in experiments, in which the clonogenic radiation survival of GSH⁻ cells was studied after treatment with MEA, support the conclusion drawn from the experiments just described, in which ssb was used as the end point. Thus, oer for the MEA-treated GSH⁺ cells was considerably larger than for similarly treated GSH⁻ cells.

IX. Radiosensitization of GSH-Deficient Cells with Misonidazole

Both the survival (Midander *et al.,* 1982) and ssb (Révész *et al.,* 1979; Révész and Edgren, 1982) assays performed to test the effect of treatment of GSH⁻ cells with MISO were concordant in indicating that either no or only a slight sensitization by this compound occurred at 8–10 mM, concentrations that resulted in a sensitization of GSH⁺ cells by a factor about 2. This dependence on endogenous GSH of the sensitizing effect of MISO is similar to the GSH dependence on the oxygen effect, discussed earlier (cf. Section VII), and suggests a similar mechanism. Sensitization by MISO has indeed been considered as an oxygen mimic (Adams and Cooke, 1969) and as "equivalent" to sensitization by oxygen (Ling *et al.,* 1980). In view of the importance of endogenous GSH in the process, depletion of GSH noted after pretreatment of the cells with MISO (Varnes *et al.,* 1980) can also be considered contributory to the increased sensitization.

X. Postirradiation Repair

Studies conducted with GSH⁻ cells on the postirradiation rejoining of radiation-induced ssb revealed a repair function of endogenous GSH not heretofore recognized (Edgren *et al.*, 1981). When GSH⁻ cells were exposed to radiation under hypoxic conditions, practically all the induced ssb were gradually rejoined within about 1 h of aerobic incubation, independently of the dose of radiation. Similar observations were made with a great number of different GSH⁺ cells (Lohman, 1968; Ormerod and Stevens, 1970). In contrast, when irradiations were performed under aerobic conditions, GSH⁻ cells failed to repair a considerable part of the induced ssb during an identical incubation period. Thus, about 30% of the ssb remained unrejoined in the GSH⁻ cells, whereas in the GSH⁺ cells, rejoining was again practically complete (Fig. 2). The failure of GSH⁻ cells to repair ssb induced by aerobic irradiation as well as do the GSH⁺ cells, was confirmed in experiments in which the cells were exposed to a radiation dose split into two equal fractions, and given with an interval of either 30 or 60 min (T. Nishidai, M. Abe, M. Edgren, and L. Révész, unpublished). During the intervals, the cells were incubated aerobically to permit rejoining of ssb induced by the first dose fraction. The total number of ssb was determined immediately after the second fraction, thus preventing rejoining of ssb induced by the latter exposure. In agreement with the data presented in Fig. 2, Fig. 3 shows that GSH⁻ cells repaired a consistently smaller proportion of the radiation-induced ssb than did the GSH⁺ cells. The data presented in the two figures appear also to be in a

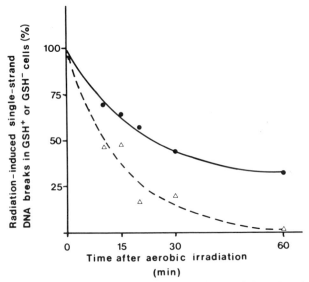

Fig. 2. Relative amount of radiation-induced ssb in GSH-proficient (△----△, GSH⁺) and GSH-deficient (●——●, GSH⁻) cells incubated for varying periods after aerobic irradiation. Means are illustrated calculated from the data in Edgren *et al.* (1981).

good quantitative agreement in demonstrating that the amount of repaired ssb after the fractionated doses was about half that found after irradiation with a single dose.

The deficient rejoining of a majority of aerobically induced ssb in GSH⁻ cells, demonstrated by these experiments, suggests that the activity of some of the enzymes involved in the repair of this particular radiation damage is dependent on GSH functioning, probably as a cofactor. The enzymes encountered in the repair of anaerobically induced damage do not show such dependence. This interpretation finds support in observations made in experiments in which GSH⁻ cells were treated with GSH, MPG, or DTT (Edgren *et al.*, 1981). After such treatment, the thiol-substituted GSH⁻ cells had the capacity to rejoin radiation-induced ssb to a fairly normal extent. Further support for the concept that the presence of GSH is essential for the rejoining of the particular aerobically induced ssb was obtained in experiments in which the irradiated GSH⁻ cells were admixed with unirradiated GSH⁻ or GSH⁺ cells, and incubated together for some time (Edgren, 1982). In the former case, the ssb rejoining capacity of the irradiated cells was not appreciably improved. In contrast,

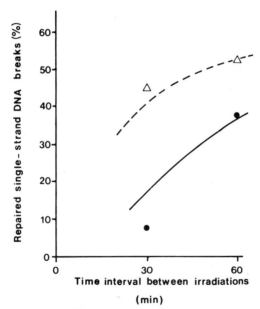

Fig. 3. The amount of ssb in GSH⁺ and GSH⁻ cells irradiated aerobically with 34 Gy split into two equal fractions, relative to the yield of ssb after irradiation with the total dose, at a single exposure. Symbols are as in Fig. 2. The time interval between the split doses was 30 or 60 min, during which period the cells were kept incubated [T. Nishidai, M. Abe, M. Edgren, and L. Révesz (unpublished)].

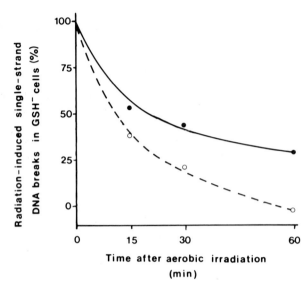

Fig. 4. Relative amount of radiation-induced ssb in GSH⁻ cells incubated for varying periods after aerobic irradiation and in the presence (upper line) of added buffer solution, unirradiated GSH⁻ cells, or misonidazole-pretreated, unirradiated GSH⁺ cells, or (lower line) added glutathione, unirradiated GSH⁺ cells, or unirradiated GSH⁻ cells pretreated with DTT. Means are presented from the data in Edgren *et al.* (1981); Edgren (1982, unpublished).

admixed GSH⁺ cells enhanced the rejoining capacity to a normal level (Fig. 4). This enhancement was inhibited, however, if GSH⁺ cells were pretreated with MISO, which decreased the GSH content to about 30% before admixture (M. Edgren, unpublished). In contrast, if the NPSH content of the unirradiated GSH⁻ cells was increased by pretreatment with DTT before admixture to the irradiated GSH⁻ cells, repair of ssb proceeded at a normal rate.

In addition to indicating the importance of NPSH and especially of GSH in the rejoining process, the experiments with the mixed cell cultures also provide evidence for a cooperation between the cells in repairing radiation damage. Such a cooperation has been considered to explain, at least in part, the increased radioresistance noted when cells were irradiated during contact with each other rather than when treated as separate units. Further experiments are in progress to test this possibility in other postirradiation repair processes such as the recovery from sublethal and potentially lethal damage.

XI. General Conclusions

Accumulated evidence, reviewed in this chapter, clearly indicates that endogenous GSH is involved in many radiation-induced chemical processes in cells, and thus represents an important factor in determining inherent cellular radiosensitivity. Participating in *radical processes,* GSH scavenges different radiation-induced radicals as well as repairing radiation-damaged key target molecules by hydrogen donation, in competition with oxygen, which may fix the damage irreversibly. Probably as a cofactor in some enzymatic reactions, GSH is also involved in some *biochemical repair processes,* in particular those leading to rejoining of ssb induced by aerobic irradiation. Glutathione may also be one of the substances exchanged between cells in close contact and may increase the resistance of cells to radiation by enhancing the repair of some radiation damage, especially in DNA. The processes in which GSH is involved can be intercepted by sulfhydryl-reactive radiation sensitizers such as MISO.

The role of GSH in these processes is largely specific and can be shared to only a minor degree by other aminothiols. This may be a result of the particular efficiency of glutathione in some radical reactions, at least with OH· radicals, in which case one carbon-centered radical is formed in addition to the sulfur-centered radical (Sjöberg *et al.,* 1982). The specificity may also be attributed to the particular spatial distribution of GSH, particularly in nucleoproteins in close contact with key target molecules.

The information available on the particular role of GSH in radiation reactions has several practical applications. For instance, the mixed glutathione–protein disulfides can be regarded as a cellular reservoir of physiological radioprotective agents. If GSH is released from this reservoir by interference, the cellular level of free GSH may increase and thus provide an increased protection of the cells against radiation. In contrast, treatment of cells by some enzyme inhibitors (e.g., buthionine sulfoximine) may block the new synthesis of GSH specifically (Griffith and Meister, 1979b). The ensuing decreased GSH level may confer on the cells an increased sensitivity to radiation and may also enhance the effect of sulfhydryl-reactive radiation sensitizers. Because the sensitivity of hypoxic cells is influenced by changes in the GSH level to a greater extent than that of oxic cells (cf. Section IV), the sensitization induced by decreasing the cellular GSH content may be particularly useful in radiotherapy to enhance specifically the effect on hypoxic radioresistant tumor cells.

References

Adams, G. E., and Cooke, M. (1969). Electron-affinic sensitization. A structural basis for chemical radiosensitizers in bacteria. *Int. J. Radiat. Biol.* **15,** 457.

Alexander, P., and Charlesby, A. (1955). Physico-chemical methods of protection against ionizing radiation. *In* "Radiobiology Symposium" (M. Bacq and P. Alexander, eds.), p. 49. Butterworth, London.

Alexander, P., Bacq, Z. M., Cousens, S. F., Fox, M., Herve, A., and Lazar, J. (1955). Mode of action of some substances which protect against the lethal effects of X-rays. *Radiat. Res.* **2,** 392.

Alexander, P., Dean, C. J., Hamilton, L. D. G., Lett, J. T., and Parkins, G. (1965). Critical structures other than DNA as sites for primary lesions of cell death induced by ionizing radiation. *In* "Cellular Radiation Biology" (M. D. Andersson, ed.), p. 241. Williams & Wilkins, Maryland.

Apontoweil, P., and Berends, W. (1978). Isolation and initial characterization of glutathione deficient mutants of E. coli K 12. *Biochim. Biophys. Acta* **399,** 10.

Bacq, Z. M., Herve, A., Lecomte, J., Fischer, P., Blavier, J., Dechamps, G., LeBihan, H., and Rayet, P. (1951). Protection contre le rayonnement X par la β-mercaptoethylamine. *Arch. Int. Physiol.* **59,** 442.

Barron, E. S. G. (1952). The effect of ionizing radiation on some systems of biological importance. *In* "Symposium on Radiobiology" (J. J. Nickson, ed.), p. 216. Wiley, New York.

Barron, E. S. G., Dickman, S., Muntz, J. A., and Singer, T. P. (1949). Studies on the mechanism of action of ionizing radiations. I. Inhibition of enzymes by X-rays. *J. Gen. Physiol.* **32,** 537.

Beutler, E., and Srivastava, S. K. (1974). GSH metabolism of the lens. *In* "Glutathione" (L. Flohe, H. Ch. Benöhr, H. Sies, H. D. Waller, and A. Wendel, eds.), p. 157. Thieme, Stuttgart.

Boyd, M. R., Stiko, A., Statham, C. N., and Jones, R. B. (1982). Protective role of endogenous pulmonary glutathione and other sulphydryl compounds against lung damage by alkylating agents. *Biochem. Pharmacol.* **31,** 1579.

Boyland, E., and Chasseaud, L. F. (1969). The role of glutathione and glutathione S-transferases in mercapturic acid biosynthesis. *Adv. Enzymol. Relat. Areas Mol. Biol.* **32,** 173.

Bridges, B. A. (1969). Sensitization of organisms to radiation by sulphydryl binding agents. *Adv. Radiat. Biol.* **3,** 123.

Bruce, A. E., and Malcham, W. H. (1965). Radiation sensitization of Micrococcus radiodurans, Sarcina lutea and Escherichia coli by p-HMB. *Radiat. Res.* **24,** 473.

Brunborg, G. (1977). Variation in the SH-content of haploid yeast and their relevance to radiosensitivity. *Int. J. Radiat. Biol.* **32,** 285.

Caspersson, O., and Révész, L. (1963). Cytochemical measurement of protein-sulphydryls in cell lines of different radiosensitivity. *Nature (London)* **199,** 153.

Chapman, W. H., and Cronkite, E. P. (1950). Further studies on the beneficial effect of glutathione on X-irradiated mice. *Proc. Soc. Exp. Biol. Med.* **75,** 318.

Dale, W. M. (1942). The effect of X-rays on the conjugated protein d-amino-acid oxidase. *Biochem. J.* **36,** 80.

Deschavanne, P. J., Midander, J., Edgren, M., Larsson, A., Malaise, E. P., and Révész, L. (1981). Oxygen enhancement of radiation induced lethality is greatly reduced in glutathione-deficient human fibroblasts. *Biomedicine* **35,** 35.

Dewey, D. L. (1963). The X-ray sensitivity of Serratia marcescens. *Radiat. Res.* **19,** 64.

Doherty, D. G., and Burnett, W. T., Jr. (1955). Protective effect of S, β-amino-ethyl-isothiouronium Br. HBr and related compounds against X-radiation death in mice. *Proc. Soc. Exp. Biol. Med.* **89**, 312.

Douglas, G. W., and Mortensen, R. A. (1956). The rate of metabolism of brain and liver glutathione in the rat studied with C-14-glycine. *J. Biol. Chem.* **222**, 581.

Edgren, M. (1982). Intercellular co-operation in repairing radiation-induced single-strand DNA breaks. *Int. J. Radiat. Biol.* **41**, 589.

Edgren, M., Larsson, A., Nilsson, K., Révész, L., and Scott, O. C. A. (1980). Lack of oxygen-effect in glutathione-deficient human cells in culture. *Int. J. Radiat. Biol.* **37**, 299.

Edgren, M., Révész, L., and Larsson, A. (1981). Induction and repair of single-strand DNA breaks after X-irradiation of human fibroblasts deficient in glutathione. *Int. J. Radiat. Biol.* **40**, 355.

Edgren, M., Modig, H., and Révész, L. (in press). Radioprotection of glutathione-deficient cells by thiol compounds. *In:* "Problems of Natural and Modified Radiosensitivity" (M. M. Konstantinova and A. M. Kuzin, eds.). Nauka, Moscow.

Elder, H. A., and Mortensen, R. A. (1956). The incorporation of labeled glycine into erythrocyte glutathione. *J. Biol. Chem.* **218**, 261.

Eriksson, S. (1974). "Metabolic Reduction of Mixed Disulphides." Ph.D. Thesis, Stockholm Univ., Sweden.

Fuchs, J. A., and Warner, H. R. (1975). Isolation of an Escherichia coli mutant deficient in glutathione synthesis. *J. Bacteriol.* **124**, 140.

Gorin, G. (1965). Mercaptan-disulphide interchange and radioprotection. *Prog. Biochem. Pharmacol.* **1**, 142.

Griffith, O. W., and Meister, A. (1979a). Glutathione: interorgan translocation, turnover and metabolism. *Proc. Natl. Acad. Sci. USA* **76**, 5606.

Griffith, O. W., and Meister, A. (1979b). Potent and specific inhibition of glutathione synthesis by buthionine sulfoximine (S-n-butyl homocysteine sulfoximine). *J. Biol. Chem.* **254**, 7558.

Harding, J. J. (1969). Glutathione-protein mixed disulphides in human lens. *Biochem. J.* **114**, 88.

Harisch, G., and Schole, J. (1974). Der Glutathionestatus der Rattenleber in Abhängigkeit vom Leberalter und von akuter Belastung. *Z. Naturforsch. C* **29**, 261.

Harrap, K. R., Jackson, R. C., Riches, P. G., Smith, C. A., and Hill, B. T. (1973). The occurrence of protein-bound mixed disulphides in rat tissues. *Biochim. Biophys. Acta* **310**, 104.

Harris, J. W., and Biaglow, J. E. (1972). Non-specific reactions of the glutathione oxidant "Diamide" with mammalian cells. *Biochem. Biophys. Res. Commun.* **46**, 1743.

Harris, J. W., and Power, J. A. (1973). Diamide: a new radiosensitizer of anoxic cells. *Radiat. Res.* **56**, 97.

Howard-Flanders, P. (1960). Effect of oxygen on the radiosensitivity of bacteriophage in the presence of sulphydryl compounds. *Nature (London)* **186**, 485.

Kosower, E. M., and Kosower, N. S. (1974). Manifestations of changes in the GSH-GSSG status of biological systems. *In* "Glutathione" (L. Flohe, H. Ch. Benöhr, H. Sies, H. D. Waller, and A. Wendel, eds.), p. 287. Thieme, Stuttgart.

Kosower, N. S., and Kosower, E. M. (1978). The glutathione status of cells. *Int. Rev. Cytol.* **54**, 109.

Larsson, A. (1981). 5-oxoprolinuria and other inborn errors related to the γ-glutamyl cycle. *In* "Transport and Inherited Disease" (N. R. Belton and C. Toothill, eds.), p. 277. MIT Press, Cambridge, Massachusetts.

Latarjet, R., and Ephrati, E. (1948). Influence protectrice de certaines substances contre l'inactivation d'un bacteriophage par les rayon X. *C. R. Seances Soc. Biol. Ses Fil.* **142**, 497.

Ling, C. C., Michaels, H. B., Epp, E. R., and Person, E. C. (1980). Interaction of misonidazole and oxygen in the radiosensitization of mammalian cells. *Int. J. Radiat. Oncol. Biol. Phys.* **6**, 583.

Lohman, P. H. M. (1968). Induction and rejoining of breaks in the deoxyribonucleic acid of human cells irradiated at various phases of the cell cycle. *Mutat. Res.* **6**, 449.

Macdougall, L. G. (1968). Red cell metabolism in iron-deficiency anemia. *J. Pediatr. (St. Louis)* **72**, 303.

Mazia, D. (1961). Mitosis and the physiology of cell division. *In* "The Cell" (J. Brachet and A. E. Mirsky, eds.), Vol. 3, p. 251. Academic Press, New York.

Meister, A. (1973). On the enzymology of amino acid transport. *Science (Washington, D.C.)* **180**, 33.

Meister, A. (1981a). Metabolism and functions of glutathione. *Trends Biochem. Sci.* **6**, 231.

Meister, A. (1981b). On the cycles of glutathione metabolism and transport. *Curr. Top. Cell. Regul.* **18**, 21.

Midander, J. (in press). Oxygen enhancement ratios for glutathione-deficient human fibroblasts determined from the frequency of radiation induced micronuclei. *Int. J. Radiat. Biol.*

Midander, J., Deschavanne, P. J., Malaise, E. P., and Révész, L. (1982). Survival curves of irradiated glutathione-deficient human fibroblasts: indication of a reduced enhancement of radiosensitivity by oxygen and misonidazole. *Int. J. Radiat. Oncol. Biol. Phys.* **8**, 443.

Modig, H. G. (1968). Cellular mixed disulphides between thiols and proteins, and their possible implication for radiation protection. *Biochem. Pharmacol.* **17**, 177.

Modig, H. G. (1973). Interaction of cysteamine with thiol and disulphide groups in deoxyribonucleoproteins. *Biochem. Pharmacol.* **22**, 1623.

Modig, H. G., and Révész, L. (1967). Non-protein sulphydryl and glutathione content of Ehrlich ascites tumor cells after treatment with the radioprotectors AET, cysteamine and glutathione. *Int. J. Radiat. Biol.* **13**, 469.

Modig, H. G., and Révész, L. (1968). Cellular sulphydryl levels and the effect of two mercaptopyridoxine derivatives with differential radioprotective action. *Arzneim. Forsch.* **18**, 1156.

Modig, H. G., Edgren, M., and Révész, L. (1971). Release of thiols from cellular mixed disulphides and its possible role in radiation protection. *Int. J. Radiat. Biol.* **22**, 257.

Ohara, H., and Terashima, T. (1970). Variation of cellular sulphydryl content during cell cycle of Hela cells and its correlation to cyclic changes of X-ray sensitivity. *Exp. Cell Res.* **58**, 182.

Ormerod, M. G., and Stevens, U. (1970). The rejoining of X-ray-induced strand breaks in the DNA of a murine lymphoma cell (L-517-8Y). *Biochim. Biophys. Acta* **232**, 72.

Patt, H. M., Tyree, E. B., Straube, R. L., and Smith, D. E. (1949). Cysteine protection against X-irradiation. *Science (Washington, D.C.)* **110**, 213.

Révész, L., and Edgren, M. (1982). Mechanisms of radiosensitization and protection studied with glutathione-deficient human cell lines. *In* "Current Radio-Oncology" (K. H. Kärcher, H. Kogelnik, and G. Reinartz, eds.), p. 235–242. Raven, New York.

Révész, L., and Modig, H. G. (1965). Cysteamine induced increase of cellular glutathione-level: a new hypothesis of the radioprotective mechanism. *Nature (London)* **207**, 430.

Révész, L., Bergstrand, H., and Modig, H. G. (1963). Intrinsic non-protein sulphydryl levels and cellular radiosensitivity. *Nature (London)* **198**, 1275.

Révész, L., Modig, H. G., and Konstantinova, M. M. (1974). Release of endogenous glutathione by exposure of cell cultures to Thiola. *Proc. Int. Symp. Thiola 2nd*, p. 12.

Révész, L., Edgren, M., and Larsson, A. (1979). Mechanisms of radiosensitivity by oxygen and misonidazole studied with glutathione deficient human fibroblasts in culture. In "Radiation Research: Proceedings of The Sixth International Congress of Radiation Research" (S. Okada, M. Imamura, T. Terashima, and H. Yamaguchi, eds.), p. 862. Jpn. Assoc. Radiat. Res., Tokyo.

Sabine, J. C. (1964). Glutathione concentration and stability in the red blood cells in various disease states, and some observations on the mechanism of action of acetylphenylhydrazine. *Br. J. Haematol.* **10,** 477.

Sinclair, W. K. (1969). Protection by cysteamine against lethal X-ray damage during the cell cycle of Chinese hamster cells. *Radiat. Res.* **39,** 135.

Sjöberg, L., Eriksen, T. E., and Révész, L. (1982). The reaction of the hydroxyl radical with glutathione in neutral and alkaline aqueous solution. *Radiat. Res.* **89,** 255.

Tanaka, Y., and Sugahara, T. (1970). Chemical radiation protection in man as revealed by chromosome aberrations in peripheral lymphocytes. *J. Radiat. Res.* **11,** 166.

Tietze, F. (1970). Disulphide reduction in rat liver. I. Evidence for the presence of nonspecific nucleotide-dependent disulphide reductase and GSH-disulphide transhydrogenase activities in the high speed supernatant fraction. *Arch. Biochem. Biophys.* **138,** 177.

Varnes, E. M., Biaglow, J. E., Koch, C. J., and Hall, E. J. (1980). Depletion of nonprotein thiols of hypoxic cells by misonidazole and metronidazole. *In* "Radiation Sensitizers" (L. W. Brady, ed.), p. 121. Masson, New York.

Vergroesen, A. J., Budke, L., and Cohen, J. A. (1964). Factors influencing the radioprotection of tissue culture cells by sulphydryl compounds. *Nature (London)* **204,** 246.

Yuhas, J. M., Spellman, J. M., and Culo, F. (1980). The role of WR-2721 in radiotherapy and/or chemotherapy. *In* "Radiation Sensitizers" (L. W. Brady, ed.), p. 303. Masson, New York.

3 Protection against Radiation-Induced Damage—Experimental Radioprotection

Hiroji Nagata

Tsutomu Sugahara

Kyoto National Hospital
Kyoto 612, Japan

I. Introduction

Chemical radiation protection in rodents was first discovered in 1949 by Patt *et al.*, and clinical application in cases of acute radiation sickness seemed to be promising. Numerous chemicals were screened in various laboratories, but clinically available chemical protectors were not discovered, as was extensively reviewed by Thomson in 1962. He concluded that although a number of compounds may be capable of efficient protection of mice when given before exposure to X or γ rays, none could be considered a practical agent for protection of humans. On the basis of synthesis, stability, and effectiveness of oral administration, as well as dose-reduction properties, *S*-(2-aminoethyl)isothiouronium (AET) would seem to be the drug of choice. However, preliminary tests of AET in humans indicated that the toxicity may be far too great.

New chemical protectors have been reported, following two different lines of research in Japan and in the United States. In Japan, an adrenochrome derivative, adrenochrome monoguanylhydrazone methanesulfonate (AMM) and a new sulfhydryl compound, 2-mercaptopropionylglycine (MPG), which are both effective in much lower doses than their toxic dose in mice, were reported by Sugahara and Tanaka (1968), Sugahara *et*

Modification of Radiosensitivity in Cancer Treatment

al. (1970), and Nagata *et al.* (1972). In the United States, after a large screening of various kinds of derivatives of cysteamine, WR-2721, *S*-2-(3-aminopropylamino)ethylphosphorothioic acid was reported by Sweeny (1971) to have a very high dose-reduction factor of 2.5 or more, thus effective even at a less toxic dose.

To make use of these chemicals in cases of cancer radiotherapy, differential protection between tumor and normal tissues has to be established. Studies along this line have been also carried out with WR-2721 and MPG. The results obtained so far are promising for the improvement of radiotherapy. Clinical studies on these chemicals will be reported in this volume by Tanaka (Chapter 5). In this chapter, experimental studies on these chemicals are reviewed, emphasizing our own research. These topics were discussed in part by Sugahara in 1973.

II. Adrenochrome Derivatives

Radiation protection with adrenochrome and its derivatives has been studied since 1949, but the protective activity has not been confirmed, as reviewed by Thomson (1962). Adrenochrome is an indole derivative of adrenaline (epinephrine) but has none of its pharmacological properties. Its derivatives have been widely used clinically as hemostatic agents but not for radiation protection, and adrenochrome itself is quite unstable. Thus, the synthesis of stable derivatives has been attempted in various laboratories. Because the first stable derivative, adrenochrome mono-semicarbazone (AMC), known as carbazochrome, has a very low water solubility, other stable and more soluble derivatives were investigated. As a result of the research, two other derivatives with a higher solubility than that of AMC are now commercially available; adrenochrome monosemicarbazone 3-sodium sulfonate (ASS) and adrenochrome monoguanylhydrazone methanesulfonate (AMM).

Protection against lethal doses of radiation with these compounds was studied over a wide range of doses. As shown in Fig. 1, the survival after irradiation was not increased linearly with the dose administered in the case of AMM. Significant protection was afforded with AMM at its optimal dose of 5 mg/kg, a very low dose as compared with LD_{50}, 2000 mg/kg. Extensive studies on radiation protection by AMM in various irradiation conditions have been carried out in mice, and the results are summarized in Table I. Data on the protection with various adrenochrome derivatives with different solubilities are shown in Table II. Protective activity seemed to be independent of the solubility of the compounds. The radiation protection by adrenochrome derivatives was confirmed, and AMM

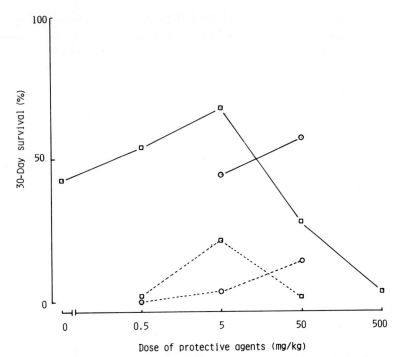

Fig. 1. Dose–response relationship of radiation protection by AMM and ASS. Mice were injected ip with AMM (□) or ASS (○) and then irradiated with either 700 (——) or 1000 R (-----) X ray. Percentage 30-day survival was plotted against drug dose.

seemed to be the most promising for clinical application because of its high solubility and low effective dose. Intravenous AMM (100–500 mg) has been used clinically as a hemostatic agent without any serious side effects.

TABLE I

Protection by AMM in Mice under Various Irradiation Conditions

Irradiation condition	DMF	Criterion	Remarks
Single dose (65 R/min)	1.32	$LD_{50/30}$	5 mg/kg ip
Single dose (~1 R/min)	1.24	$LD_{50/30}$	0.84 mg AMM/g diet
Continuous (6–10 R/h)	1.5	Survival time	0.84 mg AMM/g diet

TABLE II

X-Ray Protection by Adrenochrome Derivatives with Different Solubilities

Compound[a]	MW	Solubility (mg/ml at 0°C)	No. of mice	30-day survival (%)
AMC Na–salicylate complex	396.35	1.025	64	35.9
AMM	331.36	180	64	32.8
Adrenochrome monoguanylhydrazone nicotinate	358.37	7.0	45	8.9
ASS	322.29	15	63	6.4
None	—	—	104	3.8

[a] All compounds were given ip in a dose of 5 mg/kg in about 0.1 ml saline solution 15 min before irradiation of 900 R.

III. 2-Mercaptopropionylglycine

In the screening of sulfhydryl compounds for chemical protection, we found that a new synthetic sulfhydryl compound commercially available in Japan as a clinical drug for detoxification, which is most effective for metal poisoning [2-mercaptopropionylglycine (MPG), commercial name Thiola], protected mice against lethal doses of radiation. As shown in Fig. 2, the compound has an optimal dose of 20 mg/kg (0.5 mg/mouse) for protection, its dose-modifying factor (DMF) being 1.4. Acute LD_{50} of the drug is 2000 mg/kg ip. This is again quite different from other sulfhydryls, which usually show protection in proportion to the dose. The protection by MPG lasts for more than 3 h after a single ip administration, whereas the protection by other sulfhydryls disappears within an hour after a single administration. In addition to radiation protection, MPG is reportedly effective for protection against and to restore normal states after leukopenia induced by nitrogen mustard, in dogs and rabbits (Wakizaka *et al.*, 1960, 1961).

Chemical protection by MPG in a tumor was studied by Tsukiyama in 1976. He compared TRT_{50} (50% tumor regrowth time) of transplanted mammary tumor in C3H/He mice originating spontaneously in a C3H/He female mouse. As shown in Table III, the protective effect of the drug, as detected by TRT_{50}, was little or negligible compared with the protection as detected by LD_{50}.

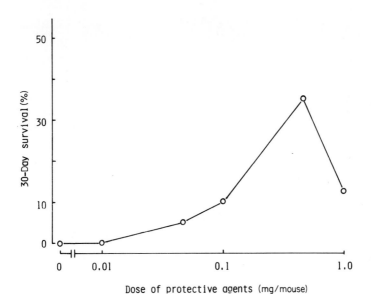

Fig. 2. Dose–response relationship of radiation protection by MPG. Experimental procedures were the same as for Fig. 1.

To obtain more efficient and less toxic protective compounds than MPG and to correlate the chemical structure and radioprotection, the related compounds shown in Fig. 3 were synthesized by Santen Pharmaceutical Co. Ltd., Osaka, and screened for their protective effect in mice. Among 15 compounds tested, only 2-mercaptopropionylglycineamide

TABLE III

TRT$_{50}$ of Transplanted Mammary Tumors after Single and Fractionated X Irradiation with and without MPG Pretreatment[a]

X-Ray dose	MPG dose (mg/kg)	TRT$_{50}$[b] (days)	DMF
40 GY × 1	0	23.4 (22.8–24.0)	1.19
40 GY × 1	20	18.8 (17.6–20.0)	
8 GY × 5	0	18.6 (18.1–19.1)	0.97
8 GY × 5	20	19.1 (18.1–20.2)	

[a] From Tsukiyama (1976).
[b] 95% Confidence limit.

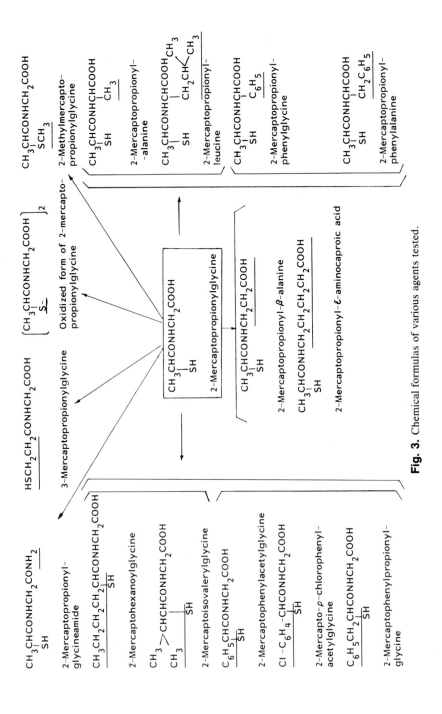

Fig. 3. Chemical formulas of various agents tested.

(MPG-amide) was shown to have comparable protection with MPG; 3-mercaptopropionylglycine (3-MPG) and S-methyl MPG had comparatively less but a significant protection, the former being more effective than the latter. Further comparisons of the protection with the three compounds were made as shown in Fig. 4.

The structural difference between MPG and 3-MPG is the position of sulfhydryls in the main chain. The latter has a structural similarity to glutathione, as far as the SH position on the carbon chain is concerned. A comparable effect to that of MPG was seen with MPG-amide in the screening experiment, but less protection in general was evident. In Fig. 4 the protection by cysteamine is plotted for comparison.

Radioprotection was further studied in cultured L cells by Mori *et al.* (1978). They compared the protective effect of various sulfhydryl compounds, including these three compounds, using colony formation and DNA strand breaks as criteria. The most effective radioprotection was obtained with cysteamine and cysteine. Cysteamine at 0.1 to 0.4 mM and cysteine at 0.4 to 2.0 mM reduced the survival of unirradiated cells but were much less toxic and potently radioprotective at higher concentrations. The next most effective radioprotection was obtained with AET, MPG-amide, and glutathione (GSH). Cytotoxicity to unirradiated cells was seen with AET at 0.1 to 0.8 mM and GSH at 1 to 4 mM, whereas

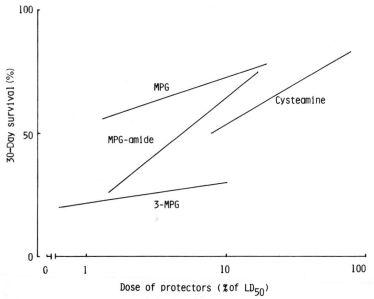

Fig. 4. Dose–response relationships of radiation protection by various protective agents.

MPG-amide showed only a slight toxicity at 0.4 to 0.8 m*M*. These chemicals were also radioprotective at higher concentrations. In contrast, MPG and 3-MPG were nontoxic and generally ineffective in protecting irradiated cells, except that MPG at concentrations around 0.02 m*M* and 3-MPG around 15 m*M* had a slightly protective action.

The protection against radiation-induced DNA single-strand breaks was also studied with cysteamine, AET, and MPG at 60 m*M,* 30 m*M,* and 0.02 m*M,* respectively. The DMFs of these chemicals for cell survival at 500-R irradiation were roughly estimated to be 3.5, 2.4, and 1.4, respec-

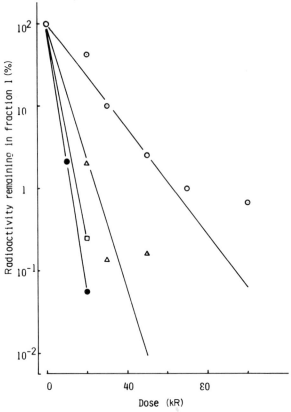

Fig. 5. Protection of X-ray-induced double-strand breaks by various agents. Mouse L cells, labeled with [³H]TdR, were irradiated with X ray in the presence of protective agents, and DNA was fractionated by neutral sucrose gradient. Because DNA from unirradiated cells sedimented at the bottom of the tube, most of the radioactivity was recovered in fraction 1. Radioactivity remaining in fraction 1 decreased with increasing X-ray doses. ●, Untreated; ○, treated with 60 m*M* cysteamine; △, treated with 30 m*M* AET; □, treated with 0.02 m*M* MPG.

tively. Significant protection for DNA single-strand breaks was observed with cysteamine and AET but not with MPG, as shown in Fig. 5. Similar results were obtained on X-ray–induced DNA double-strand breaks.

Although molecular and cellular analyses of the radioprotection by MPG were not clear enough as compared with cysteamine, the protection in mice has been confirmed repeatedly at the tissue level, and clinical applications have confirmed the protection, as reported elsewhere (Kumar, Chapter 4 this volume). Its low toxicity and effectiveness by oral administration in humans indicates that MPG is an effective radioprotector for humans.

IV. WR-2721

With extensive studies on the differential protection between normal and malignant tissues, as first reported by Yuhas and Storer in 1969, the interest in chemical protection for eventual clinical applications was renewed, as reviewed by Harris (1976). As shown in Table IV, WR-2721 has a high DMF in normal tissue (except against central nervous system lethality) but rather a low DMF in animal tumors, except for the cell-killing

TABLE IV

Protection of Mouse Tissues by WR-2721 Injected 15–30 Min before X Irradiation

End point	WR-2721 Dose (mg/kg)	DMF	References
$LD_{50/30}$	500	2.6–2.7	Harris (1976)
Skin ulceration (30 days)	500	2.4	Harris (1976)
$LD_{50/0}$ (CNS)	250, 500	1.0, 0.5	Harris (1976)
$LD_{50/7}$ (G.I.)	250, 500	1.6, 1.8	Harris (1976)
$LD_{50/120}$ (lung death)	500	3.4	Harris (1976)
Hair loss (60 days)	500	2.1	Harris (1976)
Parotid gland (acute)	400	2.5	Sodicoff et al. (1978a)
Parotid gland (late)	400	2.3	Sodicoff et al. (1978b)
Transplantability of mammary carcinoma (%)	500	1.15	Harris (1976)
EMT-6 Tumor cell killing (aerobic)	300	1.5–2.0	Harris (1976)
p388 Leukemia cell killing (mean survival time)	500–600	2.2	Harris (1976)
EMT-6 Tumor (cure)	500–600	1.3	Harris (1976)
Control of KHT sarcoma	400	1.2	Harris (1976)

TABLE V

Differential X-Ray Protection of Normal and Tumor
Tissue by WR-2721 [a,b]

Criterion[c]	Control	WR-2721	DMF
$LD_{50/5}$ (G.I.)	9.5 Gy	1.9 Gy	2.1
$ED_{50/24}$	1.8 Gy	3.8 Gy	2.09
TRT_{50} (40 Gy × 1)	6.3 days	6.24 days	0.97
TRT_{50} (80 Gy × 5)	6.84 days	6.73 days	0.98

[a] From Tsukiyama (1978).

[b] WR-2721 dose (400 mg/kg) given 30 min before X irradiation.

[c] ED, epilation dose; TRT, tumor regression time in mammary tumors in C3H/He mice.

effect on p388 leukemia cells. Although WR-2721 is toxic (i.e., acute $LD_{50/30}$ is 784 mg/kg in C57BL/6-J mice), it was suggested that this chemical might be effective at low doses because of its high DMF.

On the basis of these data, Yamanouchi Pharmaceutical Co. Ltd., Tokyo, provided the chemical for experimentation in the early 1970s. Tsukiyama (1978) confirmed the differential protection in ICR female mice and C3H mammary carcinoma, as shown in Table V.

Accumulation of WR-2721 in the rat parotid glands and short- and long-term protection of the gland were reported by Sodicoff *et al.* (1978a,b). Protection against oral radiation death in mice was also reported by Utley *et al.* (1978). On the basis of these reports, Tanaka and Sugahara (1980) did clinical trials on oral damage following radiotherapy of head and neck tumors.

It is well recognized that WR-2721 must be dephosphorylated to be active for radioprotection. Thus Purdie (1979) observed a very low DMF of 1.3 in cultured human cells. Mouse L cells, although not protected by WR-2721, were protected when incubated together with the mouse liver homogenate for 15 to 30 min (T. Mori and C. Murayama, personal communication). Chang's liver cells were found to be well protected without the liver homogenate.

With regard to the mechanisms of differential protection, differences in activation capacities in different tissues and/or in drug distribution were proposed. Yuhas (1982) emphasized the latter mechanisms; that is, solid tumors incorporated very low quantities of WR-2721 whereas most normal tissues readily incorporated the drug. The difference may not be due to differences in vascularities but rather to a particular partition coefficient of the drug and its dependence on pH. This would provide a clue for improvement of chemical radioprotectors for radiotherapy.

V. Superoxide Dismutase

Because the involvement of superoxide is one explanation of the oxygen effect in radiobiology, Petkan et al. (1975a,b) attempted radioprotection with superoxide dismutase (SOD) in mice using 30-day lethality and bone marrow stem cell survival as criteria. A small but significant DMF of 1.12 at $LD_{50/30}$ was obtained by giving 35 $\mu g/g$ body weight of SOD intravenously 1 h before X irradiation. They confirmed the protection in mouse bone marrow stem cells, demonstrating that the largest DMF of more than 2 was observed at 35 $\mu g/g$, from 20 to 100 $\mu g/g$.

Nishidai et al. (1980) made an extensive study on the radioprotective effects of SOD on murine tissues, because SOD is not only radioprotective but is also reportedly antiinflammatory by reducing superoxide released from phagocytizing leukocytes. Radiation-induced 30-day mortality, acute skin reaction, and foot deformation after 3 months were used as criteria. A dose of 1.0 mg/mouse ip of SOD was given 1 h before and after irradiation. A small but significant protection was observed in all three criteria. However, immunological complications associated with the administration of SOD, which is antigenic to the animal, have to be overcome before this enzyme can be clinically applied.

VI. Prospects

Improvement of tumor radiotherapy depends on achieving differential sensitization, either by sensitizing tumor cells or by protecting normal tissue. However, presently available sensitizers and protectors show no significant improvement. Thus experimental studies are needed on ways to protect critical normal tissue against acute effects of irradiation. Ideally the protection should be against not only acute radiation effects but also late radiation effects, including cancer induction and other tissue damage such as growth retardation, late hemorrhage, and ileus. These possibilities should be pursued more intensively, experimentally as well as clinically. Postirradiation hyperthermia was reported to reduce transformation frequency in cultured cells (Harisiadis et al., 1980).

The combination of protectors and sensitizers, if sufficiently selective, should give the best results with regard to the biologically effective dose distribution and radiation-induced late effects.

References

Harisiadis, L., Miller, R. C., Harisiadis, S., and Hall, E. J. (1980). Oncogenic transformation and hyperthermia. *Br. J. Radiol.* **53**, 479–482.

Harris, J. W. (1976). Radiation modifiers. An evaluation of recent research and clinical potential. *In* "Modification of Radiosensitivity of Biological Systems," pp. 11–28. IAEA, Vienna.

Mori, T., Horikawa, M., Nikaido, O., and Sugahara, T. (1978). Comparative studies on protective effect of various sulfhydryl compounds against cell death and DNA strand breaks induced by X-rays in culture mouse L cells. *J. Radiat. Res.* **19**, 319–335.

Nagata, H., Sugahara, T., and Tanaka, T. (1972). Radiation protection by 2-mercaptopropionylglycine in mice. *J. Radiat. Res.* **13**, 163–166.

Nishidai, T., Ono, K., Ri, N., Hiraoka, M., Takahashi, M., and Abe, M. (1980). Radioprotective effects of superoxide dismutase (SOD) on murine tissues. *Nippon Igaku Hoshasen Gakkai Zasshi* **40**, 983–990.

Patt, H. M., Tyree, E. B., Stranbe, R. L., and Smith, D. E. (1949). Cysteine protection against X-irradiation. *Science (Washington, D.C.)* **110**, 213–214.

Petkan, A., Chelack, W. S., Pleskach, S. D., Meeker, B. F., and Brady, C. M. (1975a). Radioprotection of mice by superoxide dismutase. *Biochem. Biophys. Res. Commun.* **65**, 886–893.

Petkan, A., Kelly, K., Chelack, W. S., Pleskach, S. D., Barefoot, C., and Meeker, B. E. (1975b). Radioprotection of bone marrow stem cells by superoxide dismutase. *Biochem. Biophys. Res. Commun.* **67**, 1167–1174.

Purdie, J. W. (1979). A comparative study of the radioprotective effects of cysteamine, WR-2721 and WR-1065 in cultured human cells. *Radiat. Res.* **77**, 303–311.

Sodicoff, M., Conger, A. D., Trepper, P., and Pratt, N. E. (1978a). Short-term radioprotective effects of WR-2721 on the rat parotid glands. *Radiat. Res.* **75**, 317–326.

Sodicoff, M., Conger, A. D., Patt, N. E., and Trepper, P. (1978b). Radioprotection of WR-2721 against long-term chronic damage to the rat parotid gland. *Radiat. Res.* **76**, 172–179.

Sugahara, T. (1973). Possible application of chemical radioprotectors to radiotherapy. *In* "Fraction Size in Radiobiology and Radiotherapy" (T. Sugahara, L. Révész, and O. Scott, eds.), pp. 84–93. Igaku-Shoin, Tokyo.

Sugahara, T., and Tanaka, T. (1968). Protection against whole-body X-irradiation by adrenochrome monoguanylhydrazone methansulfonate in mice. *Nature (London)* **220**, 271–272.

Sugahara, T., Tanaka, T., and Nagata, H. (1970). Protection of mice against ionizing radiations by adrenochrome monoguanylhydrazone methansulfonate; a promising agent for clinical use. *In* "Radiation Protection and Sensitization" (H. L. Morison and H. Quintiliani, eds.), pp. 401–408. Taylor & Francis, London.

Sweeny, T. R. (1971). Comment. *In* "Biological Aspects of Radiation Protection" (T. Sugahara and O. Hug, eds.), pp. 164–168. Igaku-Shoin, Tokyo.

Tanaka, Y., and Sugahara, T. (1980). Clinical experiences of chemical radiation protection in tumor radiotherapy in Japan. *In* "Radiation Sensitizers: Their Use in the Clinical Management of Cancer" (L. Brady, ed.), pp. 421–425. Masson, New York.

Thomson, J. F. (1962). "Radiation Protection in Mammals." Reinhold, New York.

Tsukiyama, I. (1976). Radioprotective effects of cysteine and α-mercaptopropionylglycine for normal and malignant tissues. *Nippon Igaku Hoshasen Gakkai Zasshi* **36**, 652–663.

Tsukiyama, I. (1978). Radioprotective effects of YM-08310 on normal and malignant tissues. *Nippon Igaku Hoshasen Gakkai Zasshi* **38**, 888–902.

Utley, J. F., King, R., and Giansanti, J. S. (1978). Radioprotection of oral cavity structure by WR-2721. *Int. J. Radiat. Oncol. Biol. Phys.* **4,** 643–647.

Wakizaka, J., Yuge, S., Mita, R., Kakuo, T., Miyamoto, T., Ichibangase, Y., Eto, Y., and Tanaka, T. (1960). An excellent effect of new drug α-thiola for leucopenia caused by antineoplastic substances. *Kurume Med. J.* **23,** 626–630.

Wakizaka, J., Yuge, S., Mita, R., Kakuo, T., Lee, M. Y., Watanabe, M., and Murakami, N. (1961). Experimental studies of the effects of thioacetoglycine derivatives on the leukopoiesis. *Kurume Med. J.* **24,** 2379–2387.

Yuhas, J. M. (1982). Present status and future directions for radioprotective drugs in radiotherapy. IAEA-SR-62, prospective methods of radiation therapy in developing countries. IAEA-TEDOC, **266,** 77–86.

Yuhas, J. M., and Storer, J. B. (1969). Differential chemoprotection of normal and malignant tissues. *J. Natl. Cancer Inst. (US)* **42,** 331–335.

4 Chemical Radiation Protection: Progress and Prospects

Ashok Kumar

Bio-Science Department
H.P. University
Summer-Hill
Simla 171005
India

I. Definition and Scope

Chemical radiation protectors are substances that, when administered to an animal or added to a culture medium under conditions of exposure to ionizing radiations, decrease significantly the effects of these radiations.

Since the 1940s, scientists the world over have studied chemical compounds that modify the effects of ionizing radiation on biological systems. Although these studies have contributed significantly to our knowledge of radiation effects, they have had little impact on cancer radiotherapy. Until recently, the generally held opinion was that no great contribution of these chemicals could be expected. Yuhas and Storer (1969) showed that S-2-(3-aminopropylamino)ethylphosphorothioic acid (WR-2721) protected normal tissues in mice but did not modify the response of the tumor tissue to radiation. Hence chemical modification is once again being evaluated, at the clinical level.

Modification of Radiosensitivity in Cancer Treatment

II. Introduction

Studies on chemical protection began in the 1940s when Dale (1942) showed that certain substances (e.g., colloidal sulfur, thiourea, formate), when added to an aqueous solution of carboxypeptidase and amino acid oxidase, decreased the inactivation of these enzymes by X rays. In 1948 Latarjet and Ephrati noted the protective effects of thioglycolic acid, tryptophan, glutathione, and cysteine in bacteriophages, even under conditions of hypoxia. However, it was only after 1949 that Patt *et al.* found that cysteine, provided protection in mammals. Among the numerous drugs studied, cysteamine and its derivatives and serotonin have been chosen as representative of compounds with a high protective activity. To obtain a higher protection with a tolerable dose, combined usage of various protectors and new derivatives of cysteamine has been extensively studied. Recently, the "first-generation" drugs, WR-2721 and *N*-(2-mercaptopropionyl)glycine (MPG) have been shown to warrant clinical therapy.

III. Progress

A. Experimental Studies *in Vivo*

Bacq *et al.* (1951) showed that the decarboxylated form of cysteine, namely 2-mercaptoethylamine (MEA, cysteamine), is an even more promising protective agent. Cysteamine reportedly provided the same protection at a dose of 150 mg/kg, compared to cysteine at 1200 mg/kg in mice. Cysteamine is more protective of the gastrointestinal (G.I.) tract than the bone marrow of mice. Cysteamine sulfate was shown to be protective against X irradiation in animals (Sorbo, 1958; Holmberg and Sorbo, 1959). Bacq and Beaumariage (1965) showed that the protective action of cysteamine in mice was optimal when administered 10 min preirradiation, whereas in rats the most favorable effects were obtained with administration 45 min preirradiation (Smoliar, 1962). Cysteamine appeared to be devoid of any therapeutic efficacy when administered in rats postirradiation, and protection in chickens was nil. Although the compound protected spermatozoa of mice and rats, it did not prevent leukopenia in mice (Bacq *et al.*, 1953; Mandl, 1959; Lüning *et al.*, 1961; Starkie, 1961; Kojima, 1961).

Cysteine, the prototype of all mammalian antiradiation agents first used by Patt *et al.* (1949), was effective if given from 5 min to 1 h preirradiation. Smith (1959) later showed that cysteine is effective in the hibernating squirrel only by the iv route, and protection was nil if given after radiation exposure. In 1966 Sakakibara *et al.* observed that cysteine protected mice from enhanced infection after X irradiation, and that the number of survivors correlated with dose of the drug. Various esters of cysteine do provide good protection (Yakovlev, 1962). Romito (1970) showed that cysteine reduced the chromosome damage of irradiated human bone marrow cells. Bacq *et al.* (1961) observed that cysteine gave local protection against depilation in young mice.

Glutathione, a tripeptide, is present within the cell and functions to maintain CoA in a reduced active form. It is a moderately good protector in mice and rats (Chapman and Cronkite, 1950), and this favorable effect has been repeatedly confirmed in various species. Doherty *et al.* (1957) classified glutathione as a nonprotective substance. Glutathione is the only known substance naturally present in sufficiently large amounts within the cell that has detectable radioprotective activity (Révész and Modig, 1965; Graevsky *et al.*, 1966; Modig and Révész, 1967).

In 1959, Arburov claimed that sodium 2,3-dimercaptopropylsulfonate, compared to other thiols, was more protective and less toxic (LD_{50} 1400 mg/kg in mice). Mono- and dimercaptoalkylcarboxylic acids have also been tested for possible radioprotective properties.

Beaumariage (1957) found that cystamine was as effective as cysteamine, has a low toxicity, and has activity when administered orally to mice and rats. In lethally irradiated rats, cystamine (146 mg/kg) afforded 60% survival. This compound is ineffective in chickens (Beaumariage *et al.*, 1966). Booz *et al.* (1965) showed that cystamine protected antibody formation in irradiated rats. Cystamine is effective in mice, rats, guinea pigs, and dogs (Makhalova *et al.*, 1966). Optimum protection was observed in mice when cystamine was given 10 min before irradiation (Bacq and Beaumariage, 1965).

Doherty and Burnett (1955) first reported that AET [S-(2-amino-ethyl)-isothiouronium bromide · HBr] at a dose of 250 mg/kg protected 88% of all mice subjected to lethal irradiation, and that this drug was more protective than cysteamine, on a molar basis. Other workers have obtained excellent results with AET in mice (Maisin *et al.*, 1960; Kakehi *et al.*, 1961; Maisin and Doherty, 1963; Zherbchenko and Zaitseva, 1969; Antoku and Sawada, 1970; Duzhenkova, 1979).

Mole *et al.* in 1950 observed that thiourea has only a limited activity, and a substantial dose (1800 mg/kg) is required. However, sodium diethyldithiocarbamate reportedly affords good protection (Lyashenko *et al.*, 1959).

The reaction of an aldehyde or ketone with cysteamine or an *N*-substituted cysteamine yields a thiazolidine. The advantage of thiazolidines is the slow release of the radioprotector activity. Thiazolidines have to be given in large doses. (Kaluszyner *et al.*, 1961; Riemschneider, 1961; Riemschneider and Hoyer, 1962).

The radioprotective action of dimethyl sulfoxide (DMSO) was first reported by Ashwood-Smith (1961) in mice. Radioprotective effects of DMSO have also been reported (Shapiro *et al.*, 1968; Farmer *et al.*, 1973).

Klayman (1973) reviewed the radioprotective effects of certain selenium-containing compounds on alcohol dehydrogenase and ribonuclease; however, these agents did not protect mammals against whole-body irradiation. Breccia *et al.* (1969) found that organoselenium compounds had a radioprotective activity in rats.

Non-sulfur-containing agents such as antioxidants also have radioprotective properties. Gorodetskii and Baraboi (1962) found that sodium gallate (60 mg/kg), a gallic acid derivative, is radioprotective in mice and rats. Its protective action has also been studied in dogs (Gorodetskii *et al.*, 1965). Similar observations were also made by Pozza and Verza (1960), who found that propyl gallate, the most active ester of gallic acid, protected 30% of the lethally irradiated mice, when the acid was given in a dose of 50 mg/kg ip.

Other nonsulfur compounds, *p*-aminoacetophenone, *p*-aminopropiophenone (PAPP), and *p*-aminobutyrophenone, reportedly are radioprotective in rats and dogs (Romantsev and Tikhomirova, 1963). Administration of PAPP dissolved in propylene glycol (PG) before irradiation has been reported to increase the survival of irradiated mice and rats (Storer and Coon, 1950; Doull *et al.*, 1959; Hasegawa and Landahl, 1967; Vacek and Sugahara, 1967).

Smith reported in 1958 that certain mitotic suppressive agents, such as trimethylcolchicinic acid methyl ether *d*-tartrate, yielded a fair degree of protection against radiation. Tranquilizers and psychotropic drugs possess only moderate antiradiation properties. Fair protection was reported for the rauwolfia alkaloid reserpine (Langendorff *et al.*, 1959).

Among the biogenic amines, serotonin (5-hydroxytryptamine; 5-HT) is a vasoconstrictor and causes increases in blood pressure, particularly in the brain. It also has a fairly active radioprotective effect in rodents (Langendorff *et al.*, 1959; van der Meer and van Bekkum, 1959; Langendorff, 1962; Maisin and Doherty, 1963; Streffer *et al.*, 1968; Chaudhuri and Langendorff, 1970; Srivastava, 1971). Mexamine (5-methoxytryptamine), a methyl ether derivative of serotonin, protects mice from the effects of whole-body irradiation (Dukor, 1962).

More recently *S*-2-(3-aminopropylamino)ethylphosphorothioic acid, commonly known as WR-2721, has been studied in numerous investigations because of its high antiradiation activity (Piper *et al.*, 1969). It was

Stromberg and co-workers (1968) who showed that WR-2721 promotes wound healing in irradiated rats. Yuhas (1969) noted that the drug protected mice against the life-shortening effects of X rays and normal irradiated tissue. A. Kumar (unpublished) also found a marked protection of various tissues of mice exposed to γ rays. Yuhas (1972) stated that when WR-2721 is administered 15 min preirradiation, resistance of the immune response to radiation injury is increased by a factor of 3.4. Harris and Phillips (1971) screened thiophosphate radioprotective compounds: Trials of S-2-(5-aminopentylamino)ethylphosphorothioic acid monohydrate, sodium hydrogen S-(2-aminoethyl)phosphorothioate (WR-638), and WR-2721 are under way.

In 1970 Sugahara et al. suggested two types of sulfhydryl protectors: (1) the naturally originating compound glutathione, which has a low toxicity, and (2) cysteamine, an artificial compound usually with high toxicity. Very high doses are required to achieve successful protection. A third type of sulfhydryl protector is MPG; this synthetic compound has a low toxicity and is effective in very low doses. Related reports on the radiation protection of mice by MPG include Tanaka and Sugahara (1970), Nagata et al. (1972), Uma Devi et al. (1979), Kumar and Bhagat (1981), and Dev et al. (1982). Cittadini et al. (1970) found radioprotective effects of hematoporphyrin in mice, when administered 30 min before irradiation. Novak (1970) showed that ip administration of 5 or 7.5 mg/kg fluoroacetate (FAC) in physiological saline affords very marked protection against the effect of ionizing radiation lasting for roughly 30–40 min to 7 h after application of the compound. He compared FAC with cysteine, cystamine, AET, and serotonin and reported that it possesses a similar radioprotective effect.

Preirradiation injection of bacterial endotoxin was shown to increase the survival of irradiated mice, dogs, sheep, and monkeys (Smith et al., 1957; Bron and Lajtha, 1966; Ainsworth and Mitchell, 1968).

In 1968 Sugahara and Tanaka reported adrenochrome monoguanylhydrazone methanesulfonate, an adrenochrome derivative, to be highly effective in providing radioprotection and proposed its possible application in radiotherapy (Sugahara, 1974). Petkau (1978) reported that the protection of X-irradiated mice by bovine superoxide dismutase (SOD) is enhanced when the enzyme is given iv both before and after the radiation exposure. He stated that this protection occurs in a dose range where hematological damage is an important contributor to animal health. The proliferative capacity of bone marrow stem cells X-irradiated in air is protected by SOD. Evidence for the potential clinical use of SOD to ameliorate the late radiation effect is mounting (Edsmyr et al., 1976).

Il'Yuchenok et al. (1979) studied toxicity and radioprotective properties of 1,3-oxazine and 1,3-thiazine derivatives. 4,4,6-Trimethyl-2-dimethylamino-4H-1,3-oxazine exerted a pronounced radioprotective action.

Sverdlov *et al.* (1979) reported extensive radioprotection by S-2-(5-aminopentylamino)ethylphosphorothioic acid monohydrate, in mice exposed to X and neutron radiation, and Kalnitskii (1979) observed that a preliminary single vaccination with *Proteus vulgaris* has a beneficial effect on radioresistance of albino mice affected by incorporated ^{137}Cs.

Pospisil *et al.* (1980) noted the promising radioprotective effect of K and Mg aspartate in male mice of a noninbred strain H. Gheorghe *et al.* (1980) observed effects of prolonged γ-irradiation at 1500 R on the radioprotected rat. Given 25 mg/kg of falcysteine 1 h before irradiation, the number of survivors doubled.

Nishimura *et al.* (1980) reported remarkable radioprotective effects of DL-5-alkylthiomethyl-5-methylhydantoin (150 mg/kg body weight), and Sverdlov *et al.* (1980) found a pronounced radioprotective effect against X and fission neutron radiation in mice given sodium S-(S-thioethyl-2-amino)thiophosphate.

Baver *et al.* (1981) and A. Kumar (unpublished) found that solcoseryl, a dialysate of calf serum, protects mice against X rays. Agrawal and Nagaratnam (1981) observed that certain flavonoids (nepitrin, suitellarein rutin, and naringen) provided protection in mice, possibly as a result of inhibition of increase in capillary permeability caused by histamine. Novikova *et al.* (1980) studied the radioprotective properties of certain heterylpyrazoles and noted that dimethylpyrazole has low toxicity and increases the survival rate of animals by 50 to 60%, in comparison with the control.

B. *In Vitro* Studies

As compared to *in vivo* studies, *in vitro* there are few studies on radiation protection.

Kohn and Gunter (1959) for the first time demonstrated protection of bacteria (*E. coli* B/r) by cysteine. They reported that maximum protection was observed when cysteine was added to the bacterial suspension 15 min before irradiation. Other workers have noted a marked protection of viruses by sulfhydryl compounds, cysteine, and cysteamine (Ginoza and Norman, 1957; Braams, 1960). Radioprotective effects of cysteamine were also observed in bacteriophages (Howard-Flanders, 1960; Hotz and Müller, 1962). Bridges (1962) reported that thiourea is an effective protective agent for bacteria (*Pseudomonas* spp.). Later on, Vergroesen *et al.* (1967) also showed that thiourea can protect mammalian cells *in vitro*.

Cramp (1969) showed radiation protection of *Shigella flexneri* by ethanol, 2-mercaptoethanol, and several polyhydric alcohols. Marcovich (1957) tested the ability of a group of alcohols, including glycerol, to protect *E. coli* K/2 irradiated while oxygen was bubbled through. Dewey (1963) later on reported protection in *Serratia marcescens* by glycerol, ethylene glycol, and ethanol. However, Erikson and Szybalski (1961) reported only glycerol to be radioprotective for eukaryotic cells.

Lohman *et al.* (1970) studied protection against X irradiation by cysteamine and glycerol on mammalian cells in tissue culture and bacteria (*E. coli* K12 AB 1157). Cysteamine protects against DNA breaks induced by irradiation in T cells and bacterial cells. In *E. coli* K12 cells, preincubation with cysteamine yielded a better protection in the stationary than in the logarithmic phase. Glycerol was found to protect mortality, as well as DNA breaks, only in T cells. Roots and Okada (1972) also reported protective action of alcohol and SH compounds against single-strand breaks in the DNA of mouse leukemia cells.

Yu and Sinclair (1970) showed that cysteamine protected against X-ray-induced mitotic delay and chromosomal aberrations in synchronized Chinese hamster cells. Stuart and Stannard in 1968 reported that although cystamine does not protect yeast or mammalian cells (Vos *et al.*, 1970), the addition of heparinized whole rat blood before irradiation led to the finding that cystamine was as protective as cysteamine, possibly as a result of cleavage of the disulfide bond. Vos *et al.* (1976) studied the protective action of cysteamine, WR-638, WR-2721, and 2-(3-aminopropylamino)ethylmercaptan (WR-1065) in a heteroploid human kidney cell line.

Nakayama and Nakamura (1978) observed radioprotective effects of 5-hydroxytryptamine (5-HT) and 5-hydroxytryptophan (5-HTP) in three mammalian cell lines: 5-HT synthesizing FM3A and 5-HT nonsynthesizing FM3A and B16 C2W. They reported that in these cells preincubation of cells for 40 min in a 5-HTP containing medium resulted in the elevation of the 5-HT content concomitantly with an increase in the radioresistance of FM3A cells.

Whillians and Hunt (1978), in rapid-mix experiments, showed that differences in incubation time of mammalian cells with cysteamine and DMSO were required to give detectable protection.

Compounds such as 5-fluorouracil (5-FU), thymidine, and flavins have been tested for their radioprotective effect against UV light (Roth and Roth, 1972; Kahn *et al.*, 1973; Kahn and Curry, 1979). Kano *et al.* (1979) reported that pretreatment of L cells with 4.5×10^{-4} *M* kerecyanin, one of the flavonoids, for 20 min provided protection against the lethal action of UV light (254 nm). The protection selectively appeared in UV-sensitive

S-phase cells, whereas the survival of less sensitive cells at the G_1–S border and in G_2 was apparently not affected by the drug.

Purdie (1979) made a comparative study of the radioprotective effects of cysteamine, WR-2721, and WR-1065 in cultured human cells and found that WR-2721 and WR-1065 had no harmful effect at concentrations of 4 and 10 mM for periods up to 3 h, whereas cysteamine was toxic if left in contact with cells for over 30 min. Increase in the concentration of protective agents did not increase the dose-reduction factor (DRF) under these conditions, except in the case of cysteamine. Extending the period of treatment before irradiation increased the DRF for WR-2721 and WR-1065.

Nagata (1980) investigated the protective effects of MPG and its derivatives on cultured mammalian cells. *In vitro* radioprotection was afforded by MPG at the dose of 0.01 to 0.1 mM, when applied 15 min prior to irradiation.

Vos *et al.* (1981) studied the radioprotection by a number of thiazolidine derivatives *in vitro:* thiazolidine, 5-methyl-2-phenylthiazolidine, 5-methylthiazolidine, *N*-propylthiazolidine, 2-phenylthiazolidine, 2-methyl-2-phenylthiazolidine, 2(2-methylphenyl)thiazolidine, 2-diethyl-2-germathiazolidine, and 2-dibutyl-2-germathiazolidine. Reproductive integrity of single cells was used as a parameter for survival after irradiation. They reported that thiazolidine had no protective effect when dissolved in culture medium, but that there was a good protective effect when thiazolidine was dissolved in rat blood. Rat blood improved the radioprotective activity of most other thiazolidine derivatives. Millar *et al.* (1981) observed that glycerol and DMSO protected Chinese hamster cells *in vitro,* irradiated in air.

C. Combined Effects of Radioprotective Drugs

Research on various chemical protectors has yet to produce a clinically applicable radioprotective drug. Compounds used in animal experiments appeared to be most effective, yet were extremely toxic in humans. Antagonists were then given attention. Different combinations of radioprotective agents with different mechanisms of action were used to decrease toxicity and increase radioprotective efficiency. Several articles have already been published describing the advantages of concomitant administration of two or more radioprotective agents (Wang and Kereiakes, 1962; Gantz and Wang, 1964; Maisin and Mattelin, 1967). The most extensively studied drug for combination use is AET. Sztanyik and Santha (1976) reported that combinations of radioprotective drugs, such as AET and cysteine, AET and methoxytryptamine (MOT), and AET and MPG, led to a most significant improvement in protective activity and diminution of toxicity. They studied the synergistic effect of AET in combination with MOT and reported that a combination of these radioprotectors in adequate proportions increased the survival of mice irradiated with lethal doses in the range of 630 to 1260 R more efficiently than when the components were given individually in larger doses. The $LD_{50/30}$ of mice treated with 150 mg/kg of AET and 12.5 mg/kg of MOT was increased from 500 ± 30 R to 1025 R (DRF = 2.05). This combination resulted in survival rates not achieved by either AET or MOT given separately.

They further reported that cysteine hydrochloride (CSH) but not AET diminishes the toxic effects of other components. The combination of AET and CSH improved the survival of mice as compared to individual administration of these drugs. An enhanced radioprotective effect in mice pretreated with a combination of 0.5 to 1.5 mM/kg of AET and 0.25 to 2.0 mM/kg of MPG, following exposure to supralethal doses of γ radiation, was observed (Sztanyik and Santha, 1976). The efficacy of radioprotection increased in proportion to the doses of the components combined. Maisin *et al.* (1976) also observed that the administration of a mixture of radioprotectors increases the degree of protection for the 30-day survival (compared with that of AET alone) but also exerts a favorable influence on the life span of mice exposed to single or repeated total-body X irradiations. However, Ghose and Pant (1981) reported that MPG combined with AET provided no additional radioprotection to peripheral blood leukocytes after 760-R γ-ray exposure. In contrast to AET, the combination was less effective than the respective dose given alone.

Newsome and Overman (1964) reported that a combination of AET and *p*-aminopropiophenone (PAPP) provided significant protection in dogs. Because AET protects animals from G.I. tract damage, it has been tested along with other drugs such as mexamine (Yarmonenko, 1965; Sztanyik and Santha, 1970), DMSO (Ashwood-Smith, 1962; Schröder and Huber, 1962), pentobarbital (Melville and Leffingwell, 1964), and cysteine (Anderson, 1962).

Mkrtchyan (1962) observed that although a mixture of cysteine and thiourea protected animals if administered preirradiation, the mixture given postirradiation hastened the death of the test animal.

Different combinations of cysteamine with other drugs have also been screened. Rothe and Grenan (1961) observed that in combination with colcemide, sodium arsenite, cadmium chloride, epinephrine, and cortisone, the radioprotection of cysteamine was enhanced. Serotonin has been successfully used in combination with sulfur-containing radioprotectors such as cysteamine, providing immediate protection of the bone marrow (Langendorff and Hagen, 1962). Serotonin with WR-638 protects the hematopoietic tissues of mouse spleen to a greater extent than the individual agents (Zaitseva *et al.*, 1969). Krasnykh *et al.* (1962) also reported that a combination of mexamine (75 mg/kg) and cysteamine (100 mg/kg) had excellent protective effects in white mice and rats.

Solov'e *et al.* (1979), using irradiated (950 R) mice, noted that the radioprotective effects of WR-2721 (administered orally) and diethyl *S*-ethylisothiuronium phosphate (inhaled) are additive, as long as these substances are administered in the small doses that provided a low radioprotective effect when the preparations were used individually.

Stoklasova *et al.* (1980) reported significantly better protection in rats treated with a mixture of cystamine and mexamine. Suroegin (1980) observed that a combination of WR-2721, *S*-ethylisothiouronium, euspiran, and mexamine, administered ip, possesses a better therapeutic efficacy than each of these protective agents ingested separately at supralethal radiation doses.

IV. Prospects

Radioprotective compounds have been used in experimental radiotherapy of cancer since 1949. However, because of their toxicity, low protective effects, and lack of a selective protection of normal tissues, they could not be applied clinically as radioprotectors.

Yuhas and Storer (1969) for the first time reported that the thiophosphate compound WR-2721 protected irradiated tissues in tumor-bearing mice but did not protect the tumor.

Harris and Phillips (1971) showed that WR-2721 protected marrow colony-forming units better than cysteamine, the DMFs being 3.0 and 1.7, respectively. Furthermore, WR-2721 protected hypoxic marrow cells only slightly, and, unlike cysteamine, entered cells by passive diffusion. Utley *et al.* (1974) also observed that in cases of EMT-6 tumor, WR-2721 was a poor protector of hypoxic cells.

Harris and Phillips (1971), Phillips *et al.* (1973), and Sigdestad *et al.* (1975) reported that WR-2721 protected tumor cells in the ascites form and therefore recommended that WR-2721 may not be useful for treating hematological neoplasms.

Phillips *et al.* (1973) reported a DMF of 1.3 for cure of solid EMT-6 carcinomas in mice. Yuhas (1973) had also shown the selective protection by WR-2721 for normal tissue, in case of a urethane-induced lung tumor system. Similar results were also obtained by Lowy and Baker (1973).

Utley *et al.* (1974) administered WR-2721 to mice 30 min before each of 10 irradiations in 12 days and obtained DMFs of 1.3 to 1.5 for skin damage and 1.7 for intestinal damage. Sigdestad *et al.* (1975) compared the protective efficacy of WR-2721 on tracts of mice irradiated with X rays or with fission neutrons. They found a relatively low protection for the X-irradiated gut (DMF = 1.6), and they obtained a similar DMF (1.6) in case of the neutron-irradiated gut.

Extensive studies on the pharmacological effects and distribution of WR-2721 revealed that it causes profound vasodilation in mice (Yuhas *et al.*, 1973), but that the cardiovascular effects in cats and dogs were not so acute (Caldwell and Heiffer, 1975).

The distribution of ^{35}S-labeled WR-2721 in normal and malignant tissues of mice and rats showed that there is a deficient absorption of the drug by a variety of solid tumors (Kollmann *et al.*, 1973; Washburn *et al.*, 1974). They suggested that WR-2721 does not penetrate the blood–brain barrier but does reach most other tissues, including the intestine and gut. Washburn *et al.* (1976) proposed that the tissue concentration of WR-2721 injected iv is more closely related to the injected dose per unit surface area than it is with the injected dose per unit body weight. They predicted that a dose of 20 mg of WR-2721 per kilogram of body weight would provide patients with the same degree of protection seen with 100 mg/kg in mice, that is, a 50–80% increase in radiation resistance.

Harris and Meneses (1978) examined the ability of WR-2721 to protect splenic T lymphocytes that responded to alloantigen in mixed-leukocyte cultures by differentiating into immunologically specific cytolytic T lymphocytes. They reported that WR-2721 provides a significant degree of protection for tissues and suggested that WR-2721 may prevent or moderate the immunosuppression that follows radiation therapy. Thus they confirmed the earlier observation of Yuhas (1972).

Sodicoff *et al.* (1979) observed the radioprotection of the rat parotid gland by WR-2721 alone (DMF = 2.4) and compared to the protection afforded when WR-2721 was given in combination with the hypoxic-cell radiosensitizer misonidazole (Ro-07-0582). They concluded that the radiosensitization of malignant tumor cells by Ro-07-0582 was compatible with that afforded without WR-2721 and did not reduce the protection of normal tissues afforded by WR-2721.

Studies on WR-2721 are under way in the United States and in Japan. Yuhas (1981) reported that a single dose as high as 740 mg/m^2 had been administered to patients without evidence of dose-limiting toxicity, and multiple-dose trials are in progress. Initial clinical trials involving WR-2721 in combination with cyclophosphamide or *cis*-platinum are in progress in various institutions.

Tanaka (1981) reported that in Japan the drug WR-2721 was named Amifostine, and the phase II study showed that side effects were all but nil in doses up to 2.0 mg/kg/day (60 mg/m^2). Liver function tests revealed normal ranges. The protective effects in the course of radiotherapy for carcinoma of the oral cavity showed a DMF of about 1.7 in grade 1, 1.3 in grade 2. In this group, the occurrence of xerostomia (52.9%) was decreased markedly compared with radiotherapy alone (73.3%). Fosteamine also protected to some extent the occurrence of fibrosis in the lung after radiotherapy for cancer.

V. Conclusion

Chemical protectors combined with radiosensitizers for treatment of patients with a malignancy have undergone extensive study. In various laboratories the world over, investigations are under way to obtain effective, low-toxicity compounds that will be synergistically functional in the protection of patients from lethal radiation.

References

Agrawal, O. P., and Nagaratnam, A. (1981). *Toxicon* **19**, 201.

Ainsworth, E. J., and Mitchell, F. A. (1968). *Radiat. Res.* **34**, 669.

Anderson, D. R. (1962). *Chem. Abstr.* **57**, 2543.

Antoku, S., and Sawada, S. (1970). *J. Radiat. Res.* **11**, 70.

Arburov, S. J. (1959). *Pharmazie* **14**, 132.

Ashwood-Smith, M. J. (1961). *Int. J. Radiat. Biol.* **3**, 41.

Ashwood-Smith, M. J. (1962). *Int. J. Radiat. Biol.* **5**, 201.

Bacq, Z. M., and Beaumariage, M. L. (1965). *Arch. Int. Pharmacodyn. Ther.* **153**, 457.

Bacq, Z. M., Herve, A., Lecomte, J., Fischer, P., Blavier, J., Decamps, G., Lebihan, H., and Rayet, P. (1951). *Arch. Int. Physiol.* **59**, 442.

Bacq, Z. M., Herve, A., and Scherber, F. (1953). *Arch. Int. Pharmacodyn. Ther.* **94**, 93.

Bacq, Z. M., Beaumariage, M. L., and Radiojevic, D. (1961). *Bull. Acad. R. Med. Belg.* **1**, 519.

Baver, D., Locker, A., Grigoriadis, P., Goslar, H. G., and Jaeger, K. H. (1981). *Biochem. Exp. Biol.* **15**, 147.

Beaumariage, M. L. (1957). *C. R. Seances Soc. Biol. Ses Fil.* **5**, 1788.

Beaumariage, M. L., van Canegham, P., and Bacq, Z. M. (1966). *Strahlentherapie* **131**, 342.

Booz, G., Simar, L. J., and Betz, E. H. (1965). *Int. J. Radiat. Biol.* **9**, 429.

Braams, R. (1960). *Radiat. Res.* **12**, 113.

Breccia, A., Badiello, R., Trenta, A., and Matti, M. (1969). *Radiat. Res.* **38**, 483.

Bridges, B. A. (1962). *Radiat. Res.* **17**, 801.

Bron, J. W., and Lajtha, L. T. (1966). *Br. J. Radiol.* **39**, 382.

Caldwell, R. W., and Heiffer, M. H. (1975). *Radiat. Res.* **62**, 62.

Chapman, W. II., and Cronkite, E. P. (1950). *Proc. Soc. Exp. Biol. Med.* **75**, 318.

Chaudhuri, J. P., and Langendorff, H. (1970). *In* "Radiation Protection and Sensitization" (H. L. Morison and H. L. Qumtiliani, eds.), p. 376. Taylor & Francis, London.

Cittadini, G., Lanfredini, L., and Mancini, G. (1970). *In* "Radiation Protection and Sensitization" (H. L. Morison and H. L. Quintiliani, eds.), p. 335. Taylor & Francis, London.

Cramp, W. A. (1969). *Int. J. Radiat. Biol.* **15**, 227.

Dale, W. M. (1942). *Biochemistry* **36**, 80.

Dev, P. K., Goyal, P. K., and Kumar, S. (1982). *Radiobiol. Radiother. (Berlin)* **23**, 173–177.

Dewey, D. L. (1963). *Radiat. Res.* **19**, 64.

Doherty, D. G., and Burnett, W. T., Jr. (1955). *Proc. Soc. Exp. Biol. Med.* **89**, 312.

Doherty, D. G., Burnett, W. T., Jr., and Shapiro, R. (1957). *Radiat. Res.* **7**, 13.

Doull, J., Phak, V., and Brois, S. J. (1959). *Radiat. Res.* **11**, 439.

Dukor, P. (1962). *Strahlentherapie* **117**, 330.

Duzhenkova, N. A. (1979). *Radiobiologiya* **19**, 604.

Edsmyr, F. W., Huber, W., and Menander, K. B. (1976). *Curr. Ther. Res.* **19**, 198.

Erikson, R. L., and Szybalski, W. (1961). *Biochem. Biophys. Res. Commun.* **4**, 258.

Farmer, P. S., Leung, C., and Lui, E. M. K. (1973). *J. Med. Chem.* **16**, 411.

Gantz, J. A., and Wang, R. I. H. (1964). *J. Nucl. Med.* **5**, 606.

Gheorghe, N., Boeresci, I., and Sandulescu, T. (1980). *Rev. Roum. Morphol. Embryol. Physiol.* **17**, 77.

Ghose, A., and Pant, R. D. (1981). *J. Radiat. Res.* **22**, 381.

Ginoza, W., and Norman, A. (1957). *Nature (London)* **179**, 520.

Gorodetskii, A. A., Baraboi, V. A., and Cherentskii, V. P. (1965). *Chem. Abs.* **63**, 18617.

Graevsky, E. Y., Konstantinova, M. M., Nekraskova, I. V., Sokolova, O. M., and Tarasenko, A. (1966). *Nature London* **212**, 475.

Harris, J. W., and Meneses, J. J. (1978). *Int. J. Radiat. Oncol. Biol. Phys.* **4**, 437.

Harris, J. W., and Phillips, T. L. (1971). *Radiat. Res.* **46**, 362.

Hasegawa, A. J., and Landahl, H. D. (1967). *Radiat. Res.* **31**, 389.

Holmberg, B., and Sorbo, B. (1959). *Nature London* **183**, 832.

Hotz, G., and Müller, A. (1962). *Z. Naturforsch.* **176**, 34.

Howard-Flanders, P. (1960). *Nature London* **186**, 485.

Il'Yuchenok, T. Yu., Frigilova, L. M., Shadurskii, K. S., Lepekhin, V. P., Ignatova, L. A., and Unikovskii, B. V. (1979). *Farmakol. Toksikol. (Moscow)* **42**, 643.

Kahn, G., and Curry, M. C. (1979). *Arch. Dermatol.* **109**, 510.

Kahn, G., Curry, M. C., and Dustin, R. (1973). *Dermatologica* **147**, 97.

Kakehi, H., Ichikawa, H., and Nakano, M. (1961). *Radioisotopes* **10**, 240.

Kalnitskii, S. A., Ponomarena, T. V., and Shubik, V. M. (1979). *Radiobiologiya* **19**, 246.

Kaluszyner, A., Czerniak, P., and Bergmann, E. D. (1961). *Radiat. Res.* **14**, 23.

Kano, E., Miyakoshi, J., Ikebuchi, M., Yamagata, K., and Sugahara, T. (1979). *Radiat. Res.* **77**, 547.

Klayman, D. L. (1973). *In* "Organic Selenium Compounds, Their Chemistry and Biology" (D. L. Klayman and W. H. H. Günther, eds.), p. 727. Wiley, New York.

Kohn, H., and Gunter, S. E. (1959). *Radiat. Res.* **11**, 732.

Kojima, K. (1961). *Chem. Abstr.* **55**, 27645.

Kollmann, G., Yuhas, J., Leon, S., and Shapiro, B. (1973). *Radiat. Res.* **55**, 603 (Abstr.)

Krasnykh, I. G., Zherebchenko, P. G., Murashova, V. S., Suvorov, N. N., and Sorokina, N. P. (1962). *Radiobiologiya* **2**, 298.

Kumar, A., and Bhagat, R. M. (1981). *Radiobiol. Radiother.* (Berlin) **22**, 635–638.

Langendorff, H. (1962). *Eff. Ioniz. Radiat. Immune Processes Sci. Pap. Int. Symp.*, p. 281.

Langendorff, H., and Hagen, U. (1962). *Strahlentherapie* **117**, 321.

Langendorff, H., Melching, J., and Ladner, H. A. (1959). *Strahlentherapie* **108**, 57.

Latarjet, R., and Ephrati, E. (1948). *C. R. Seances Soc. Biol. Ses Fil.* **142**, 497.

Lohman, P. H. M., Vos, O., van Sluis, C. A., and Cohen, J. A. (1970). *Biochim. Biophys. Acta* **224**, 339.

Lowy, R. O., and Baker, D. G. (1973). *Acta Radiol.* **12**, 425.

Lüning, K. G., Frölen, H., and Nelson, A. (1961). *Radiat. Res.* **14**, 813.

Lyashenko, V. D., Pekkerman, S. M., Semenov, L. F., and Simon, I. B. (1959). *Tiolvye Soedin. Med. Tr. Nauchn. Konf.*, p. 276.

Maisin, J. R., and Doherty, D. G. (1963). *Radiat. Res.* **19**, 474.

Maisin, J. R., and Mattelin, G. (1967). *Nature (London)* **214**, 207.

Maisin, J. R., Novelli, G. D., Doherty, D. G., and Congdon, C. C. (1960). *Int. J. Radiat. Biol.* **2**, 281.

Maisin, J. R., Collier, M. L., and Mattelin, G. (1976). *In* "Modification of Radiosensitivity of Biological System" (International Atomic Energy Agency), p. 89. Vienna.

Makhalova, O. K., Mozzhukhin, A. S., and Bertash, V. I. (1966). *Radiobiologiya* **6**, 883.

Mandl, A. M. (1959). *Int. J. Radiat. Biol.* **1**, 131.

Marcovich, H. (1957). *Ann. Inst. Pasteur (Paris)* **93**, 456.

Melville, G. S., Jr., and Leffingwell, T. P. (1964). *Chem. Abstr.* **61**, 10980.

Millar, B. C., Sapora, O., Fielden, E. M., and Loverock, P. S. (1981). *Radiat. Res.* **86**, 506.

Mkrtchyan, R. G. (1962). *Chem. Abstr.* **56**, 6334.

Modig, H. G., and Révész, L. (1967). *Int. J. Radiat. Biol.* **13**, 469.

Mole, R. H., Philbot, J. St. L., and Hodges, G. R. V. (1950). *Nature (London)* **166**, 515.

Nagata, H. (1980). *J. Exp. Med.* **27**, 15.

Nagata, H., Sugahara, T., and Tanaka, T. (1972). *J. Radiat. Res.* **13**, 163.

Nakayama, T., and Nakamura, W. (1978). *Int. J. Radiat. Biol.* **34**, 81.

Newsome, J. R., and Overman, R. R. (1964). *Radiat. Res.* **21**, 520.

Nishimura, A., Hashimoto, M., Konno, K., Ohta, Y., Tahara, S., and Nishimura, H. (1980). *Z. Naturforsch.* **35**, 726.

Novak, L. (1970). *In* "Radiation Protection and Sensitization" (H. L. Morison and M. Quintiliani, eds.), p. 335. Francis & Taylor, London.

Novikova, A. P., Postovskii, Ya., Puchkova, S. M., Chechulina, L. A., and Tuzhilkova, T. N. (1980). *Khim. Farm. Zh.* **14**, 46.

Patt, H. M., Tyree, E. B., Straube, R. L., and Smith, D. E. (1949). *Science (Washington, D.C.)* **110**, 113.

Petkau, A. (1978). *Photochem. Photobiol.* **28**, 765.

Phillips, T. L., Kane, L., and Utley, J. F. (1973). *Cancer (Philadelphia)* **32**, 528.

Piper, J. R., Stringbellow, C. R., Jr., Elliot, R. D., and Johnson, T. P. (1969). *J. Med. Chem.* **12**, 236.

Pospisil, M., Netikova, J., Pipalova, I., and Mikeska, J. (1980). *Folia Biol. (Prague)* **26**, 53.

Pozza, F., and Verza, G. (1960). *Boll. Soc. Ital. Biol. Sper.* **36**, 1120.

Purdie, J. W. (1979). *Radiat. Res.* **77**, 303.

Révész, L., and Modig, H. (1965). *Nature (London)* **207**, 430.

Riemschneider, R. (1961). *Z. Naturforsch.* **16B**, 75.

Riemschneider, R., and Hoyer, G. A. (1962). *Z. Naturforsch.* **17B**, 765.

Romantsev, E. F., and Tikhomirova, M. V. (1963). *Radiobiologiya* **3**, 126.

Romito, S. (1970). *Chem. Abstr.* **73**, 84419.

Roots, R., and Okada, S. (1972). *Int. J. Radiat. Biol.* **21**, 329.

Roth, D., and Roth, D. M. (1972). *J. Invest. Dermatol.* **58**, 233.

Rothe, W. E., and Grenan, M. M. (1961). *Science (Washington, D.C.)* **133**, 888.

Sakakibara, T., Miyamoto, S., Aizawa, K., Nagoya, T., and Toshioka, T. (1966). *Chem. Abstr.* **65**, 18967.

Schröder, E., and Huber, R. (1962). *Acta Biol. Med. Ger.* **9**, 62.
Shapiro, W., Tansy, M. F., and Elkin, S. (1968). *J. Pharm. Sci.* **57**, 1725.
Sigdestad, C. P., Connor, A. M., and Scott, R. M. (1975). *Radiat. Res.* **62**, 267.
Smith, D. E. (1959). *Radiat. Res.* **10**, 335.
Smith, W. W. (1958). *Science (Washington D.C.)* **127**, 340.
Smith, W. W., Alderman, I. M., and Gillespie, R. E. (1957). *Am. J. Physiol.* **191**, 124.
Smoliar, V. (1962). *C. R. Seances Soc. Biol. Ses Fil.* **156**, 1202.
Sodicoff, M., Conger, A. D., Pratt, N. E., Sinesi, M., and Trepper, P. (1979). *Radiat. Res.* **80**, 348.
Solv'e, V., Yu, A., and Zherebchenko, P. G. (1979). *Radiobiologiya* **19**, 143.
Sorbo, B. (1958). *Acta Chem. Scand.* **12**, 1990.
Srivastava, P. N. (1971). *In* "Biological Aspects of Radiation Protection" (T. Sugahara and O. Hug, eds.), p. 157. Igaku-Shoin, Tokyo.
Starkie, C. M. (1961). *Int. J. Radiat. Biol.* **3**, 609.
Stoklasova, A., Krizala, J., and Ledrina, M. (1980). *Strahlentherapie* **156**, 205.
Storer, J. B., and Coon, J. M. (1950). *Proc. Soc. Exp. Biol. Med.* **74**, 202.
Streffer, C., Langendorff, H., and Allert, U. (1968). *Strahlentherapie* **135**, 76.
Stromberg, L. R., McLaughlin, M. M., and Donati, R. M. (1968). *Proc. Soc. Exp. Biol. Med.* **129**, 140.
Sugahara, T. (1974). *In* "Fraction Size in Radiobiology and Radiotherapy" (L. Revesz, O. Scott, and T. Sugahara, eds.), p. 84. Igaku-Shoin, Tokyo.
Sugahara, T., and Tanaka, T. (1968). *Nature (London)* **220**, 271.
Sugahara, T., Tanaka, Y., Nagata, H., Tanaka, T., and Kano, E. (1970). *Proc. Int. Symp. Thiola*, p. 267.
Suroegin, E. V. (1980). *Radiobiologiya* **20**, 746.
Sverdlov, A. G., Bogatyren, A. V., Nikanorova, N. G., Timoshenko, S. I., and Kalmykova, G. I. (1979). *Radiobiologiya* **19**, 293.
Sverdlov, A. G., Grachev, S. A., Bondarev, A. N., Bogatyereu, A. V., Nikanorova, N. G., Timoshenko, S. J., Kalmykova, G. I., and Krasotskaya, G. I. (1980). *Radiobiologiya* **20**, 143.
Sztanyik, L. B., and Santha, A. (1970). *In* "Radiation Protection and Sensitization" (H. L. Morison, and M. Quintiliani, eds.), p. 325. Francis & Taylor, London.
Sztanyik, L. B., and Santha, A. (1976). *In* "Modification of Radiosensitivity of Biological Systems," p. 47. International Atomic Energy Agency, Vienna.
Tanaka, T., and Sugahara, T. (1970). *J. Radiat. Res.* **11**, 166.
Tanaka, Y. (1981). *In* "Prospective Methods of Radiotherapy in Developing Countries," p. 35. International Atomic Energy Agency, Vienna.
Uma Devi, P., Saini, M. R., Saharan, B. R., and Bhartiya, H. C. (1979). *Radiat. Res.* **80**, 214.
Utley, J. F., Phillips, T. L., Kane, L. J., Wharam, M. D., and Wara, W. M. (1974). *Radiology (Easton, Pa.)* **110**, 213.
Vacek, A., and Sugahara, T. (1967). *Proc. Soc. Exp. Biol. Med.* **124**, 356.
van der Meer, C., and van Bekkum, D. W. (1959). *Int. J. Radiat. Biol.* **1**, 5.
Vergroesen, A. J., Budke, L., and Vos, O. (1967). *Int. J. Radiat. Biol.* **13**, 77.
Vos, O., Grant, G. A., and Budke, L. (1970). *Int. J. Radiat. Biol.* **18**, 111.
Vos, O., Budke, L., and Grant, G. A. (1976). *Int. J. Radiat. Biol.* **30**, 433.
Vos, O., Budke, L., Fatome, M., and Vanhoodonk, C. (1981). *Int. J. Radiat. Biol.* **39**, 291.
Wang, R. I. H., and Kereiakes, J. G. (1962). *Acta Radiol.* **52**, 99.
Washburn, L. D., Carlton, J. E., Hayes, R. L., and Yuhas, J. M. (1974). *Radiat. Res.* **59**, 475.

Washburn, L. D., Rafter, J. J., and Hayes, R. L. (1976). *Radiat. Res.* **66,** 100.

Whillians, D. W., and Hunt, J. W. (1978). *Br. J. Cancer* **37** (Suppl. 3), 38.

Yakovlev, V. G. (1962). *Chem. Abstr.* **56,** 1724.

Yarmonenko, S. P. (1965). *Zh. Obshch. Biol.* **26,** 501.

Yu, C. K., and Sinclair, W. K. (1970). *Radiat. Res.* **43,** 357.

Yuhas, J. M. (1969). *J. Gerontol.* **24,** 251.

Yuhas, J. M. (1972). *Cell. Immunol.* **4,** 256.

Yuhas, J. M. (1973). *J. Natl. Cancer Inst.* (*US*) **50,** 69.

Yuhas, J. M. (1981). *In* "Prospective Methods of Radiotherapy in Developing Countries," International Atomic Energy Agency, Vienna.

Yuhas, J. M., and Storer, J. B. (1969). *J. Natl. Cancer Inst.* (*US*) **42,** 331.

Yuhas, J. M., Tennant, R. W., Hanna, M. G., and Clayp, N. K. (1973). *In* "Radionuclide Carcinogenesis" (C. L. Sanders, R. H. Busch, J. E. Bullov, and D. P. Mahalam, eds.), p. 312. US Atomic Energy Cmsion., Washington, D.C.

Zaitseva, K. K., Zherebchenko, P. G., and Zaitseva, T. G. (1969). *Radiobiologiya* **9,** 236.

Zherbchenko, P. G., and Zaitseva, T. G. (1969). *Radiobiologiya* **9,** 701.

5 Clinical Experiences with a Chemical Radioprotector in Tumor Radiotherapy: WR-2721

Yoshimasa Tanaka

Department of Radiology
Kansai Medical University
Moriguchi 750, Japan

I. Introduction

Since cysteine was found by Patt *et al.* (1949) to protect lethally irradiated rats, sulfhydryl compounds that provide protection of laboratory animals against lethal doses of ionizing radiations have also been given much attention. The SH compounds have been the most extensively investigated, and β-aminoethylisothiouronium (AET) and cysteamine have been selected as being representative of those drugs that are highly protective. However, clinical application is limited, as the toxicity of these compounds is high.

In a series of experiments to reevaluate radioprotective agents with low toxicity, we found that 2-mercaptopropionylglycine (MPG) and adrenochrome monoguanylhydrazone methanesulfonate (AMM) have a potent radioprotector effect in a dose far below their toxic doses in both mice and humans (Sugahara and Tanaka, 1968; Sugahara *et al.*, 1970, 1977; Nagata *et al.*, 1972; Sugahara, 1973). Recently, the development of effective

Modification of Radiosensitivity in Cancer Treatment
Copyright © 1984 by Academic Press Japan, Inc.
All rights of reproduction in any form reserved.
ISBN 0-12-676020-9

$$\left[\begin{array}{c} {}^{+}NH_3 \cdot C \cdot NH \cdot C \underset{\underset{\displaystyle NH}{\|}}{\overset{}{}} \quad OH \\ \end{array} \right] CH_3SO_3^{-} H_2O$$

$$C_{11}H_{17}N_5O_5S \cdot H_2O: 349.37$$

thiophosphate derivatives of cysteamine, namely WR-2721 [*S*-2-(3-amino-propylaminoethyl)phosphorothioate] by the U.S. Army Medical Research and Development Commands, led to a reevaluation of these compounds and their potential in radiotherapy (Yuhas and Storer, 1969; Yuhas, 1981). Initial investigations by Yuhas and Storer (1969) indicated that WR-2721 provided a considerable degree of radioprotection to normal tissues. This compound provided excellent protection for normal tissues (DMF = 2–2.5) but little protection for the transplanted tumor. Thus this drug may have a differential protection *in vivo* and may be useful for improving the therapeutic ratio in cancer radiotherapy. In Japan, this compound was manufactured by the Yamanouchi Pharmaceutical Co. Ltd. with the commercial name Amifostine (YM-08310), and the phase II study has been completed. The results of animal and chemical experiments in Japan are summarized herein.

II. Studies on a Chemical Protector with a Low Toxicity

A. Protective Effects in Mice with MPG and AMM

Since 1963 MPG has been prescribed in Japan as a detoxifying drug with a wide range of clinical applications and is particularly effective for metal poisoning. This compound is manufactured and sold by the Santen Pharmaceutical Co. Ltd., Osaka, under the commercial name Thiola (Sugahara *et al.*, 1977).

Protection against a lethal dose of ^{60}Co γ ray with MPG has been studied extensively in mice. Male dd/Y mice obtained from Funabashi Farms were used at 60 days of age. The percentage of 30-day survivals of mice irradiated with graded doses and given an ip dose of MPG 15 min before irradiation are shown in Fig. 1. Contrary to expectations, the MPG dose of 0.5 mg/mouse was more effective than 1.0 mg/mouse. The dose-modifying factors (DMF) based on $LD_{50/30}$ are 1.4 and 1.22 for the doses of 0.5 and 1.0 mg, respectively. To confirm the higher effectiveness of 0.5

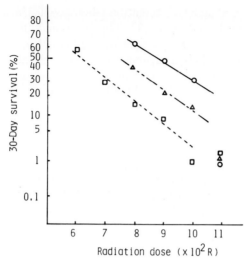

Fig. 1. Dose–survival relationship for mice given MPG 15 min before irradiation. MPG 0.5 mg/mouse (DRF 1.4, ○) or 1.0 mg/mouse (DRF 1.22, △) was administered ip. □, Control.

mg/mouse, the doses of MPG from 0.01 to 1.0 mg/mouse were tested for protection, and the percentage of 30-day mortality of mice thus treated are shown in Fig. 2. Maximum protection was observed in a dose of 0.5 mg/mouse. This dose corresponds approximately to 20 mg/kg body weight.

Protection in mice using such a low dose was confirmed in later experiments done for a comparison with other compounds (Nagata *et al.*, 1972; Sugahara *et al.*, 1977). The protective effects of MPG lasted for more than 3 h after a single ip administration. The mechanisms of such prolonged protection remain to be elucidated.

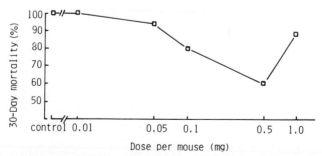

Fig. 2. Thirty-day percentage mortality of mice given various doses of MPG 30 min before irradiation (1000 R).

Mice are protected against irradiation when given AMM in a low dose of 5 mg/kg ip, and the DMF is 1.32. The combined effect of MPG with AMM was studied in mice by giving 20 mg/kg ip of MPG 30 min and 5 mg/kg ip of AMM 15 min before irradiation. This combined administration resulted in a higher survival rate than was seen with a single treatment with MPG. The DMF of the combined treatment was estimated to be about 1.6.

B. Clinical Applications of MPG and AMM

Cervical cancer patients given radiotherapy were treated with MPG in a dose already recognized to be safe for humans being treated for liver diseases and for metal intoxications. The cancer patients receiving fractionated radiotherapy were divided at random into two groups.

Patients in one group were given MPG 250 mg iv in a 20% glucose solution 15–30 min before each irradiation, and those in the other group served as the untreated controls. Also before each irradiation, 100 mg of AMM were administered. All patients receiving whole-pelvis irradiation through two parallel opposing fields using a 6-MeV Linac by the conventional fractionation method in a dose of 150 rads, 5 days/week, the total tumor dose being about 6000 rads in the case of radiotherapy alone, or 4050 rads in postoperative cases.

Peripheral blood cell counts and blood cell cultures for chromosome study were performed at various intervals and at 1 or 2 weeks after the last exposure.

Chromosome preparations were performed according to the method of Moorhead et al. (1961) with some modification. The culture time was 50 h in all cases (Tanaka and Sugahara, 1970). Differences in the leukocyte counts and aberration yields between the treated and untreated groups were statistically significant near the end of the therapy, as shown in Table I. The effect on the leukocyte counts was confirmed by a double-blind test carried out with the collaboration of eight hospitals in Japan.

In the case of AMM, the increases in the percentage of cells with an acentric fragment and in the percentage of cells with dicentrics and rings in protected and control patients are shown in Figs. 3 and 4, respectively. The nonlinear increases in the incidence are in good accord with the results of Tamura et al. (1970). The increase in chromosome aberrations was inhibited in the drug-treated patients. With the χ^2 test, the difference was statistically significant ($p < .05$) at 3000 rads and 1 week after radiotherapy for dicentrics and rings. It should be noted that this depression was not apparent at 1000 rads, that is, 10 days after the start of the radiotherapy.

TABLE I

Leukocyte Counts and Incidence of Chromosome Aberrations
Close to the End of Radiotherapy in Treated and
Control Patients

	MPG + X[a]	AMM + X	X Alone
White blood cells			
Number of cases	16	18	15
Leukocyte counts	$4500^b \pm 580^c$	4300 ± 650^c	3500 ± 380^c
Lymphocyte counts	$45.3^b \pm 8.8^c$	43.2 ± 9.2^c	29.4 ± 11.6^c
(% of control)			
Chromosome aberrations			
Number of cases	9	6	5
Total number of cells scored	525	450	420
Cells with acentric fragments (%)	8.6^b	—	14.1
Cells with dicentrics (%)	7.1^b	8.2^b	11.0

[a] $X = $ X irradiation (5000 rads).
[b] $p < .05$.
[c] Mean $\pm$ SD.

In clinical studies, the most important problem is to see whether or not these drugs have a protective effect against late injuries as well as acute radiation effects. Cervical cancer patients given radiotherapy were examined for injuries to the bowel such as ileus symptoms and bleeding. All

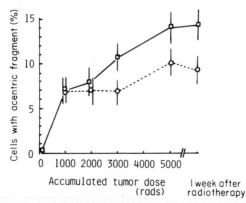

Fig. 3. Percentage of cells with acentric fragment in peripheral lymphocyte during and after radiotherapy, 150 rads/day, five times/week. □———□, Control patients; O-----O, protected patients (AMM 100 mg iv within 20 min before irradiation).

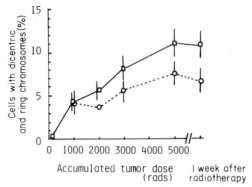

Fig. 4. Percentage of cells with dicentric and ring chromosomes in peripheral lymphocyte during and after radiotherapy. For symbols, see Fig. 3.

those patients at 5 years posttreatment had received a total dose of 6000 rads. Treated groups with MPG compared with X-treated alone revealed no significant difference in survival, but there were fewer complications. Namely, 236 patients with no chemical protector treatment had 11 various side effects (4.7%) related to bowel injuries, and in 48 patients who had been given MPG, only one (2.1%) had side effects, as shown in Table II.

Chemical protection by SH compounds in mice and humans is summarized in Table III (Sugahara *et al.*, 1977). Glutathione has been widely used in Japan, and protection against radiation-induced leukopenia has been reported (Sugahara *et al.*, 1977). The doses effective for humans were very low compared with the effective dose in mice. In comparison with these compounds, MPG and AMM can be given to humans in a dose comparable to that effective for both species. As reported by Sugahara (Sugahara, 1973; Sugahara *et al.*, 1977), protection for humans was demonstrated not only in leukocyte counts that have large individual and physiological variations, but also in the yield of chromosome aberrations

TABLE II

Number of Late Injuries of the Bowel
after Radiotherapy[a]

	Number of patients	Number of bowel injuries
MPG not given	236	11 (4.7%)
MPG given	48	1 (2.1%)

[a] Late injuries consist of ileus symptom, bleeding no operation; 6000 rads irradiated.

TABLE III

Chemical Radiation Protection in Mice and Humans

Compound	Biological features	Mice				Humans	
		Toxicity (LD_{50}, mg/kg)	Protective dose (mg/kg)	DMF	Administered dose (mg/kg)	Leukopenia protection	Chromosomal aberration protection
Cysteine	Natural	1500	1200 iv	1.42	n.d.[a]	—	—
Glutathione	Natural	4000	4000 ip	1.28	200	yes	no
			1600 ip	1.12	—	—	—
Cysteamine	Toxic	275	150 ip	1.45	200–400	yes	no
AET	Toxic	690	400 ip	2.15	100–200	yes	no
WR-2721	Toxic	550	400 ip	2.60	100–200	yes	no
MPG	Nontoxic	1400	20 ip	1.40	250	yes	yes
AMM	Nontoxic	—	50 ip	1.32	100	yes	yes

[a] n.d., not done.

in peripheral lymphocytes. Chromosome aberrations are a rather consistent parameter for radiation effects in humans and can be used for biological dosimetry.

III. Radioprotective Effects of WR-2721 (YM-08310) in Japan

A. Experimental Results in Mice (Tanaka and Sugahara, 1980)

1. The Distribution of [¹⁴C]YM-08310 in Tissues

The distribution pattern of [¹⁴C]YM-08310 in normal and tumor tissue (MM-2 mouse mammary tumor) following single iv administration in a dose of 100 mg/kg to C3H mice was studied. The drug was found in the majority of the tissues such as the salivary gland, kidney, lung, and small intestine at higher levels than in the blood and plasma, within 30 min after injection (Tanaka and Sugahara, 1980). The drug was transferred into

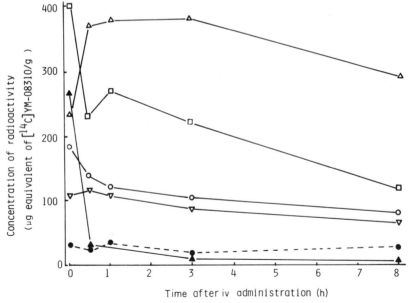

Fig. 5. Concentration of radioactivity in various body tissues after a single iv administration (100 mg/kg) to C3H mice of [¹⁴C]YM-08310. △, Salivary gland; □, kidney; ○, lung; ▽, small intestine; ●, plasma; ▲, tumor (1 cm³).

tumor tissue and testes at very low levels, and was not found in the central nervous system, as shown in Fig. 5. An initial high level in the kidney fell rapidly with time, thereby suggesting a rapid excretion. Figure 6 shows the radioactivity in tissues after 21 daily repeated administrations. The tissue levels of the drug were four to eight times higher compared with the levels after one administration, after which the levels reached a plateau. The mouse mammary tumor had a low concentration with only a minimal increase over a 21-day period. This correlated with the low level of radioprotection demonstrated in this tumor.

Whole-body autoradiograms of mice 3 min, 30 min, 1 h, and 3 h after injection of 100 mg/kg of [^{14}C]YM-08310 are shown in Fig. 7. Radioactivity was higher in salivary gland and intestinal mucosa, thus corresponding to the radioprotection by this drug (Fig. 5, Fig. 7). On the contrary, at 3 min the mammary tumor and brain showed very little drug concentration. At 30 min there appeared to be a slight increase in density in the periphery of the mammary tumor, but concentrations in the center of the tumor mass were lower than levels in the circulating blood.

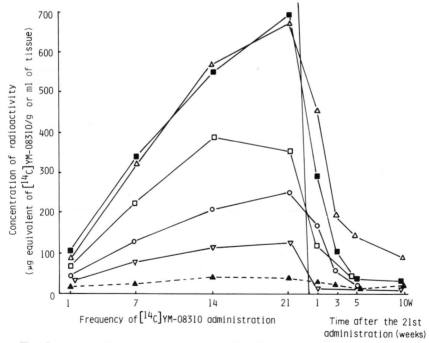

Fig. 6. Concentration of radioactivity in various body tissues after daily repeated iv administrations (100 mg/kg) to C3H mice of [^{14}C]YM-08310. △, Salivary gland; ■, spleen; □, kidney; ○, pancreas; ▽, small intestine; ▲, tumor.

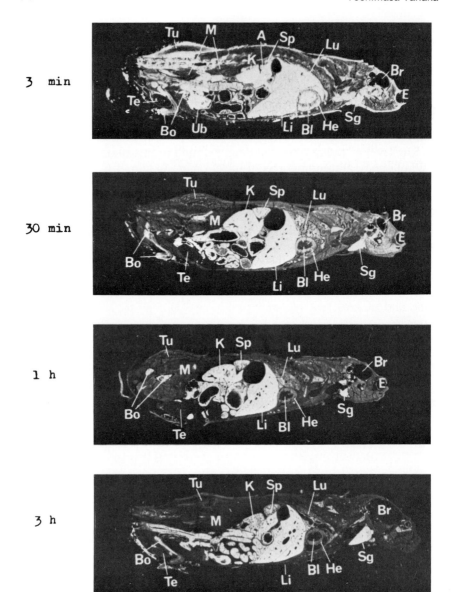

Fig. 7. Autoradiograms showing the distribution over time of radioactivity (740 μCi/kg) after a single iv administration of [^{14}C]YM-08310 (100 mg/kg) in a male mouse bearing the MM-2 mouse mammary tumor. A, Adrenal; Bl, blood; Bo, bone; Br, brain; E, eyeball; He, heart; K, kidney; Li, liver; Lu, lung; M, muscle; Sg, salivary glands; Sp, spleen; Te, testicle; Tu, tumor; Ub, urinary bladder.

2. *Radioprotection of the Tumor and Normal Tissues by YM-08310 in Mice*

The radioprotective effects by YM-08310 were determined over a wide range of normal and tumor tissues. The compound was dissolved in distilled water and 400 mg/kg given ip prior to irradiation (Table IV). The maximum protective effects against whole-body lethality secondary to bone marrow damage were obtained when YM-08310 was injected 60 min before irradiation. The degree of protection was dose dependent; that is, there appeared to be an increasing dose-modifying factor when the dose of YM-08310 was increased in the range of 20 to 300 mg/kg.

Esophageal damage by irradiation was measured by esophageal $LD_{50/30}$, using C57BL mice. The DMF value obtained for esophageal death for air-breathing animals was 1.5; it was 1.7 for animals breathing oxygen at 1 atm.

Pulmonary damage was measured by pulmonary $LD_{50/160}$. The DMF value in case of pulmonary death while breathing air was 1.2.

Delay in regrowth, using the sarcoma 180 as a function of radiation alone and of radiation combined with treatment of YM-08310 prior to exposure, was also studied. There was no statistical difference in delay in regrowth between the two groups.

From animal studies, the degree of protection that can be achieved by YM-08310 is not uniform in each organ (Phillips *et al.*, 1973). It may be concluded that YM-08310 shows significant protection for bone marrow, skin, mucous membranes, salivary glands, and the small intestine. This

TABLE IV

Radioprotection of Normal Tissues by YM-08310 in
C57BL Mice

Mode	$LD_{50/30}$ (rads)	$LD_{50/160}$ (rads)	DMF
Whole-body lethality			
Air	583	—	—
Air + YM-08310	1230	—	2.1
Esophageal lethality			
Air	2600	—	—
Air + YM-08310	3850	—	1.5
Oxygen (1 atm)	2120	—	—
Oxygen + YM-08310	3625	—	1.7
Pulmonary lethality			
Air	—	1500	—
Air + YM-08310	—	1820	1.2

compound appears to have potential effectiveness for treatment of head and neck cancer and of abdominal malignancies, as well as with hemibody and whole-body irradiation, where its significant bone marrow protection will be important, as described by Phillips (1982).

B. Clinical Applications of YM-08310 in Tumor Radiotherapy

1. Results of the Phase II Study

The phase II study was completed in Japan with the collaboration of eight hospitals (Tanaka and Sugahara, 1980). Immediately before use, YM-08310 was dissolved in saline solution; it was then slowly injected iv 30 min before irradiation.

a. Side effects. Side effects seen with 2.0 mg/kg/day (60 mg/m²) of this drug are shown in Table V. Slight fever occurrence in 10.5% (eight), nausea in 5.2% (four), but sometimes the effect could hardly be distinguished from the effects caused by the radiation therapy itself. These side effects were not so serious and disappeared with cessation of administration of the drug. Onset of side effects usually occurred the first week after irradiation but rarely the second week or later on. Liver function tests were within normal limits during and after radiotherapy, and elevations of serum GOT and GPT observed in a few patients was slight and transient.

b. Evaluation of YM-08310 (Table VI). In the phase II study there were 17 cases of head and neck tumors, 10 of lung cancer, and 6 of breast cancer. This treatment was evaluated to be remarkably effective in 5, moderately effective in 15, not so effective in 7, and ineffective in 7.

TABLE V

Frequencies of Side Effects with
YM-08310

Side effect	Number of cases (%)
Slight fever	8 (10.5)
Exanthema	7 (9.2)
Nausea	4 (5.2)
Diarrhea	1 (1.3)
Vomiting	1 (1.3)
Total no. of patients with side effects	12 (15.7)
Total no. of patients	76 (100)

2. Radioprotection of the Oral Cavity by YM-08310

a. Radioprotection from death due to oral radiation (Goepp, 1962, 1967). The findings of a high concentration of [^{14}C]YM-08310 in mouse salivary glands led to studies of possible radioprotection of these glands from radiation. Irradiation was given to the heads of C57BL mice. The field extended from the tip of the nose to the base of the neck. The weight loss was progressive, amounting to about 50% at the time of death, 10–15 days after irradiation. The mice were given YM-08310, 450 mg/kg ip, 30 min before a single exposure to radiation, the dose of which ranged from 1500 to 3000 rads. The $LD_{50/20}$ occurred in nontreated groups at 2100 rads. In animals treated with YM-08310, this occurred at 3000 rads. Here, the DMF was 1.4. Utley (1978) also showed that the dose required to induce "radiation oral death syndrome" increased by a factor of 2.1 in BALB/c mice, when WR-2721 was given 30 min before irradiation of the head. The salivary flow in mongrel dogs following doses of 1000 to 3000 rads was inhibited, in both the presence and absence of WR-2721.

b. Protective effects to the oral mucosa in radiotherapy. The most serious problem was a mucositis of the oral cavity. The intense mucosal reaction frequently forced a discontinuation of the planned radiotherapy for patients with carcinoma of the maxillary antrum and oral cancer.

Stomatitis usually begins with reddening of the oral mucosa (grade 1), followed by gradual development of furred patches (grade 2, patchy mucosa) that become confluent to cover the entire area affected (grade 3, confluent mucosa). Table VII shows the mean radiation doses at which oral mucositis of grades 1, 2, and 3 occurred. More pronounced reactions of the oral mucosa occurred in those receiving combined radiosensitizer–radiation regimens (BrdU + 5-FU), as compared to those given X irradiation alone. In 17 patients with carcinoma of the maxillary antrum, YM-

TABLE VI

Estimation of Effectiveness of YM-08310 in Various Types of Carcinoma

Type of carcinoma	Remarkable	Moderate	Poor	None	Unknown	Total	Effectiveness (%)
Head and neck tumor	1	6	1	2	7	17	70.0
Lung cancer	0	4	0	2	4	10	66.6
Breast cancer	1	1	1	1	2	6	50.0
Uterine cancer	2	2	4	0	24	32	50.0
Others	1	2	2	1	2	8	50.0
Total	5	15	7	7	39	73	58.9

TABLE VII

Treatment Plan and Onset of Mucositis

Onset by grade[a]	Treatment group			DMF	
	I BrdU + 5-FU + X	II X Alone	III YM-08310 + X	II/I	III/II
1	1125 ± 335 rads (n = 49)	1750 ± 374 rads (n = 15)	2950 ± 380 rads (n = 17)	1.6	1.7
2	1687 ± 395 rads (n = 44)	3850 ± 810 rads (n = 15)	4869 ± 425 rads (n = 17)	2.3	1.3
3	2612 + 660 rads (n = 25)	—	—	—	—

[a] Grade 1: erythema, edema; grade 2: patchy mucosa, petechiae; grade 3: confluent mucosa, slight bleeding.

08310 (2.0 mg/kg/day) was injected iv 30 min before irradiation. Onsets of grades 1 and 2, expressed as the mean radiation dose, were at 2950 and 4869 rads, respectively. Here, the DMF (YM-08310 + X/X alone) was 1.7 in Grade 1 and 1.3 in Grade 2.

c. Protective effects against radiation-induced xerostomia. Radiation treatment decreases salivation, causing mastication difficulties. Radiation-induced xerostomia in patients treated for head and neck malignancy has been widely described clinically. Salivary flow rate decreases when the major salivary glands are included in the radiation fields.

The degree of xerostomia was determined by the following criteria at 3 to 4 months after irradiation:

Severe   very dry mouth (+ + +) and mastication difficulties (+ +)
Moderate dry mouth (+ +), mastication difficulties (+)
Slight   dry mouth (+), mastication difficulties (−)

In the groups treated with YM-08310, the occurrence of xerostomia (52%; 11 of 17) decreased markedly compared with X rays alone (73.3%; 11 of 15), as shown in Table VIII.

d. Protective effects against lung fibrosis. Patients receiving irradiation to the lungs were given YM-08310. The following four criteria were used to grade the degree of lung fibrosis on the X rays 3 months after the treatment:

Grade 0 No change
Grade 1 Less intensity than the ribs
Grade 2 Same intensity as the ribs
Grade 3 Same intensity as the liver

TABLE VIII

Occurrence of Xerostomia under Different
Treatment Conditions

Extent of xerostomia	Treatment group[a]		
	BrdU + 5-FU + X[b]	X Alone[c]	YM-08310 + X[d]
Severe	10 (20.4)	3 (20)	1 (5.9)
Moderate	16 (32.7)	4 (26.7)	4 (23.5)
Slight	18 (36.7)	4 (26.7)	4 (23.5)
None	5 (10.2)	4 (26.7)	8 (47.1)

[a] Percentage of total given in parentheses.
[b] $n = 49$, mean radiation dose 4500 ± 326 rads.
[c] $n = 15$, mean radiation dose 5500 ± 453 rads.
[d] $n = 17$, mean radiation dose 5900 ± 459 rads.

The intensity of lung fibrosis on the X rays reached fairly constant levels 3 or 4 months after radiotherapy. Changes at 3 to 4 months after irradiation were compared with findings in case of X-ray therapy alone and in those patients given YM-08310. The incidence of pulmonary fibrosis proved to be closely related to factors such as NSD (nominal standard dose), field size, and age. Relation between NSD and field size was plotted in each case, as shown in Fig. 8. The changes on the X rays were grade 2 in the case of X irradiation combined with YM-08310.

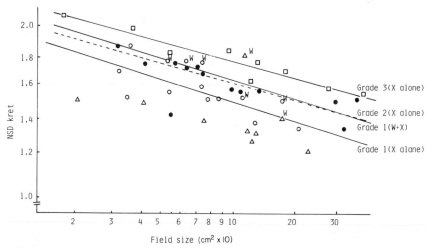

Fig. 8. Relation between NSD and field size in the treatment of lung fibrosis. △, Grade 0 (no change); ○, grade 1; ●, grade 2; □, grade 3; o^W, WR-2721 plus X irradiation.

IV. Discussion

Conditions required for the use of radioprotective agents in tumor radiotherapy include the following: (1) potent radioprotective effects and low toxicity, (2) differential normal tissue protection, (3) protective effects against both early and late injuries, (4) protective effects against both single and fractionated irradiation, and (5) protection against toxic effects of chemotherapeutic agents.

Since cysteine was found to have protective effects, AET and cysteamine with a higher DMF were developed; however, these agents were not effective (Sugahara, 1973).

Yuhas *et al.* (1969) and Yuhas (1981) demonstrated that WR-2721 has outstanding protective effects of DMF 2.0 or more in a wide range of normal tissues. The protective effects of this compound in normal and malignant tumors in mice are summarized in Table IX (Yuhas, 1981). Injection of WR-2721 increased the resistance of the hematopoietic tissues by a factor of 2.7 and of the skin by a factor of 2.4, but yielded little protection in cases of transplanted mammary carcinoma in mice. Well-oxygenated ascites tumor cells characterized p338 leukemia, with its high DMF value (Table IX).

TABLE IX

Comparative Protection of Tumors and Normal Tissues in Mice
by WR-2721

Tumor	DRF	Normal tissue	DRF	References
Mammary carcinoma	1.15	Skin	2.4	Yuhas and Stover (1969)
		Bone marrow	2.7	Yuhas and Stover (1969)
Lung adenoma	1.0	Lung	1.7	Yuhas (1972, 1973)
		Skin	2.1	Yuhas (1972, 1973)
EMT-6	1.0–1.3	Skin	2.1	Phillips *et al.* (1973)
p338 Leukemia	2.2	Bone marrow	2.2–3.0	Phillips *et al.* (1973)
		Esophagus	1.4	Phillips *et al.* (1973)
		Lung	1.2	Phillips *et al.* (1973)
EMT-6				
Aerated cell	1.5–2.0	—	—	Utley *et al.* (1974)
Anoxic cell	1.2–1.5	—	—	Utley *et al.* (1974)
KHT Sarcoma	1.2	Skin	2.0	Lowy and Baker (1973)
Lung adenoma	1.0	Skin	1.7	Echoles (1973)
Mammary carcinoma	1.0	Skin	1.7	Echoles (1973)

The following mechanisms are suggested for the differential protection afforded by WR-2721 (Yuhas, 1981).

1. The tumor lacks vascularity, particularly in the central portion; hence transfer of the drug into the tumor is often poor. Accumulation of [^{14}C]WR-2721 was seen only in the peripheral highly vascularized area of the tumor.
2. The protective effects of WR-2721 may be insufficient for hypoxic cells compared with well-oxygenated cells. Cell membrane permeability of WR-2721 is also reportedly different between normal and hypoxic cells.

Radioprotectors with a low toxicity are required for clinical application (Sugahara, 1973; Sugahara *et al.*, 1977). Protection by AMM and MPG was compared with sulfhydryl compounds such as cysteamine and WR-2721, as shown in Fig. 9. The doses are expressed as a percentage of the LD$_{50}$, because the LD$_{50}$ values of these compounds differ markedly (Sugahara, 1973). Cysteamine and MPG showed comparable protection, but MPG was more effective in a lower dose.

Late injury frequently develops following curative radiation therapy (Tanaka and Sugahara, 1980). With megavoltage radiation, the skin and soft tissues can withstand the early effects of radiation. High doses of radiation are required to control many radioresistant tumors, and here, late tissue atrophy and fibrosis sometimes occur. It is well known that radiation injury to vascular and connective tissue structures takes the

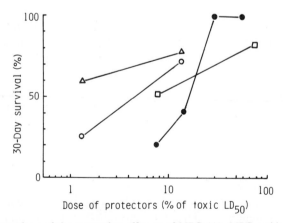

Fig. 9. Comparison of the protective efficacy of MPG (△), MPG-amide (○), WR-2721 (●), and cysteamine (□) in mice as represented by the percentage of 30-day survival after 1000 rads whole-body irradiation of ^{60}Co γ rays. Doses of the compounds are indicated as a percentage of acute LD$_{50}$.

form of late radiation tissue damage. Therefore, radioprotection of vascular and connective tissues could increase normal tissue tolerance, or, accordingly, could allow for transfer of larger doses to malignant tumors, for a given level of late tissue injury.

Utley *et al.* (1981) reported that WR-2721 protects against acute and chronic radiation injury to vessels, skin, and muscle in rats. Here, the injury was evaluated by measuring tissue blood flow. As reported in our experiments, MPG suppressed the occurrence of late injury after radiotherapy for cervical cancer.

These results indicate that an increased therapeutic gain can be expected when these drugs are used concomitantly with clinical radiation therapy.

For clinical application, the potential of these drugs must be studied with regard to selective normal tissue protection when small doses are delivered just before a series of daily radiation fractionations. Three factors have to be considered (Yuhas, 1981): (1) chronic toxicity of the drug, (2) ability of the drug to offer protection in the low-dose range, when given repeatedly, and (3) inability of the drug to protect tumors, even with repeated administrations.

The possibility that WR-2721 can protect the solid tumor when the treatments are given in daily fractionations has to be considered, as a solid tumor can reoxygenate or change physiologically. Echoles (1973) studied this problem in mammary tumors growing in BALB/c mice. Mice were given daily localized X rays, with and without the injection of 200 mg/kg of WR-2721 before each treatment, and there was no indication of a protective influence of WR-2721 (Fig. 10).

Yuhas (1979) found that WR-2721 protected against chemotherapeutically induced toxicity. He postulated that the differential uptake seen for WR-2721 in normal tissues as compared to tumors could yield a differential protection of normal tissue against alkylating agent toxicity. He also demonstrated that chemotherapeutic agent distribution was uniform between tumor and normal tissue, whereas WR-2721 concentrations were much higher in normal tissue. Phillips (1982) also found that WR-2721 protects bone marrow colony-forming units (CFUs) against *cis*-platinum, cyclophosphamide, nitrogen mustard, and BCNU, but that it did not significantly protect the EMT-6 tumor from these agents, as judged by regrowth of the tumor.

In Japan in March 1982, a group of radiotherapists started a randomized double-blind clinical trial (phase III study) on the radioprotective effect of WR-2721 (supported by Yamanouchi Pharmaceutical Co. Ltd.). Protection against radiation-induced oral mucositis in the head and neck of cancer patients, and diarrhea, leukopenia, subjective symptoms and so

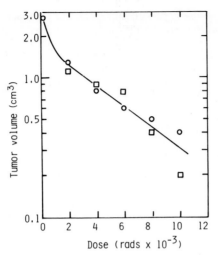

Fig. 10. Volume of mammary tumors growing in BALB/c mice on the day after completion of a 10-fraction X-ray course. ○, Mice given an injection of saline before each exposure; □, mice given 200 mg/kg of WR-2721 before each exposure. From Echoles (1973).

on, in cases of lower abdominal malignancies are the major events being studied. Tumor response and incidence and severity of the side effects are slated for comparison in blind tests (1983–1984).

It would appear that extensive combinations of radiation, hypoxic sensitizers, cytotoxic chemotherapy, and radioprotectors may yield significant improvement in the therapeutic ratio and in the control of tumors (Yuhas *et al.,* 1977; Phillips, 1982).

Acknowledgments

I am grateful to Dr. T. Sugahara at Kyoto National Hospital and Professor J. M. Yuhas of the University of Pennsylvania for permission to use their data.

References

Echoles, F. S. (1973). "Normal and Malignant Tissue Response to Fractionated Radiation Exposure and the Radioprotective Drug WR-2721." Ph.D. Dissertation, Univ. of Florida, Gainesville.

Goepp, R. A. (1962). Pathological study of oral radiation death in mice. *Radiat. Res.* **16,** 833–845.

Goepp, R. A. (1967). The use of parenteral chemicals for protection against oral radiation death in mice. *Radiat. Res.* **31,** 149–155.

Lowy, R. O., and Baker, D. G. (1973). Effects of radioprotective drugs on the therapeutic ratio for mouse tumor system. *Acta Radiol.* **12,** 425–433.

Moorhead, P. S., Nowell, P. C., Mellman, W. M., Batlips, D. H., and Hunerford, D. A. (1961). Chromosome preparations of leucocyte cultured from human peripheral blood. *Exp. Cell Res.* **20,** 613–616.

Nagata, H., Sugahara, T., and Tanaka, T. (1972). Radiation protection by 2-mercaptopropionylglycine in mice. *J. Radiat. Res.* **13,** 163–166.

Patt, H. M., Tyree, E. B., and Straube, R. L. (1949). Cysteine protection against X-irradiation. *Science (Washington, D.C.)* **110,** 213–214.

Phillips, T. L. (1982). Radiation sensitizers and protectors. *In* "Cancer Principles and the Practice of Oncology" (V. T. De Vita, ed.), pp. 1822–1836. Lippincott, Philadelphia.

Phillips, T. L., Kane, L., and Utley, J. F. (1973). Radioprotection of tumor and normal tissues by thiophosphate compounds. *Cancer (Philadelphia)* **32,** 528–535.

Sugahara, T. (1973). Possible application of chemical radioprotectors to radiotherapy. *In* "Fraction Size in Radiobiology and Radiotherapy" (T. Sugahara, ed.), pp. 84–93. Igaku-Shoin, Tokyo.

Sugahara, T., and Tanaka, T. (1968). Protection against whole body X-irradiation by adrenochrome monoguanyl hydrazone methansulfonate in mice. *Nature (London)* **220,** 271–272.

Sugahara, T., Tanaka, T., and Nagata, H. (1970). Protection of mice against ionizing radiations by adrenochrome monoguanylhydrazone methansulfonate; a promising agent for clinical use. *In* "Radiation Protection and Sensitization" (H. L. Horoson, ed.), pp. 401–408. Taylor & Francis, London.

Sugahara, T., Horikawa, M., Hikita, M., and Nagata, H. (1977). Studies on a sulfhydryl radioprotector of low toxicity. *In* "Radioprotection" (A. Locker, ed.), pp. 53–61. Birkhäuser, Basel.

Tamura, H., Sakurai, M., and Sugahara, T. (1970). A study of time and radiation dependent changes in the frequency of lymphocytes with chromosome aberrations in the circulation following multiple exposures of the pelvis to gamma-irradiation. *Blood* **36,** 43–51.

Tanaka, Y., and Sugahara, T. (1970). Chemical radiation protection in man as revealed by chromosome aberrations in peripheral lymphocytes. *J. Radiat. Res.* **11,** 166–168.

Tanaka, Y., and Sugahara, T. (1980). Clinical experiences of chemical radiation protection in tumor radiotherapy in Japan. *In* "Radiation Sensitizer, Their Use in the Clinical Management of Cancer" (L. Brady, ed.), pp. 421–425. Masson, New York.

Utley, J. F. (1978). Radioprotection of oral cavity structures by WR-2721. *Int. J. Radiat. Oncol. Biol. Phys.* **4,** 643–647.

Utley, J. F., Phillips, T. L., Kane, L. T., Wharamn, M. D., and Wara, W. M. (1974). Differential radioprotection of euoxic and hypoxic mouse mammary tumors by Thiophosphate compounds. *Radiology (Easton, Pa.)* **110,** 213–216.

Utley, J. F., Quinn, C. A., White, F. C., Seaver, N. A., and Bloor, C. M. (1981). Protection of normal tissue against late radiation injury by WR-2721. *Radiat. Res.* **85,** 408–415.

Yuhas, J. M. (1972). Improvement of lung tumor radiotherapy through differential chemoprotection of normal and tumor tissue. *J. Natl. Cancer Inst. (US)* **48,** 1255–1257.

Yuhas, J. M. (1973). Radiotherapy of experimental lung tumors in the presence and absence of a radioprotective drug, S-2-(3-aminopropylamino) ethylphosphorothioic acid (WR-2721). *J. Natl. Cancer Inst. (US)* **50,** 69–78.

Yuhas, J. M. (1979). Differential protection of normal and malignant tissues against the cytotoxic effects of mechlorethamine. *Cancer Treat. Rep.* **63,** 971–976.

Yuhas, J. M. (1981). On the potential application of radioprotective drugs in solid tumor radiotherapy. *In* "Radiation-Drug Interactions in Cancer Management" (G. Sokol, ed.), pp. 113–135. Wiley, New York.

Yuhas, J. M., and Storer, J. B. (1969). Differential chemoprotection of normal and malignant tissues. *J. Natl. Cancer Inst.* (*US*) **42,** 331–335.

Yuhas, J. M., Yurconic, M., Kligerman, M., West, G., and Peterson, D. F. (1977). Combined use of radioprotective and radiosensitizing drugs in experimental radiotherapy. *Radiat. Res.* **70,** 433–443.

PART THREE

Hypoxic Cell Sensitizers

6 Molecular Mechanism of Radiosensitization by Nitro Compounds

Tsutomu Kagiya
Takeshi Wada[1]
Sei-ichi Nishimoto
Department of Hydrocarbon Chemistry
Faculty of Engineering, Kyoto University
Kyoto 606, Japan

I. Introduction

Since Adams and Dewey (1963) found that N-ethylmaleimide enhances the radiation damage of hypoxic cells, radiosensitizing abilities of various electron-affinic organic compounds have been studied. Aromatic and heterocyclic nitro compounds, especially nitroimidazole derivatives such as

---

[1] Present address: Osaka University of Economics and Law, Osaka 581, Japan.

misonidazole and metronidazole, are effective for radiosensitizing hypoxic cells (Hall and Roizin-Towle, 1975; Stratford, 1982).

A reaction mechanism of hypoxic-cell radiosensitization involving repair inhibition of damaged intracellular molecules by electron-affinic compounds was proposed at an early stage of the investigations (Adams and Cooke, 1969): The cation radical and electron are produced in a target molecule following ionization processes by the direct absorption of radiation energy, and the damaged molecule is repaired by charge neutralization with the electron. This repair reaction is inhibited by electron-affinic compounds as a result of their preferential capturing of the electron. This mechanism was supported by electron spin resonance (ESR) and pulse radiolysis studies of the radiation-induced reaction of DNA-related compounds, in a solid state. An alternative mechanism of the free-radical fixation by sensitizer was also proposed (Willson and Emmerson, 1970; Greenstock *et al.*, 1970; Adams *et al.*, 1972). The free radical produced in a molecule forms a bond with the sensitizer, either by direct or by indirect action, and irreversible damage ensues. This mechanism is the same as that suggested for the oxygen effect and also for the nitroxyls.

However, in biochemical reactions, most of the damage to the target molecule is the result of reactions with active chemical species produced by the radiolysis of water, as most cells have a high water content.

In this chapter a molecular mechanism of radiosensitization by electron-affinic nitro compounds is discussed, mainly on the basis of the results of the radiation-induced chemical studies of DNA-related compounds in aqueous solutions.

In Section II the general aspects of the radiation chemistry of organic compounds in the absence and presence of oxygen in aqueous solution are shown in order to demonstrate characteristic differences between radiation chemical reactions in hypoxic and oxic cells. The effects of nitro compounds on the radiolysis yields of DNA-related compounds in aqueous solutions are described in Section III. In Section IV the retardation effects of misonidazole on the radiation chemical processes of DNA-related compounds are shown along with the reaction characteristics of misonidazole with hydroxyl radical ($\cdot$OH) and hydrated electron (e_{aq}^-) produced by the radiolysis of water. The promotion of radiation-induced oxidation of thymine into thymine glycol (TG) by nitro radiosensitizers in deoxygenated solution and the relations between the activity of nitro compound for the thymine glycol formation and the enhancement activity measured *in vitro* are described in Section V. Finally, the protection against radiation-induced damage of thymine by a sulfhydryl compound of glutathione and the ability of electron-affinic compounds to decompose the intracellular radioprotector are described in Section VI.

II. General Aspects of the Radiation Chemistry of Organic Compounds in Aqueous Solution

Because the water content in most cells is high (75–90%), the effects of radiation on the cells will be closely related to the radiation-induced chemical reaction of a target molecule in aqueous solution. For a better understanding of the chemical reactions involved in the enhancement of radiation-induced damages of hypoxic cells by a sensitizer, it is necessary to characterize radiation-induced chemical reactions occurring in the presence and absence of oxygen, in aqueous solutions of organic compounds.

In deoxygenated aqueous systems, most of the radiation-related energy is absorbed by the water molecule, and various ions (H_2O^+, e_{aq}^-) and the electronically excited water molecule (H_2O^*) are produced as the primary species, within an extremely short period (10^{-15} sec).

$$H_2O \xrightarrow{\hspace{1cm}} H_2O^+, e^-, H_2O^* \tag{1}$$

The intermediate H_2O^+ and H_2O^* give ·OH and H· by the decompositions, and e^- reacts with water molecules to give hydrated electron (e_{aq}^-) during 10^{-13} to 10^{-12} sec.

$$H_2O^+ \xrightarrow{\hspace{1cm}} H^+ + \cdot OH \tag{2}$$

$$H_2O^* \xrightarrow{\hspace{1cm}} H\cdot + \cdot OH \tag{3}$$

$$e^- + nH_2O \xrightarrow{\hspace{1cm}} e_{aq}^- \tag{4}$$

Mutual recombinations of ·OH and H· give H_2 and H_2O_2 molecules within 10^{-8} to 10^{-7} sec.

$$2 \, H\cdot \xrightarrow{\hspace{1cm}} H_2 \tag{5}$$

$$2 \, \cdot OH \xrightarrow{\hspace{1cm}} H_2O_2 \tag{6}$$

When neutral water is irradiated with 1 daGy of γ ray or an electron beam with energy lower than 1 MeV, about 5 μmol of H_2O decompose along with the formation of a short-lived active species; ·OH (2.7 μmol), e_{aq}^- (2.7 μmol), H· (0.55 μmol), and stable molecules; H_2O_2 (0.75 μmol), H_2 (0.45 μmol): [$G(-H_2O) = 5.0$, $G(\cdot OH) = 2.7$, $G(e_{aq}^-) = 2.7$, $G(H\cdot) = 0.55$, $G(H_2O_2) = 0.75$, $G(H_2) = 0.45$].

Three typical radical reactions of ·OH and H· occur with organic substances: (1) hydrogen abstraction from saturated alkyl compounds (RH) [Eqs. (7) and (8)], (2) addition reaction to unsaturated groups ($R^1{=}R^2$) [Eqs. (9) and (10)], and (3) recombination with the radicals formed by the hydrogen abstraction [Eq. (11)], respectively.

$$RH + \cdot OH \longrightarrow R\cdot + H_2O \tag{7}$$

$$RH + H\cdot \longrightarrow R\cdot + H_2 \tag{8}$$

$$R^1{=}R^2 + \cdot OH \longrightarrow \cdot R^1R^2OH \tag{9}$$

$$R^1{=}R^2 + H\cdot \longrightarrow \cdot R^1R^2H \tag{10}$$

$$R\cdot + \cdot OH \longrightarrow ROH \tag{11}$$

In contrast; e_{aq}^- acts as a nucleophilic reagent and can add to electrophilic organic compounds (RH, $R^1{=}R^2$) [Eqs. (12) and (13)]. The anion radical thus formed will undergo subsequent decomposition and protonation into radicals [Eqs. (14) and (15)].

$$RH + e_{aq}^- \longrightarrow RH^{\bar{\cdot}} \tag{12}$$

$$R^1{=}R^2 + e_{aq}^- \longrightarrow \cdot RR^{2-} \tag{13}$$

$$RH^{\bar{\cdot}} \longrightarrow R^1 + R''H^- \tag{14}$$

$$\cdot R^1{-}R^{2-} + H^+ \longrightarrow \cdot R^1R^2H \tag{15}$$

It follows that both oxidation by $\cdot OH$ and reductions by $H\cdot$ and e_{aq}^- are involved in the radiation-induced reactions of organic compounds in the absence of oxygen in aqueous solution.

Unstable radicals such as $R\cdot$, $\cdot R^1R^2OH$, and $\cdot R^1R^2H$ undergo a variety of radical recombinations [Eqs. (16)–(21)], disproportionations [Eqs. (22) and (23)], and decompositions [Eq. (25)] to form various products.

$$R\cdot + R\cdot \longrightarrow RR \tag{16}$$

$$R\cdot + \cdot R^1R^2OH \longrightarrow RR^1R^2OH \tag{17}$$

$$R\cdot + \cdot R^1R^2H \longrightarrow RR^1R^2H \tag{18}$$

$$\cdot R^1R^2OH + \cdot R^1R^2H \longrightarrow HR^2R^1R^1R^2OH \tag{19}$$

$$2\,\cdot R^1R^2OH \longrightarrow HOR^2R^1R^1R^2OH \tag{20}$$

$$2\,\cdot R^1R^2H \longrightarrow HR^2R^1R^1R^2H \tag{21}$$

$$2\,\cdot R^1R^2OH \longrightarrow R^1R^2(OH)_2 + R^1{=}R^2 \tag{22}$$

$$2\,\cdot R^1R^2H \longrightarrow HR^1R^2H + R^1{=}R^2 \tag{23}$$

$$\cdot R^1R^2OH + \cdot R^1R^2H \longrightarrow HR^1R^2OH + R^1{=}R^2 \tag{24}$$

$$\left.\begin{array}{l} R\cdot \\ \cdot R^1R^2OH \\ \cdot R^1R^2H \end{array}\right\} \longrightarrow \text{decomposition products} \tag{25}$$

In aqueous solution containing oxygen, reducing species $H\cdot$ and e_{aq}^- react easily with oxygen [Eqs. (26) and (27)]. Superoxide radical anion

(O_2^-) thus formed reacts with H^+ to give hydroperoxyl radical ($\cdot OOH$) [Eq. (28)].

$$H\cdot + O_2 \longrightarrow \cdot OOH \tag{26}$$

$$e_{aq}^- + O_2 \longrightarrow O_2^- \tag{27}$$

$$O_2^- + H^+ \longrightarrow \cdot OOH \tag{28}$$

Because of its lower reactivity, $\cdot OOH$ is considered to be an inactive species for most of the organic substances, including DNA-related compounds (Cadet and Teoule, 1978) and amino acids (Bielski and Shiue, 1979).

Therefore, $\cdot OH$ should be the only species reactive for most of the organic substances in the presence of oxygen in aqueous solution. The oxygen molecule reacts easily with $R\cdot$, $\cdot R^1R^2OH$, and $\cdot R^1R^2H$ produced by the reactions shown in Eqs. (7)–(10) to form various oxidation products via peroxyl radicals [Eq. (25)].

$$R\cdot + O_2 \longrightarrow ROO\cdot \tag{29}$$

$$\cdot R^1R^2OH + O_2 \longrightarrow R^2(OH)R^1OO\cdot \tag{30}$$

$$\cdot R^1R^2H + O_2 \longrightarrow R^2HR^1OO\cdot \tag{31}$$

Because many types of radicals formed during these oxidative decompositions can promote the oxidation of organic compounds with oxygen, the mechanism of oxygen sensitization is considered to involve a chain reaction of DNA-related compounds.

III. Reactivity of DNA-Related Compounds toward Various Active Species Produced by the Radiolysis of Water

We determined apparent reactivities of DNA-related compounds toward the mixture of active species, $G(e_{aq}^-) = 2.7$; $G(H\cdot) = 0.55$; $G(\cdot OH) = 2.7$, produced by the radiolysis of water, under the deoxygenated conditions listed in Table I. The overall reactivities of DNA bases for active species e_{aq}^-, $H\cdot$, and $\cdot OH$ decrease in the order:

thymine (1.81) > cytosine (1.10) > adenine (0.43)

and those of thymine derivatives are (Kagiya et al., 1982) as follows:

thymidylic acid (2.76) ≥ thymidylyl(3′ → 5′)thymidine (2.51) >
thymidine (2.14) > thymine (1.81)

These results indicate that thymine is the most reactive base for the active species, e_{aq}^-, $H\cdot$, $\cdot OH$, produced by the radiolysis of water, and that

TABLE I

G Values for Conversions of DNA-Related Compounds (DRC) in the Absence (G_{do}) and Presence (G_m) of Misonidazole (MISO) in Deoxygenated Aqueous Solutions[a]

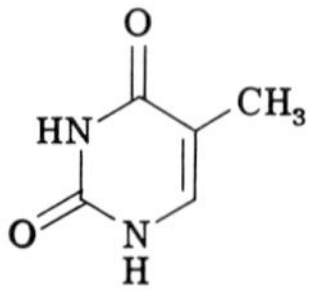

1 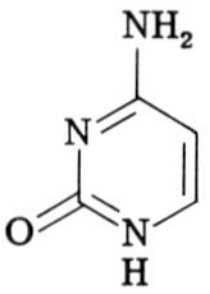   **2** 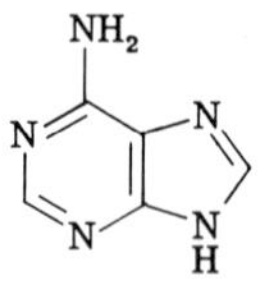   **3**

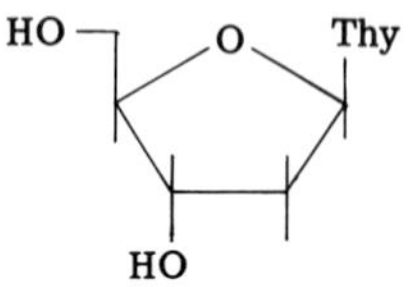

4 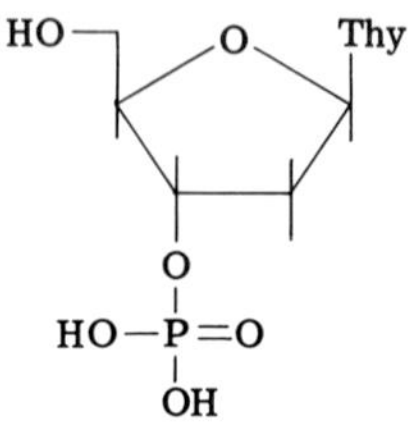   **5** 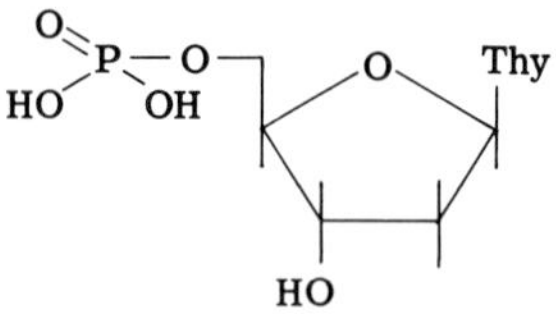   **6**

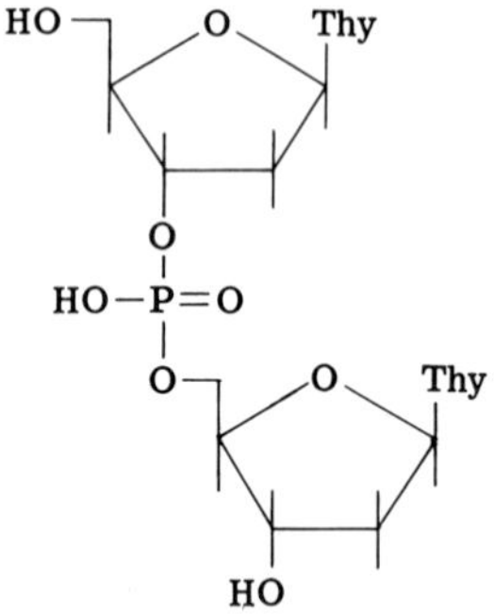

7

DRC	G_{do}	G_m	G_m/G_{do}
Thymine (**1**)	1.81	1.59	0.88
Cytosine (**2**)	1.10	1.00	0.91
Adenine (**3**)	0.43	0.30	0.70
Thymidine (**4**)	2.14	1.6	0.75
3′-Thymidylic acid (**5**)	2.51	—	—
3′-Thymidylic acid[b]	0.36	—	—
5′-Thymidylic acid (**6**)	2.76	1.51	0.55
5′-Thymidylic acid[b]	0.14	—	—
Thymidylyl(3′ → 5′)thymidine (**7**)	2.51	—	—

[a] $[DRC]_0 = 1$ mM, $[MISO]_0 = 0.1$ mM, pH 7.0, γ-irradiation dose rate $= 38$ daGy/h, time $= 0.5–5$ h at room temperature.
[b] G value for i-PO$_4$ release.

the destruction of thymine is enhanced slightly by bonding with deoxyribose (thymidine) or deoxyribose phosphate (5′-thymidylic acid). However, G values for phosphoric acid release from thymidylic acids are one-tenth to one-twentieth that for base destruction (see also Raleigh et al., 1973a,b, 1974). Thus it seems that thymine destruction can be a model reaction of the radiation-induced reaction of DNA in deoxygenated water.

To clarify details of the chemical reactions of DNA bases, we carried out an analytical study of the radiation-induced destruction of thymine as a typical DNA base in deoxygenated and N_2O-saturated aqueous solutions (Table II) (Wada et al., 1982a).

TABLE II

G Values for Thymine Conversion and Formations of Major Products in Deoxygenated (G_{do}) and N_2O-Saturated (G_{N_2O}) Aqueous Solutions[a]

Product	$G_{do}{}^{b}$	$G_{N_2O}{}^{b}$	G_{N_2O}/G_{do}
Thymine glycol (**1**)	0.13 (0.07)	0.28 (0.09)	2.2
N^1-Formyl-N^2-pyruvylurea (**2**)	0.11 (0.06)	0.08 (0.03)	0.7
5-Hydroxymethyluracil (**3**)	0.14 (0.08)	0.49 (0.15)	3.5
5-Hydroxy-5,6-dihydrothymine (**4**)	0.07 (0.04)	0.18 (0.06)	2.6
6-Hydroxy-5,6-dihydrothymine (**5**)	0.08 (0.04)	0.12 (0.04)	1.5
5-Methylbarbituric acid (**6**)	0.09 (0.05)	0.08 (0.03)	0.9
5,6-Dihydrothymine (**7**)	0.28 (0.15)	0.07 (0.02)	0.3
Unidentified compounds	0.91 (0.50)	1.87 (0.59)	2.1
Thymine conversion	1.81	3.17	1.8

[a] $[Thy]_0 = 1$ mM, pH 7.0.
[b] The value in parentheses denotes the ratio of the G value for product formation to that for thymine conversion.

The G value for thymine conversion (1.81) is about one-third that for the formation of total active species, and one-half of the converted thymine could not be identified by the UV detector of a high-performance liquid chromatograph (HPLC). One of the main products is 5,6-dihydrothymine (15% based on thymine conversion) as a reduction product, and various oxidation products (35%) are formed under deoxygenated conditions. The reduction product 5,6-dihydrothymine (Thy-H$_2$) is formed by the reactions of double bond in thymine with H· ($G = 0.55$) and/or a pair of e_{aq}^- ($G = 2.7$) and H$^+$.

$$\text{Thy} + \text{H·} \ (\text{or } e_{aq}^-, \text{H}^+) \longrightarrow \text{·Thy—H} \tag{32}$$

$$\text{·Thy—H} + \text{H·} \ (\text{or } e_{aq}^-, \text{H}^+) \longrightarrow \text{Thy}\!\!<^{\text{H}}_{\text{H}} \tag{33}$$

The redox product 5- or 6-hydroxy-5,6-dihydrothymine results from the following two routes:

$$\text{·Thy—H} + \text{·OH} \longrightarrow \text{Thy}\!\!<^{\text{OH}}_{\text{H}} \tag{34}$$

$$\text{Thy} + \text{·OH} \longrightarrow \text{·Thy—OH} \tag{35}$$

$$\text{·Thy—OH} + \text{H·} \ (\text{or } e_{aq}^-, \text{H}^+) \longrightarrow \text{Thy}\!\!<^{\text{OH}}_{\text{H}} \tag{36}$$

Thymine glycol is produced by the ·OH addition to the unsaturated group.

$$\text{·Thy—OH} + \text{·OH} \longrightarrow \text{Thy}\!\!<^{\text{OH}}_{\text{OH}} \tag{37}$$

5-Methylbarbituric acid corresponds to a dehydrogenation product of 6-hydroxy-5,6-dihydrothymine, N^1-formyl-N^2-pyruvylurea to a dehydrogenation product of thymine glycol.

$$\text{Thy}\!\!<^{\text{H}}_{\text{OH}} + 2 \ \text{·OH} \longrightarrow \text{Thy}\!\!<^{\text{H}}_{\text{O}} + 2 \ \text{H}_2\text{O} \tag{38}$$

$$\text{Thy-(OH)}_2 + 2 \ \text{·OH(or 2 ·H)} \longrightarrow \text{product} + 2 \ \text{H}_2\text{O(or 2 H}_2) \tag{39}$$

5-Hydroxymethyluracil is produced by hydrogen abstraction and ·OH addition at the methyl group of thymine.

$$\text{Ura—CH}_3 + \text{·OH(or ·H)} \longrightarrow \text{Ura—CH}_2\text{·} + \text{H}_2\text{O(or H}_2) \tag{40}$$

$$\text{Ura—CH}_2\text{·} + \text{·OH} \longrightarrow \text{Ura—CH}_2\text{OH} \tag{41}$$

To elucidate the reaction of thymine with ·OH, the radiation-induced reaction of thymine was carried out in N$_2$O-saturated solution. The conversion of e_{aq}^- to ·OH in aqueous solution is generally carried out using N$_2$O.

$$\text{N}_2\text{O} + e_{aq}^- \longrightarrow \text{·OH} + \text{OH}^- + \text{N}_2 \tag{42}$$

Thus the predominant active species in the solution saturated previously by N_2O is $\cdot OH$ ($G = 5.4$) and $H\cdot$ ($G = 0.55$). As listed in Table II, in the radiation-induced reaction of aqueous thymine solution in the presence of N_2O, the G value for total conversion of thymine is 3.17, which is less than double the value (1.81) in deoxygenated solution. This result may be attributed to the lower reactivity of $\cdot OH$ than that of e_{aq}^- toward thymine.

The yield of a hydroxythymine derivative, thymine glycol, is 2.15 times as large as that in deoxygenated solution, total hydroxy-5,6-dihydrothymines 2.0 times, and 5-hydroxymethyluracil 3.5 times, respectively. These increases in G value are attributed to the increase in $\cdot OH$ concentration by the reaction in Eq. (42).

In contrast, G values for the formation of 5-methylbarbituric acid and N^1-formyl-N^2-pyruvylurea did not vary. 5,6-Dihydrothymine decreases to one-fourth, because the reaction of thymine with a pair of e_{aq}^- and H^+ [Eqs. (32) and (33)] would not be involved in this system.

When the aqueous solution containing sodium formate is irradiated, $\cdot OH$ and $H\cdot$ are converted to reducing species of $CO_2^{\overline{\cdot}}$ by the reactions with formate anions [Eqs. (43) and (44)].

$$HCO_2^- + \cdot OH \longrightarrow H_2O + CO_2^{\overline{\cdot}} \tag{43}$$

$$HCO_2^- + H\cdot \longrightarrow H_2 + CO_2^{\overline{\cdot}} \tag{44}$$

Thus the species reacting with thymine are these reducing species, e_{aq}^- ($G = 2.7$) and $CO_2^{\overline{\cdot}}$ ($G = 3.1$) in the presence of sodium formate, and $CO_2^{\overline{\cdot}}$ ($G = 5.6$) and e_{aq}^- ($G = 0.2$) in the presence of N_2O as well as sodium formate [Eqs. (42)–(44)].

We studied the radiation-induced reaction of thymine in deoxygenated and N_2O-saturated solutions containing sodium formate in order to characterize the reactivities of e_{aq}^- and $CO_2^{\overline{\cdot}}$ toward thymine (Wada et al., 1982b; see also Loman and Ebert, 1970).

As listed in Table III, G values for thymine conversion and dihydrothymine formation and the yield of product **3** decrease, whereas product **1** increases with N_2O saturation in the presence of sodium formate. These results indicate that the reactivity of $CO_2^{\overline{\cdot}}$ is smaller than that of e_{aq}^- for the conversion of thymine into dihydrothymine.

$$Thy + 2\ CO_2^{\overline{\cdot}} + 2\ H^+ \longrightarrow Thy{\Large\langle}^H_H + CO_2 \tag{45}$$

The increased product **3** and the decreased product **1** by N_2O saturation may be attributed to the formations of carboxylic acid derivatives of thymine.

$$Thy + CO_2^{\overline{\cdot}} \longrightarrow \cdot Thy{-}CO_2^- \tag{46}$$

$$\cdot Thy{-}CO_2 + \cdot Thy{-}H \longrightarrow Thy{\Large\langle}^H_{CO_2^-} + Thy \tag{47}$$

TABLE III

G Values for Thymine Conversion [G(-Thy)] and
Dihydrothymine Formation [G(DHT)] and the Yields of Products
1–3 in Deoxygenated and N_2O-Saturated Aqueous Solutions
Containing Sodium Formate[a]

Solution		Deoxygenated sodium formate solution	N_2O-Saturated sodium formate solution
Active species $\begin{bmatrix} G(e_{aq}^-)^b \\ G(CO_2^-)^b \end{bmatrix}$		2.7	0.2
		3.1	5.6
G(-Thy)		2.7	2.1
G(DHT)		1.3	1.0
Product			
1		0.9	2.2
2		0.7	0.7
3		1.7	0.9

[a] Yields given as relative peak height in HPLC. Dose = 0–152 daGy,
$[Thy]_0 = 1.0$ mM.
[b] G Value for active species calculated from the available rate constants and
concentrations: [sodium formate]$_0$ = 0.1 M, $[N_2O]_0$ = 26 mM.

We determined the effects of oxygen on the radiation-induced reaction
of thymine in order to compare the reaction characteristics of thymine
destruction under hypoxic conditions with those under oxic conditions.
The results are listed in Table IV.

TABLE IV

G Values for Thymine Conversion and Formations of
Major Products in Deoxygenated (G_{do}) and Aerated (G_{aer})
Aqueous Solutions[a]

Products	G_{do}	G_{aer}	G_{aer}/G_{do}
Thymine glycol	0.13	1.00	7.7
5-Hydroxymethyluracil	0.14	0.03	0.2
N^1-Formyl-N^2-pyruvylurea	0.11	0.58	5.3
5-Methylbarbituric acid	0.09	0.26	2.9
5-Hydroxy-5,6-dihydrothymine	0.07	0.00	0.0
6-Hydroxy-5,6-dihydrothymine	0.08	0.02	0.3
5,6-Dihydrothymine	0.28	0.00	0.0
Unidentified compounds	0.91	0.51	0.6
Thymine conversion	1.81	2.40	1.3

[a] $[Thy]_0 = 1$ mM, pH 7.0.

The overall thymine conversion and the yields of oxidation products in aerated solution are much larger than those under deoxygenated conditions. The yields of oxidation products such as thymine glycol (7.7 times), N^1-formyl-N^2-pyruvylurea (5.2 times), and 5-methylbarbituric acid (2.9 times) increased, whereas those of reduction and redox products such as dihydrothymine (0) and hydroxy-5,6-dihydrothymines (one-third) decreased. These results indicate that oxygen sensitization in radiotherapy is caused by the enhancements of the reactions of thymine to form these oxidation products.

IV. Retardation Effects of Nitro Compounds on the Radiation-Induced Reactions of DNA-Related Compounds and Their Chemical Behavior in Deoxygenated Aqueous Solution

We studied the effects of misonidazole as a typical radiosensitizer on the radiolysis of some DNA-related compounds in deoxygenated aqueous solutions. The radiolysis yields (G values) of DNA-related compounds in the absence and presence of misonidazole are summarized in Table I. The yields of various DNA-related compounds decreased to 10 to 60% with the addition of misonidazole (10 mol%). The total G value for thymine conversion also decreased 10–40% with the addition of various nitro compounds (additive/thymine = 0.2), as shown in Table V.

TABLE V

G Values for Thymine Conversion G(-Thy) in the Presence of various Nitro Compounds in Deoxygenated Aqueous Solution[a]

Compounds	G(-Thy)$_{add}$	G(-Thy)$_{add}$/G(-Thy)$_{none}$
None	1.68	1.00
Duroquinone	0.97	0.58
Nitroxime	1.45	0.86
Nitrofurazone	1.14	0.68
3,4-Dinitrobenzoic acid	1.53	0.91
5-Nitro-2-furoic acid	1.20	0.71
4-Nitroacetophenone	1.50	0.89
Misonidazole	1.35	0.80
Desmethylmisonidazole	1.47	0.88
2-Nitroimidazole	1.47	0.88
Metronidazole	1.25	0.74

[a] [Thy]$_0$ = 500 μM, [additive]$_0$ = 100 μM, dose = 114 daGy, pH 7.0.

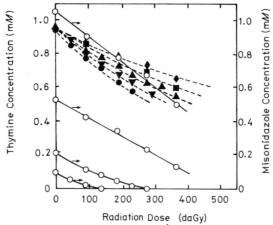

Fig. 1. Radiation-induced conversions of thymine ($\bigcirc$) and misonidazole in deoxygenated aqueous solution. Misonidazole concentrations (mM): $\blacklozenge$ (1.06); $\blacksquare$ (0.53); $\blacktriangle$ (0.22); $\blacktriangledown$ (0.10); $\bullet$ (0). The arrows indicate the corresponding vertical axis.

To clarify the role and behavior of nitro compounds in the radiation-induced thymine reactions in aqueous solution, the conversions of thymine and misonidazole were determined under deoxygenated conditions. As shown in Fig. 1, the concentrations of thymine and misonidazole decreased with irradiation. The G value for thymine conversion decreased, while that for misonidazole conversion increased, with the increased initial concentration of misonidazole. At the 0.5 molar ratio of misonidazole to thymine, the decreasing rates of thymine and misonidazole are comparable (1.1 μmol/daGy) as follows:

$[Miso]_0/[Thy]_0$	0.00	0.10	0.22	0.53	1.06
$G(-Thy)$	1.8	1.6	1.3	1.0	0.9
% Decrease of $G(-Thy)$	—	11	28	44	50
$G(-Mis)$	—	0.8	1.0	1.1	1.5

Similar tendencies of the thymine and misonidazole conversions were observed in N_2O-saturated aqueous solutions.

$[Miso]_0/[Thy]_0$	0.0	0.1	0.5	1.0
$G(-Thy)$	3.2	2.7	2.4	1.8
% Decrease of $G(-Thy)$	0	16	25	44
$G(-Miso)$	—	0.8	1.7	2.2

These results indicate that the decrease in the G value for thymine conversion by the addition of misonidazole is due to their competitive reactions with ·OH. As shown in Fig. 2, misonidazole and 2-nitroimidazole decompose with the same rate ($G = 4$) to release HNO_2 along with a small amount of HNO_3 in the radiation-induced reaction in N_2O-saturated aqueous solution (Wada *et al.*, 1981).

Stoichiometry for the reaction of nitroimidazole with ·OH indicates that one nitroimidazole reacts with ·OH to release 0.5 HNO_2. These results lead to the following scheme:

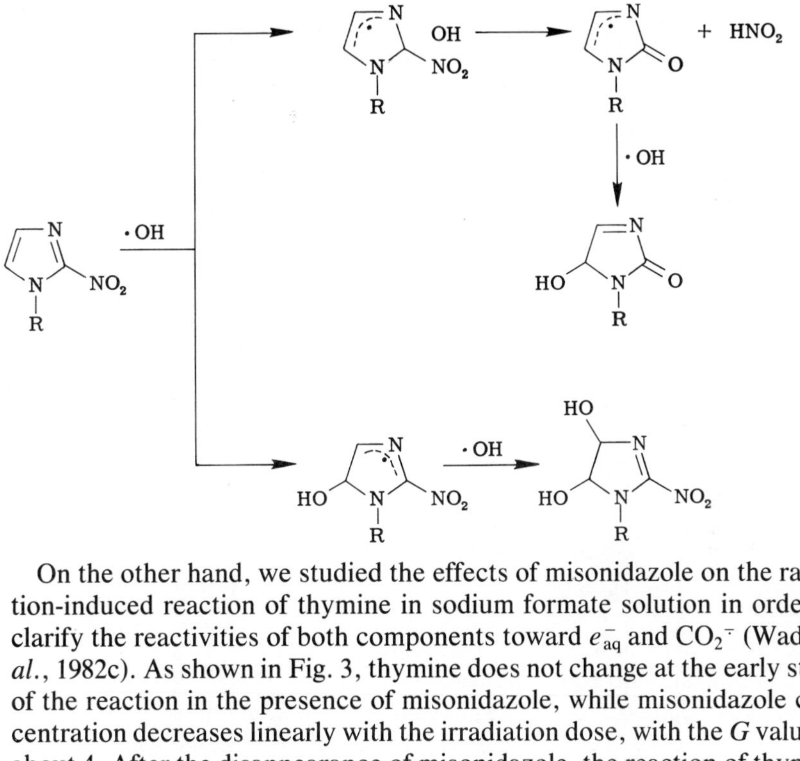

On the other hand, we studied the effects of misonidazole on the radiation-induced reaction of thymine in sodium formate solution in order to clarify the reactivities of both components toward e_{aq}^- and CO_2^- (Wada *et al.*, 1982c). As shown in Fig. 3, thymine does not change at the early stage of the reaction in the presence of misonidazole, while misonidazole concentration decreases linearly with the irradiation dose, with the G value of about 4. After the disappearance of misonidazole, the reaction of thymine with the reducing species [$G(e_{aq}^-) = 2.7$ and $G(CO_2^-) = 2.7$] was initiated with the rate of 2.7 μmol/daGy at [Miso]$_0$/[Thy]$_0$ = 0–0.2.

These results indicate that the reaction of thymine with the reducing species produced by the radiolysis of water is inhibited completely by misonidazole as a result of its preferential reaction with these species.

On the basis of these studies, it is concluded that the retardation effect of misonidazole in the radiation-induced reaction of thymine in deoxygenated aqueous solution is a result of the competitive reaction of misonida-

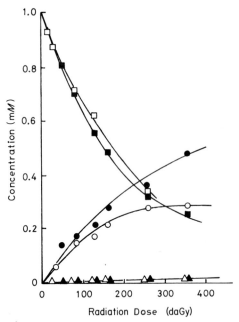

Fig. 2. Radiation-induced reactions of misonidazole and 2-nitroimidazole in N_2O-saturated aqueous solution: (□) misonidazole, (■) 2-nitroimidazole, (○, ●) HNO_2, (△, ▲) HNO_3, [nitro compound]$_0$ = 1 mM, pH 7.0.

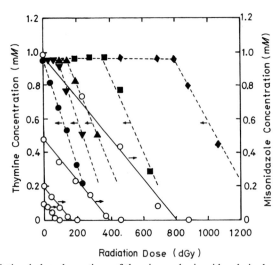

Fig. 3. Radiation-induced reactions of thymine and misonidazole in deoxygenated aqueous solution containing sodium formate. [Thy]$_0$ = 1 mM (○), [MIS]$_0$ = 0–0.9 mM (◆, 0.98; ■, 0.48; ▲, 0.20; ▼, 0.09; ●, 0). The arrows indicate the corresponding vertical axis.

zole with ·OH and to the preferential one with e_{aq}^-. The reduction products of misonidazole (see also Whillans and Whitmore, 1981) seem to exert a minor effect on the radiation-induced reaction of thymine with these reducing species.

To characterize the stoichiometry for the reaction of misonidazole with the reducing species, the relation between the amount of misonidazole reduced and the yields of reducing species (e_{aq}^- and CO_2^-) is determined, as shown in Fig. 4. This result indicates that misonidazole and 2-nitroimidazole react with four and six reducing species, respectively, per molecule.

The radiation-induced reductions of various N^1-non-substituted and N^1-substituted nitroimidazoles were also studied in order to characterize the stoichiometries for the reductions of these compounds (Kagiya et al., 1983).

As shown in Table VI, the G value for the reduction of N^1-non-substituted nitroimidazoles such as 2-nitroimidazole is about 0.9, whereas the N^1-substituted compounds such as misonidazole have a G value of 1.4. Furthermore, the ratio of the total G value for the formation of the reducing species to the conversion of nitroimidazoles is 6 for N^1-non-substi-

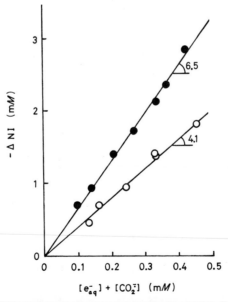

Fig. 4. Relations of total yield of reducing species ($[e_{aq}^-]$ and $[CO_2^-]$) with amounts of (○) decomposed misonidazole and (●) 2-nitro-imidazole ($-\Delta NI$) in deoxygenated aqueous solution containing sodium formate.

TABLE VI

G Values for the Reduction of Nitroimidazole Derivatives [$G(-NI)$] in Deoxygenated Aqueous Solution Containing Sodium Formate (0.1 M)[a]

	2-Nitroimidazole	5-Nitroimidazole

N¹-Non-substituted — 1 (2-Nitroimidazole structure); 2, 3, 4 (5-Nitroimidazole structures)

N¹-Substituted — 5, 7 (2-Nitroimidazole structures); 6, 8 (5-Nitroimidazole structures)

Nitroimidazole	$G(-NI)$	$G_t/G(-NI)$[b]	Product (G value)
N¹-Non-substituted			
2-Nitroimidazole (**1**)	0.92	6.5	2-Aminoimidazole (0.88)
4(5)-Nitroimidazole (**2**)	0.96	6.2	4(5)-Aminoimidazole[c]
2-Methyl-4(5)-nitroimidazole (**3**)	0.91	6.5	4(5)-Amino-2-methyl-imidazole
4(5)-Methyl-5(4)-nitroimidazole (**4**)	0.86	6.9	4-Amino-5-methyl-imidazole (0.75)
N¹-Substituted			
1-Methyl-2-nitroimidazole (**5**)	1.42	4.2	3-Methyl-4,5-dihydro-imidazolyl-4-oxime
1-Methyl-5-nitroimidazole (**6**)	1.40	4.3	—
Misonidazole (**7**)	1.42	4.2	—
Metronidazole (**8**)	1.52	3.9	—

[a] Dose = 0–418 daGy, [nitroimidazole]$_0$ = 0.5 mM, pH 7.0.
[b] $G_t = G(e_{aq}^-) + G(CO_2^-) = 5.95$.
[c] Characterized by colorimetric reaction.

tuted nitroimidazoles and 4 for the N^1-substituted compounds, respectively.

It should be noted that the formations of aminoimidazoles as a reduction product for N^1-non-substituted nitroimidazoles and 4,5-dihydroimidazolyl oxime for N^1-substituted ones were observed by HPLC and ^{13}C-NMR spectroscopy.

On the basis of these studies, the following reaction scheme is proposed for the reduction of N^1-non-substituted nitroimidazoles by hydrated electrons in aqueous solution:

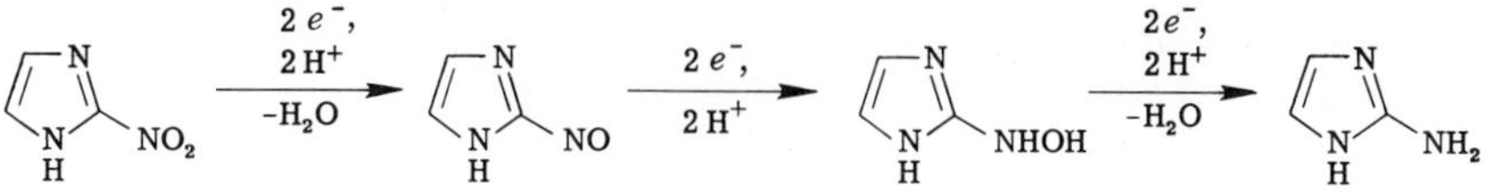

$$(51)$$

In contrast to N^1-non-substituted nitroimidazoles, oxime derivatives are obtained for N^1-substituted ones by the isomerization of hydroxyaminoimidazole as a four-electron-reduction product.

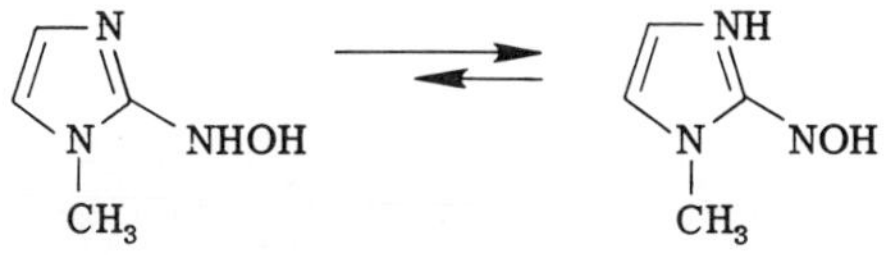

$$(52)$$

V. Role of Nitro Compounds in the Promotion of the Radiation-Induced Oxidation of Thymine in Deoxygenated Aqueous Solution

To clarify the role of nitro compounds in radiosensitization, we studied the effect of misonidazole on the yields of various products derived from thymine by the radiation-induced reaction in deoxygenated aqueous solution (Wada *et al.*, 1982a).

Although thymine conversion decreased slightly with the addition of 10% misonidazole, the yields of oxidation products, particularly thymine glycol, increased markedly while those of reduction products and unidentified compounds decreased. It should be noted that the G value (0.82) for the thymine glycol formation, which was enhanced in the presence of a small amount of misonidazole in deoxygenated solution, is comparable to that (1.00) obtained in aerated solution. Thus, misonidazole probably acts as a promoter for the selective oxidation of thymine to yield mainly thymine glycol under deoxygenated conditions, in a manner similar to that

TABLE VII

G Values for Thymine Conversion and Formations of Major
Products in the Absence and Presence of Misonidazole in
Deoxygenated (G_{do}, G_m) and Aerated (G_{aer}) Aqueous Solutions[a]

Products	G_{do}	G_m	G_m/G_{do}	G_{aer}
Thymine glycol	0.13	0.82	6.3	1.00
5-Hydroxymethyluracil	0.14	0.08	0.6	0.03
N^1-Formyl-N^2-pyruvylurea	0.11	0.14	1.3	0.58
5-Methylbarbituric acid	0.09	0.10	1.1	0.26
5-Hydroxy-5,6-dihydrothymine	0.07	0.00	0.0	0.00
6-Hydroxy-5,6-dihydrothymine	0.08	0.04	0.5	0.02
5,6-Dihydrothymine	0.28	0.13	0.5	0.00
Unidentified compounds	0.91	0.28	0.3	0.51
Thymine conversion	1.81	1.59	0.9	2.40

[a] $[\text{Thy}]_0 = 1.0$ mM, $[\text{MISO}] = 0.1$ mM, pH 7.0, γ-irradiation dose rate = 38
daGy/h, time 2 h.

with oxic conditions. Decrease in the formation of reduction products is
also attributed to the preferential reaction of misonidazole with e_{aq}^- analogous to oxygen.

We investigated correlations between the activities of a variety of nitroimidazoles for thymine glycol formation in deoxygenated solution and
the corresponding enhancement of activities *in vitro,* using V79-379A
cells (Adams *et al.*, 1979). As shown in Fig. 5, the concentration of various nitroimidazoles required to give an enhancement ratio of 1.6 decreased with increases in the G value for thymine glycol (TG) formation.

This evidence led to the conclusion that the G value for thymine glycol
formation can be used as a radiation chemical measure for the radiosensitizing activity of these compounds *in vitro.* The radiation chemical measure of the activities for thymine glycol formation was determined for 20
nitro derivatives of imidazole, furan, and benzene and quinione derivatives in deoxygenated thymine solution.

The G value for thymine glycol formation is dependent on the type of
nitro compound, increasing along a sigmoidal curve with the increase in
one-electron reduction potential $[E(A/A^{\bar{\cdot}})]$ of these compounds (Fig. 6).
The same relation has been obtained with regard to the enhancement of
the activity of nitroimidazoles in radiosensitization. Nitro- and dinitro-
benzoic acid derivatives showed the highest activity among the nitro compounds with the same one-electron reduction potential.

In the radiation-induced reaction of thymine in deoxygenated aqueous
solution, thymine reacts with ·OH produced by the radiolysis of water

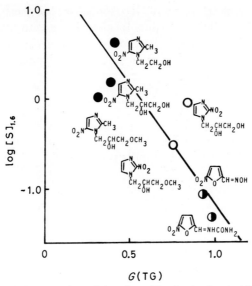

Fig. 5. Relationship between the activity of sensitization *in vitro* test (V79-379A cell) and that in radiation chemical study: (○) 2-nitroimidazoles; (●) 5-nitroimidazoles; (◑) nitrofurans.

($G = 2.7$). Nitro compounds can one-electron oxidize the intermediate radical ·Thy—OH, which is an adduct between thymine and ·OH, into the corresponding carbonium ion +Thy—OH (Whillans and Adams, 1975; Wada *et al.*, 1982a). This is analogous to the reaction of radicals with

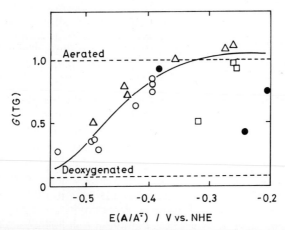

Fig. 6. Relationship between one-electron reduction potential (volt versus normal hydrogen electrode) of nitro compounds and G value for thymine glycol (TG) formation in deoxygenated solution: (○) nitroimidazoles; (□) nitrofurans; (△) nitrobenzenes; (●) quinones.

certain metal cations (Holian and Garrison, 1966; Varghese, 1975; Asmus *et al.*, 1978). The +Thy—OH thus formed reacts with OH⁻ to produce thymine glycol as follows:

$$\cdot\text{Thy—OH} + \text{RNO}_2 \longrightarrow +\text{Thy—OH} + \text{RNO}_2^{\overline{\cdot}} \tag{53}$$

$$+\text{Thy—OH} + {}^-\text{OH} \longrightarrow \text{Thy}\!\!<^{\text{OH}}_{\text{OH}} \tag{54}$$

VI. Suppression of Sulfhydryl Compounds by Misonidazole in Radiosensitization

Intracellular sulfhydryl compounds such as glutathione (GSH) act as radioprotectors for cells (Edgren *et al.*, 1980; Deshavanne *et al.*, 1981). Glutathione reacts with free radicals produced in the intracellular target molecules, to repair the damaged site by hydrogenation [Eq. (56)], and the resulting glutathione radicals react mutually to produce oxidized glutathione, GSSG [Eq. (57)] (Adams *et al.*, 1968).

$$\text{R}\cdot + \text{GSH} \longrightarrow \text{RH} + \text{GS}\cdot \tag{56}$$

$$2\,\text{GS}\cdot \longrightarrow \text{GSSG} \tag{57}$$

where R· and GSH denote target molecule radical and glutathione, respectively.

The effects of glutathione on the thymine conversion and thymine glycol formation were studied in the absence and presence of misonidazole in

TABLE VIII

G Values for Thymine Conversion [*G*(-Thy)], Thymine Glycol Formation [*G*(TG)], and Dihydrothymine Formation [*G*(DHT)] in the Presence and Absence of GSH and Misonidazole (MISO) in Deoxygenated Aqueous Solution[a]

	$[\text{Add}]_0/[\text{Thy}]_0$	G(-Thy)	G(TG)	G(DHT)	G(TG)/G(-Thy)
None	—	1.40	0.10	0.22	0.07
MISO	0.4	1.06	0.54	0.06	0.51
MISO	1.0	0.77	0.43	0.03	0.56
GSH	1.0	0.96	0.00	0.43	0.00
MISO + GSH	0.4	0.62	0.25	0.03	0.40
	1.0				
MISO + GSH	1.0	0.46	0.22	0.00	
	1.0				0.48

[a] $[\text{Thy}]_0 = 0.5$ m*M*, pH 7.0.

deoxygenated solution. As is seen in Table VIII, GSH decomposes with a high G value in aqueous solution to give GSSG and GH. The G value for GSH decomposition is almost equal that for $\cdot$OH formation (5.4) and double that for GSSG formation in N_2O-saturated solution. This indicates that an almost quantitative hydrogen abstraction of GSH by $\cdot$OH occurs as follows:

$$2 \text{ GSH} + 2 \cdot\text{OH} \longrightarrow \text{GSSG} + 2 \text{ H}_2\text{O} \tag{58}$$

Because GSH also decomposes with the G value of 3.3 to give GSSG ($G = 1.3$) in sodium formate aqueous solution, it reacts with e_{aq}^- ($G = 2.7$) and CO_2^- ($G = 3.3$) as follows:

$$2 \text{ GSH} + 2 \, e_{aq}^- + 2 \text{ H}^+ \longrightarrow \text{GSSG} + 2 \text{ H}_2 \tag{59}$$

$$2 \text{ GSH} + 2 \text{ CO}_2^- + 2 \text{ H}^+ \longrightarrow \text{GSSG} + \text{CO}_2 + 2 \text{ H}_2 \tag{60}$$

On the other hand, GSSG reacts with e_{aq}^- and H^+ to form GH ($G = 0.9$ in deoxygenated solution), by the following reactions.

$$\text{GSSG} + 4 \, e_{aq}^- + 2 \text{ H}^+ \longrightarrow 2 \text{ G}\cdot + 2 \text{ SH}^- \tag{61}$$

$$\text{G}\cdot + \text{GSH} \longrightarrow \text{GH} + \text{GS}\cdot \tag{62}$$

$$\text{SH}^- + \text{H}^+ \longrightarrow \text{H}_2\text{S} \tag{63}$$

Because the G value for thymine conversion in the presence of GSH is about two-thirds that in the absence of GSH, thymine may compete with GSH for the reactions with $\cdot$OH, H$\cdot$, and e_{aq}^- as follows:

$$\text{Thy} + \cdot\text{OH} \longrightarrow \cdot\text{Thy---OH} \tag{35}$$

$$\text{Thy} + \text{H}\cdot \text{ (or } e_{aq}^-, \text{ H}^+) \longrightarrow \cdot\text{Thy---H} \tag{32}$$

$$2 \text{ GSH} + 2 \cdot\text{OH} \longrightarrow \text{GSSG} + 2 \text{ H}_2\text{O} \tag{58}$$

$$2 \text{ GSH} + 2 \text{ H}\cdot (2 \, e_{aq}^-, \text{ H}^+) \longrightarrow \text{GSSG} + 2 \text{ H}_2 \tag{59}$$

Glutathione acts as a hydrogen donor to the radical intermediate $\cdot$Thy---OH and $\cdot$Thy---H thus formed.

$$2 \cdot\text{Thy---OH} + 2 \text{ GSH} \longrightarrow 2 \text{ Thy}{\overset{\text{OH}}{\underset{\text{H}}{\diagdown}}} + \text{GSSG} \tag{60}$$

$$2 \cdot\text{Thy---H} + 2 \text{ GSH} \longrightarrow 2 \text{ Thy}{\overset{\text{H}}{\underset{\text{H}}{\diagdown}}} + \text{GSSG} \tag{61}$$

In the thymine–misonidazole–GSH system, thymine conversion decreases much more efficiently than conversions in both the thymine–misonidazole and thymine–GSH systems because of the competitive reactions of $\cdot$OH, H$\cdot$, and e_{aq}^- with both misonidazole [Eqs. (48)–(51)] and GSH [Eqs. (58) and (59)]. The activity of misonidazole to promote thymine glycol formation was reduced by the preferential reaction of ·Thy—OH with GSH [Eq. (60)]. Similarly, the decreased formation of dihydrothymine is attributable to the reaction of e_{aq}^- with misonidazole. These results demonstrate the important role of GSH in reducing radiosensitizing efficiency.

Bridges (1960) observed that N-ethylmaleimide is also effective for hypoxic radiosensitization. Because this compound reacts completely in a few minutes with GSH, the scavenging reaction of sulfhydryl compounds can also play an important role in the radiosensitization. It was also reported that diethylmaleate can enhance the radiosensitivity of hypoxic cells by chemically suppressing intracellular glutathione (Harris, 1979; Bump and Brown, 1982). These radiosensitizers, although not promoting oxidation of thymine in deoxygenated solution, do suppress the action of SH compounds as hydrogen donors in the repair of damaged molecules.

The suppression of thiols by nitro compounds such as misonidazole and metronidazole has been observed only under hypoxic conditions *in vitro* (Varnes *et al.*, 1980). Although metronidazole does not react with sulfhydryl compounds in aqueous solution, both the concentrations of metronidazole and cysteine decrease rapidly in the presence of ferrous sulfate (Willson and Searle, 1975). These results indicate that electron-affinic compounds can exert radiosensitizing effects by suppressing intracellular radioprotectors under the catalytic action of metal cations contained in organisms.

VII. Conclusion

In light of the foregoing results, we propose a molecular mechanism of nitro compounds for the radiosensitization of hypoxic cells that involves (1) increase in the oxidative damage of DNA to give hydroxy compounds under deoxygenated conditions and (2) suppression of intracellular radioprotectors of sulfhydryl compounds. Because both the oxidation of DNA and the reaction with glutathione occur via electron transfer to nitro compounds, the radiosensitizing activity of these compounds would increase with increases in the electron affinity.

References

Adams, G. E., and Cooke, M. S. (1969). Electron-affinic sensitization. I. A structural basis for chemical radiosensitizers in bacteria. *Int. J. Radiat. Biol.* **15,** 457–477.
Adams, G. E., and Dewey, D. L. (1963). Hydrated electrons and radiobiological sensitization. *Biochem. Biophys. Res. Commun.* **12,** 473–477.

Adams, G. E., McNaughton, G. S., and Michael, B. D. (1968). Pulse radiolysis of sulphy-dryl compounds. Part 2. Free radical "repair" by hydrogen transfer from sulphydryl compounds. *Trans. Faraday Soc.* **64**, 902–910.

Adams, G. E., Greenstock, C. L., van Hemmen, J. J., and Willson, R. L. (1972). Radical oxidation mechanisms in cellular radiosensitization: electron transfer in the pulse radioly-sis of aqueous nucleotide solutions. *Radiat. Res.* **49**, 85–95.

Adams, G. E., Clarke, E. D., Flockhart, I. R., Jacobs, R. S., Sehmi, D. S., Stratford, I. J., Wardman, P., Watts, M. E., Parrick, J., Wallance, R. G., and Smithen, C. E. (1979). Structure-activity relationships in the development of hypoxic cell radiosensitizers. I. Sensitization efficiency. *Int. J. Radiat. Biol.* **35**, 133–150.

Asmus, K. D., Deeble, D. J., Garner, A., Idriss Ali, K. M., and Scholes, G. (1978). Chemi-cal aspects of radiosensitization: reaction of sensitizers with radicals produced in the radiolysis of aqueous solutions of nucleic acid components. *Br. J. Cancer.* **37** (Suppl. III), 46–49.

Bielski, B. H. J., and Shiue, G. G. (1979). Reaction rates of superoxide radicals with the essential amino acids. *Ciba Found. Symp.* **65**, 43–56.

Bridges, B. A. (1960). Sensitization of Escherichea coli to Gamma-Radiation-irradiation by N-ethylmaleimide. *Nature (London)* **188**, 415.

Bump, E. A., and Brown, J. M. (1982). The use of drugs which deplete intracellular glu-tathione as radiosensitizers of hypoxic tumor cells in vitro. *Int. J. Radiat. Oncol. Biol. Phys.* **8**, 439–442.

Cadet, J., and Teoule, R. (1978). Comparative study of oxidation of nucleic acid components by hydroxyl radicals, singlet oxygen, and superoxide anion radicals. *Photochem. Photo-biol.* **28**, 665–667.

Deshavanne, P. J., Midander, J., Edgren, M., Larson, A., Malaise, E. P., and Révész, L. (1981). Oxygen enhancement of radiation-induced lethality is greatly reduced in glu-tathione deficient human fibroblasts. *Biomedicine* **35**, 35–37.

Edgren, M., Larsson, A., Nilsson, K., Révész, L., and Scott, O. C. A. (1980). Lack of an oxygen effect in glutathione-deficient human cells in culture. *Int. J. Radiat. Biol.* **37**, 299–306.

Greenstock, C. L., Adams, G. E., and Willson, R. L. (1970). Electron transfer studies of nucleic acid derivatives in solutions containing radiosensitizers. *In* "Radiation Protection and Sensitization" (H. Moroson and M. Quintiliani, eds.), pp. 65–71. Taylor & Francis, London.

Hall, E. J., and Roizin-Towle, L. (1975). Hypoxic sensitizers: radiobiological studies at the cellular level. *Radiology (Easton, Pa.)* **117**, 453–457.

Harris, J. W. (1979). Mammalian cell studies with Diamide. *Pharmacol. Ther.* **7**, 375–384.

Holian, J., and Garrison, W. M. (1966). Radiation-induced oxidation of cytosine and uracil in aqueous solution of copper (II). *Nature (London)* **212**, 394–395.

Kagiya, T., Nishimoto, S., Nakamichi, K., Ide, H., and Shimidzu, T. (1982). Radiation-induced reactions of thymine, thymidine and thymidine-5'-monophosphate in aqueous solutions. *Nucleic Acids Res.* **S–11**, 241–244.

Kagiya, T., Ide, H., Nishimoto, S., and Wada, T. (1983). Radiation-induced reduction of nitroimidazole derivatives in aqueous solution. *Int. J. Radiat. Biol.* (in press).

Loman, H., and Ebert, M. (1970). The radiation chemistry of thymine in aqueous solution. Some reactions of the thymine-electron adduct. *Int. J. Radiat. Biol.* **18**, 369–379.

Raleigh, J. A., Greenstock, C. L., and Kremers, W. (1973a). Chemical radiosensitization of phosphate ester cleavage. *Int. J. Radiat. Biol.* **23**, 457–467.

Raleigh, J. A., Greenstock, C. L., Whitehouse, R., and Kremers, W. (1973b). Radiosensiti-zation of phosphate release from 3'- and 5'-nucleotides: correlation between chemical change and biological inactivation. *Int. J. Radiat. Biol.* **24**, 595–603.

Raleigh, J. A., Whitehouse, R., and Kremers, W. (1974). Effect of oxygen and nitroaromatic cell radiosensitizers on radiation-induced phosphate release from 3'- and 5'-nucleotides: a model for nucleic acids. *Radiat. Res.* **59,** 453–465.

Stratford, I. J. (1982). Mechanism of hypoxic radiosensitization and the development of new sensitizers. *Int. J. Radiat. Oncol. Biol. Phys.* **8,** 391–398.

Varghese, A. J. (1975). Sensitization of thymine and uracil to ionizing radiation by p-nitroacetophenone. *Int. J. Radiat. Biol.* **28,** 477–484.

Varnes, M. E., Biaglow, J. E., Koch, C. J., and Hall, E. J. (1980). Depletion of non protein thiols of hypoxic cells by misonidazole and metronidazole. *In* "Radiation Sensitizers" (L. W. Brady, ed.), pp. 121–124. Masson, New York.

Wada, T., Ide, H., Okubo, H., and Kagiya, T. (1981). Studies on the action mechanism of electron-affinic radiosensitizers. III. Radiation-induced degradation of nitro-compounds in aqueous solutions. *J. Radiat. Res.* **22,** 62–63.

Wada, T., Ide, H., Nishimoto, S., and Kagiya, T. (1982a). Radiation-induced hydroxylation of thymine sensitized by nitro-compounds in N_2O-saturated aqueous solution. *Chem. Lett.* No. 7, 1041–1044.

Wada, T., Ide, H., Nishimoto, S., and Kagiya, T. (1982b). Radiation-induced reduction of thymine in aqueous solution. *Int. J. Radiat. Biol.* **42,** 215–221.

Wada, T., Ide, H., Nishimoto, S., and Kagiya, T. (1982c). The influence of misonidazole on radiation-induced reductions of DNA bases. *J. Radiat. Res.* **23,** 34–35.

Whillans, D. W., and Adams, G. E. (1975). Electron transfer oxidation of DNA radicals by paranitroacetophenone. *Int. J. Radiat. Biol.* **28,** 501–510.

Whillans, D. W., and Whitmore, G. F. (1981). The radiation reduction of misonidazole. *Radiat. Res.* **86,** 311–314.

Willson, R. L., and Emmerson, P. T. (1970). Reaction of triacetoneamine-N-oxyl with radiation-induced radicals from DNA and deoxyribonucleotides in aqueous solution. *In* "Radiation Protection and Sensitization" (H. L. Morison, and M. Quintiliani, eds.), pp. 73–79. Taylor & Francis, London.

Willson, R. L., and Searle, A. J. F. (1975). Metronidazole (Flagyl): iron catalysed reaction with sulphydryl groups and tumour radiosensitisation. *Nature (London)* **255,** 498–500.

7 A New Hypoxic-Cell Radiosensitizer Containing the Oxidized Sulfur Group instead of the Nitro Group: 2-Mercaptoimidazole Derivatives

Seiichi Inayama

Pharmaceutical Institute
School of Medicine, Keio University
Tokyo 160, Japan

Tomoyuki Mori

Department of Radiology
School of Medicine, Tokai University
Kanagawa 259-11, Japan

I. Introduction

Considerable efforts have been made to develop effective drugs that would sensitize hypoxic radioresistant cells in tumor tissues (Adams *et al.*, 1976a; Fowler *et al.*, 1976). Among a variety of heterocyclic compounds containing the nitro group, misonidazole [1-(2-hydroxy-3-methoxypropyl)-2-nitroimidazole] (**9**) is one of the most effective radiosensitizers for hypoxic cells (Adams *et al.*, 1976a; Fowler *et al.*, 1976) and is currently under clinical evaluation (Disch *et al.*, 1977). However, because of its neurotoxicity and, to some extent, its mutagenicity (attributable to the nitro group), the clinical applicability at doses sufficient to produce optimum sensitization is limited (Brown and Wardman, 1980).

We turned our attention to the design and synthesis of a series of imidazole derivatives containing oxidized sulfur groups, in place of the nitro group, in the hope of obtaining improved radiosensitizing compounds. The radiosensitizing ability of a compound is related to its electron affinity, and such is regarded as the criterion for choosing a particular hypoxic-cell radiosensitizer (Adams *et al.*, 1976b). In our studies of a quantitative structure–activity relationship of antitumor mitomycin derivatives using molecular orbital (MO) calculation, the lowest unoccupied MO (LUMO) was found to be indispensable as a parameter (Inayama and Ohsaka, 1980). Here, we present recent advances in our work with some 2-mercaptoimidazole derivatives with potential value as radiosensitizers (Inayama *et al.*, 1981).

II. Synthesis of New Derivatives

As shown here, several new 2-mercaptoimidazole derivatives containing thiol (**1**), sulfide (**2** and **5**), sulfoxide (**3** and **6**), and sulfone moieties (**4** and **7**) were chosen as candidates for hypoxic-cell radiosensitizers. The radiosensitizing activities of these compounds were then compared with those of the well-known mononitro- (**9**) (misonidazole) and dinitroimidazole derivatives (**10**) (Agrawal *et al.*, 1979), of which the latter has been

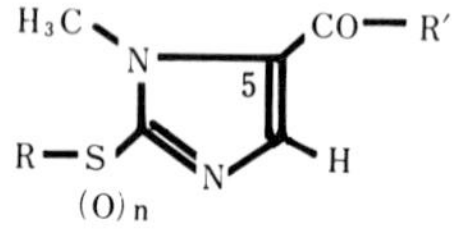

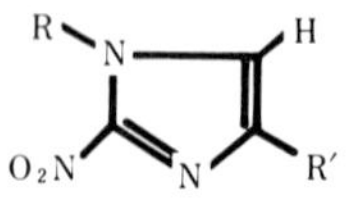

(**1**) KIH-1   (R=H ,   R'=OCH$_3$, n=0)   (**9**) misonidazole

(**2**) KIH-2   (R=CH$_3$, R'=OCH$_3$, n=0)   R=CH$_2$CH(OH)CH$_2$OCH$_3$

(**3**) KIH-3   (R=CH$_3$, R'=OCH$_3$, n=1)   R'=H

(**4**) KIH-4   (R=CH$_3$, R'=OCH$_3$, n=2)

(**5**) KIH-10 (R=CH$_3$, R'=NH$_2$,   n=0)   (**10**) 2,4-dinitroimidazole-1-ethanol

(**6**) KIH-11 (R=CH$_3$, R'=NH$_2$,   n=1)   R=CH$_2$CH$_2$OH

(**7**) KIH-12 (R=CH$_3$, R'=NH$_2$,   n=2)   R'=NO$_2$

(**8**) KIH-5   (R=CH$_3$, C$_5$-H)

shown by our group to act as a most potent radiosensitizer (Mori *et al.*, 1981; Shibata *et al.*, 1981). The electron affinities (EA) of these mercaptoimidazole derivatives shown in Fig. 1 were calculated in terms of the LUMO by the CNDO/2 method (Pople, 1970) on a HITAC 8800/8700 computer in the Tokyo University Computer Center. The geometries of the designed molecules were determined from X-ray–diffraction data

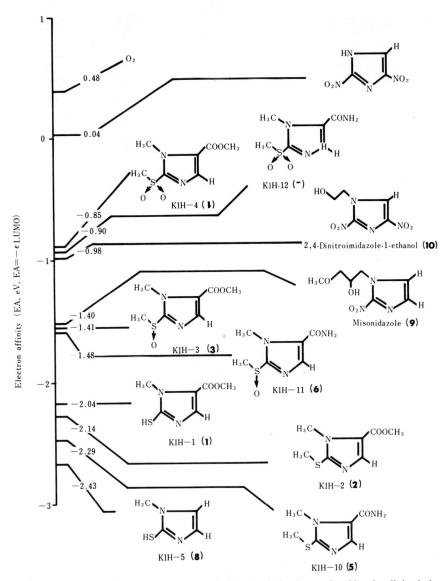

Fig. 1. Electron affinities of 2-mercaptoimidazole derivatives, misonidazole, dinitroimidazole derivatives, and oxygen, estimated on the basis of LUMO calculated by using CNDO/2 method.

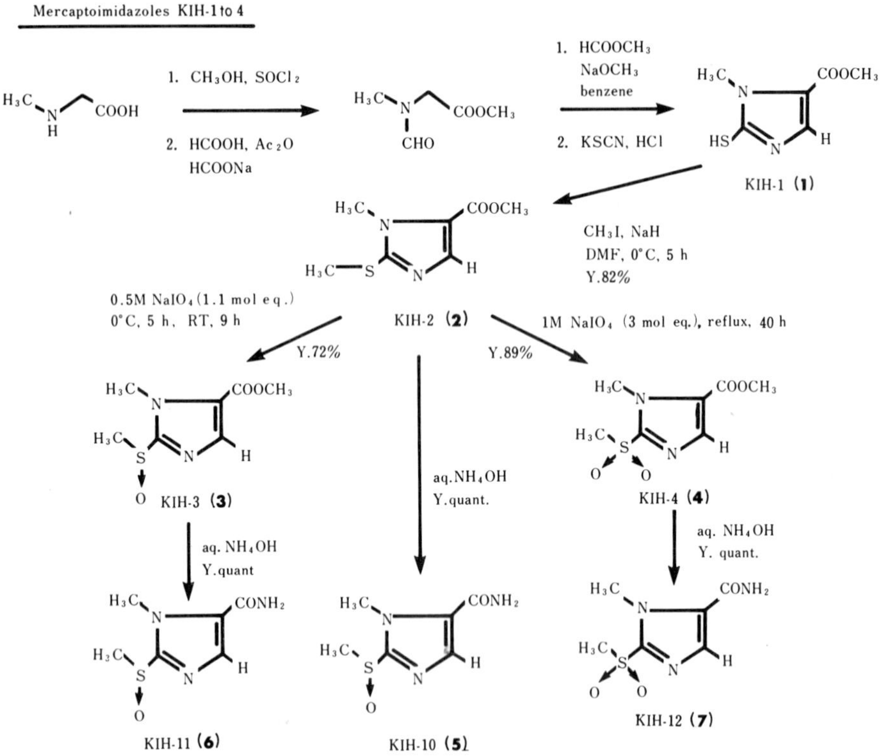

Mercaptoimidazoles KIH-1 to 4

Scheme 1. Syntheses of 2-mercaptoimidazoles.

from the methyl sulfoxide derivative **3** (KIH-3; 1-methyl-2-methylsulfinyl-5-methoxycarbonylimidazole) and from the Cambridge Crystallographic Data File (CCDF) on compounds having similar structures. The methylsulfinyl- (**3**) (EA = −1.41 eV) and the methylsulfonyl- (**4**) (EA = −0.85 eV) derivatives, being derived from methylthioether (**2**), would be expected to show a radiosensitization similar to that of misonidazole (**9**) (EA = −1.40 eV), respectively, in that the electron affinity is considered to be an essential factor in the expression of radiosensitization with these non-nitro compounds.

The imidazole derivatives just mentioned (**2**, **3**, and **4**) were synthesized from thiol (**1**) (Link and Bernauer, 1972) as follows. Methylation of thiol (**1**) (methyl iodide, sodium hydride, dimethylformamide, 0°C, 5 h) resulted in methylthioimidazole (**2**) in a yield (Y) of 82%. Selective oxidation of **2** was achieved with 0.5 M sodium metaperiodate solution (1.1 mol eq, 0°C, 5 h; room temperature (RT), 9 h) to produce methylsulfinylimidazole (**3**) in a 72% yield, and with 1 M sodium metaperiodate solution (3 mol eq, reflux, 40 h) to afford methylsulfonylimidazole (**4**) in an 89% yield. The structure and purity were confirmed by NMR, IR, and MS spectroscopic analyses in each case. These synthetic routes and physical data are summarized in Scheme 1 and Table I, respectively.

III. Methods of Evaluation

The 2-mercaptoimidazole derivatives (**1**, **2**, **3**, **4**, and **8**), as well as misonidazole (**9**) and 2,4-dinitroimidazole-1-ethanol (**10**) for comparison, were evaluated by a modified experimental method for the *in vitro* testing as radiosensitizers (Shibata *et al.*, 1981). The survival curves of the drug-treated or untreated HeLa S3 cells irradiated by ^{60}Co γ rays in the presence and absence of oxygen are shown in Fig. 2. Compounds **1**, **2**, and **3** were dissolved in ethanol or Tween 80. The dinitroimidazole derivative (**10**) had about a 10-fold greater radiosensitization than did misonidazole (**9**), paralleling their electron affinities (-0.98 and -1.40 eV) (Mori *et al.*, 1981; Shibata *et al.*, 1981). Methylsulfonylimidazole (**4**) and methyl-sulfinylimidazole (**3**) were expected to exhibit a similar sensitization corresponding to electron affinities comparable to the nitro compounds **10** and **9**, respectively, but such activity was not detected in the hypoxic screening system used.

The failure to observe radiosensitization with the mercaptoimidazoles might be mainly due to the water insolubility and also possibly to the inevitable usage of the cosolvent Tween 80, which is toxic to cells.

Therefore, the attempt was made to modify these lipophilic 2-mercaptoimidazole compounds in order to gain greater water solubility. Replacement of the methoxycarbonyl function in compounds **2**, **3**, and **4** by the carbamoyl group was intended to meet the following minimum requirements:

1. Improved hydrophilicity of the new compounds (**5**, **6**, and **7** were essentially soluble in water)
2. Minor change of the electron affinity (compound **5**, EA = -2.29 eV; **6**, EA = -1.48 eV; **7**, EA = -0.09 eV) (see Fig. 1)
3. Simple alteration of the ester function in compounds **2**, **3**, and **4**

Thus, ammonolysis of the methoxycarbonyl-2-mercaptoimidazoles afforded, in quantitative yield, the corresponding carbamoyl derivatives **5**, **6**, and **7**, respectively. The physical data of these amides (**5**, **6**, and **7**) are shown in Table I in comparison with those of the original esters (**2**, **3**, and **4**).

TABLE I

Physical Data for 2-mercaptoimidazole Derivatives[a]

Compound	Formula	mp (°C)	¹H-NMR (ppm)	IR (cm⁻¹)			MS (m/z), M⁺ (%) MW Found (calculated)
KIH-1 (1)	$C_6H_8N_2O_2S$	199–200	3.73 (s, 3 H)	3085	1723	740	M⁺ 172 (100)
			3.97 (s, 3 H)	3000	1480		172.0310
							(172.0307)
KIH-2 (2)	$C_7H_{10}O_2N_2S$	46–47	7.83 (s, 1 H)	2870	1300		M⁺ 186 (100)
			2.27 (s, 3 H)	1718			186.0419
							(186.0462)
			3.78 (s, 3 H)	1348			
			3.82 (s, 3 H)				
			7.70 (s, 1 H)				
KIH-3 (3)	$C_7H_{10}O_3N_2S$	70–72	3.17 (s, 3 H)	1725			M⁺ 202 (31)
			3.90 (s, 3 H)	1060			202.0480
							(202.0411)
			4.27 (s, 3 H)				
			7.80 (s, 1 H)				
KIH-4 (4)	$C_7H_{10}O_4N_2S$	106–107	3.43 (s, 3 H)	1730	1133		M⁺ 218 (100)
			3.93 (s, 3 H)	1314			218.0356
							(218.0361)
			4.27 (s, 3 H)	1300			
			7.73 (s, 1 H)	1140			
KIH-10 (5)	$C_6H_9N_3OS$	164–165	2.57 (s, 3 H)	3350	1620		M⁺ 171 (100)
			3.75 (s, 3 H)	3161	1315		171.0445
							(171.0465)
			7.10–7.83 (m, 2 H)	1680			
			7.67 (s, 1 H)				
KIH-11 (6)	$C_6H_9N_3O_2S$	186–188	3.07 (s, 3 H)	3350	1630		M⁺ 187 (30)
			4.07 (s, 3 H)	3175	1020		187.0393
							(187.0414)
			7.33–8.00 (m, 1 H)	1690			
			7.78 (s, 1 H)				
KIH-12 (7)	$C_6H_9N_3O_3S$	178–180	3.43 (s, 3 H)	3400	1620		M⁺ 203 (49)
			4.12 (s, 3 H)	3185	1315		203.0363
							(203.0240)
			7.33–8.33 (m, 2 H)	1690	1130		
			7.22 (s, 1 H)				

[a] Abbreviations: ¹H-NMR, Chemical shifts (ppm) of the proton nuclear magnetic resonance signals measured in deuterochloroform for **1**, **3**, and **4**; in deuteropyridine for **2**; and in deuterodimethyl sulfoxide for **5**, **6**, and **7**, with tetramethylsilane as an internal standard. IR, Stretching vibrations in the infrared spectra (cm⁻¹) determined in KBr pellets. MS, Molecular ion fragments (m/z). M⁺, Relative intensity observed in the mass spectra. Molecular weights observed (and calculated) corresponding to the compositions determined by high-resolution mass spectroscopy.

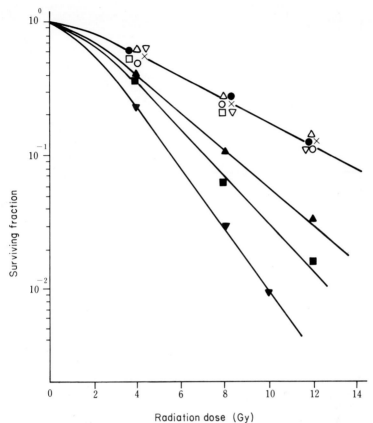

Fig. 2. Radiation survival curves of HeLa S3 cells to ^{60}Co γ rays for 5-methoxycarbonyl-2-mercaptoimidazoles (all in N$_2$, all 5 mM): **1** ($\triangledown$), **2** ($\bigcirc$), **3** ($\triangle$), **4** ($\square$), and **8** (X). Shown also for comparison: misonidazole (**9**) (1 mM, in N$_2$, $\blacktriangle$); 2,4-dinitroimidazole-1-ethanol (**10**) (1 mM, in N$_2$, $\blacksquare$); N$_2$, no drug ($\bullet$); aerobic, no drug ($\blacktriangledown$).

This replacement, however, failed to produce radiosensitizing activity in the *in vitro* screening test with the cell suspension hypoxic system, as mentioned before (Fig. 3). To confirm whether different test conditions would reflect a radiosensitization efficiency (Wardman, 1982)[1], we attempted to reevaluate the carbamoyl compound **3** (KIH-3) (most likely to be a radiosensitizer), with a newly devised hypoxic chamber (M. Furukawa, I. Kaneko, S. Yoshikawa, T. Sugahara, E. Kano, unpublished) in

---

[1] During the preparation of this paper, Wardman pointed out the need for a greater appreciation of the chemical and biochemical properties of both the compounds and the test organisms used.

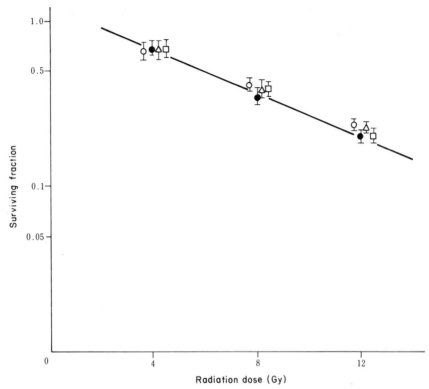

Fig. 3. Radiation survival curves of HeLa S3 cells to ⁶⁰Co γ rays for 5-carbamoyl compounds (all hypoxic, all 5 mM): **5** (○), **6** (△), **7** (□). Hypoxic, no drug (●).

which confluent cells (Chinese hamster V79 line) adhered in a monolayer on the surface of the glass plate (Nakano *et al.*, 1982).

As shown in Fig. 4, the candidate compound exhibited significant radiosensitizing activity in this hypoxic screening system. The dose-modifying effects of KIH-3 (**3**) and misonidazole (**9**) were thus calculated to be 1.75 and 2.0, respectively, under the hypoxic-cell conditions. This discrepancy in the hypoxic radiosensitizing effectiveness of the compound seems to be attributable to the cell lines or the hypoxic conditions, with special reference to the growth phases of the cell culture (Nakano *et al.*, 1982). Further studies to elucidate these factors are in progress. Cytotoxicity of **3** at 1.0 mM concentration was not observed during 7 days of incubation at 37°C under oxygenic conditions. The possible inhibitory effect of **3** against potentially lethal damage recovery is also being extensively investigated.

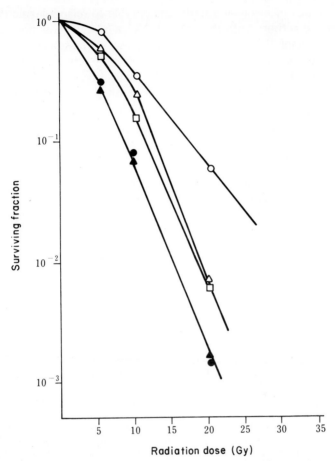

Fig. 4. Radiation survival curves of Chinese hamster V79 cells (confluent) to ^{60}Co γ rays for KIH-3 (**3**). (○) Hypoxic, (△) hypoxic + 1 mM KIH-3, (□) hypoxic + 1 mM misonidazole (**9**), (●) aerobic, (▲) aerobic + 1 mM KIH-3.

IV. Conclusion

New non-nitro imidazole derivatives containing the oxidized sulfur group were designed and synthesized to screen hypoxic radioresistant cells and to be used in place of the radiosensitizing nitroimidazoles. The electron affinity of these mercaptoimidazole derivatives, such as sulfoxide (**3**) (KIH-3) and sulfone (**4**) (KIH-4) was determined by adaptation of the lowest unoccupied molecular orbital (LUMO) estimated by molecular orbital (MO) calculation using the CNDO/2 method, and were expected to have properties of electron affinity comparable to misonidazole (**9**). Radiosensitizing activity with the hypoxic HeLa S3 cells was not detected with those lipophilic compounds or with the water-soluble carbamoyl derivatives prepared by replacement of the methoxycarbonyl function (**5, 6,** and **7**). Attempts to use KIH-3 with Chinese hamster V79 confluent cells in a newly devised hypoxic chamber resulted in a comparable sensitization to misonidazole, as expected from the electron affinity.

Acknowledgments

We thank Dr. H. Hori of Keio University, C. Murayama of Tokai University, and Dr. I. Kaneko of the Institute of Physical and Chemical Research for close cooperation in this work. These studies were supported in part by Grants-in-Aid from the Ministry of Science and Technology for Research on Peaceful Usage of Nuclear Energy (radiosensitizer), and from the Ministry of Education, Science and Culture, Japan.

References

Adams, G. E., Denenkamp, J., and Fowler, J. F. (1976a). Biological bases of radiosensitization by hypoxic-cell radiosensitizers. *Chemotherapy (Basel)* **7,** 187–206.

Adams, G. E., Flockhart, L. R., Smithen, C. E., Stratford, I. J., Wardman, P., and Watts, M. E. (1976b). Electron-affinic sensitization VII. A correlation between structures, one-electron reduction potentials, and efficiencies of nitroimidazoles as hypoxic cell radiosensitizers. *Radiat. Res.* **67,** 9–20.

Agrawal, K. C., Millar, B. C., and Neta, P. (1979). Radiosensitization of hypoxic mammalian cells by dinitroimidazoles. *Radiat. Res.* **78,** 532–541.

Brown, J. M., and Wardman, P. (1980). Partition coefficient as a guide to the development of radiosensitizers which are less toxic than misonidazole. *Radiat. Res.* **82,** 171–190.

Disch, S., Saunders, M. I., Lee, M. E., Adams, G. E., and Flockhart, I. R. (1977). Misonidazole—A Drug for trial in radiotherapy and oncology. *Br. J. Cancer* **35,** 567–579.

Fowler, J. F., Adams, G. E., and Denekamp, J. (1976). Radiosensitizers of hypoxic cells in solid tumors. *Cancer Treat. Rep.* **3,** 227–256.

Inayama, S., and Ohsaka, T. (1980). Structure-activity relationship of antitumor mitosanes using semiempical molecular orbital calculation. *Abstr. Int. Symp. Med. Chem. 7th,* p. 23.

Inayama, S., Hori, H., Ohsaka, T., Mori, T., and Shibata, C. (1981). An approach to the design and synthesis of mercaptoimidazole derivatives containing oxidized sulfur based on electron affinity sensitization. *Gann* **72,** 156–159.

Link, H., and Bernauer, K. (1972). Über die Synthese der *Pilocarpus*-Alkaloide Isopilosin und Pilocarpin, sowie die absolute konfiguration des (+)-Isopilosins. *Helv. Chim. Acta* **55,** 1053–1062.

Mori, T., Shibata, C., Ohizumi, Y., Maezawa, H., Ushiro, S., Hori, H., and Inayama, S. (1981). Hypoxic cell sensitizer: *in vitro. Gann no Rinsho* **27,** 1424–1452.

Nakano, K., Itoh, K., Kaneko, I., Hori, H., Shibata, T., and Inayama, S. (1982). Hypoxic radiosensitization of mercaptoimidazoles. *Abstr. Annu. Meet. Jpn. Assoc. Radiat. Res. 25th.* J. Rad. Res. **24,** 41.

Pople, J. A. (1970). ''Approximate Molecular Orbital Theory.'' McGraw-Hill, New York.
Shibata, C., Hori, H., Inayama, S., and Mori, T. (1981). Radiosensitizing effect of 2,4-dinitroimidazole-1-ethanol and its cytotoxicity in HeLa S3 cells. *Strahlentherapie* **157,** 481–485.
Wardman, P., Anderson, R. F., Hodgkiss, R. J., Parrick, J., Smithen, C. E., Wallace, R. G., and Watts, M. E. (1982). Radiosensitization by non-nitro compounds. Int. J. Radiat. Oncol. Biol. Phys., **8,** 399–401.

8 Design, Synthesis, and Activity of New Hypoxic-Cell Sensitizers: Spermine and Spermidine Amides Having Nitro Groups

Eiichi Fujita

Institute for Chemical Research
Kyoto University
Kyoto 611, Japan

Tomoyuki Mori

Department of Radiation Oncology
School of Medicine, Tokai University
Kanagawa 259-11, Japan

I. Design and Synthesis

One of the authors (E.F.) has been interested in the synthesis of naturally occurring amides with polyamines (especially spermine and spermidine) and of polyamine-containing compounds, as these compounds have potential biological and/or physiological activity.

Polyamines interact with DNA, and the binding of polyamines to nucleic acids seems to involve a noncovalent linkage between the basic groups of the polyamine and the highly acidic phosphate groups of the nucleic acid, or conversely to involve noncovalent linkage between the ammonium ion of the polyamine salt and the phosphate anion of the sodium or potassium salt. Spermine (1) and spermidine (2) stabilize and protect DNA, by their binding. Thus, spermine (1) and spermidine (2) are

Modification of Radiosensitivity in Cancer Treatment

important substances for DNA; they interact readily with DNA and have a charge–charge affinity. As a hypoxic-cell sensitizer has to make contact with nucleic acids in the cancer cells, we designed a molecule containing spermine (**1**) or spermidine (**2**).

$$H_2N-(CH_2)_3-NH-(CH_2)_4-NH-(CH_2)_3-NH_2$$

1

$$H_2N-(CH_2)_3-NH-(CH_2)_4-NH_2$$

2

It may be desirable for the hypoxic-cell sensitizer to contain portion(s) to be inserted into the DNA molecule. Some aromatic compounds bind to nucleic acids by intercalation, that is, the insertion of a flat molecule between the base pairs of a double helix. Becker and Dervan (1979) reported that bis(methidium)spermine (BMSp) (**3**), in which two intercalating monomers of ethidium bromide (EB) (**4**), connected by a spermine link, are incorporated into the same molecule, can bind nucleic acids with a free energy approaching the sum of the free energies of the monomeric constituents resulting in substantial increases in both binding affinity and specificity. They suggested that both EB moieties in BMSp simultaneously intercalate. Therefore we arranged molecules with two benzene rings at both ends of spermine (**1**) or spermidine (**2**) as the benzene ring is a simple, flat molecule.

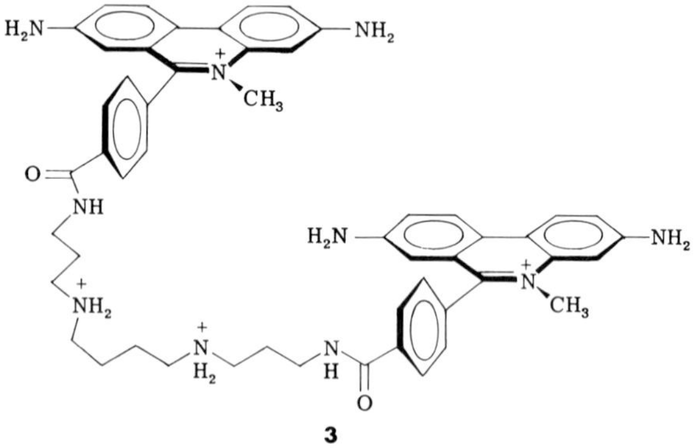

3

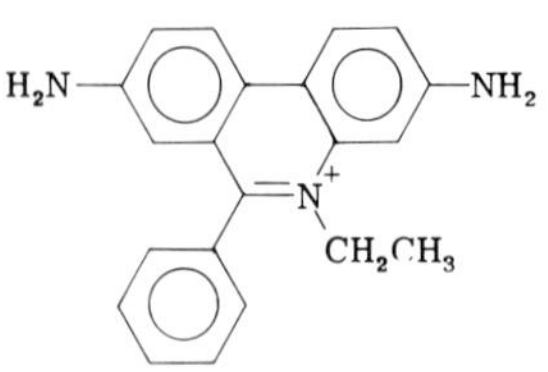

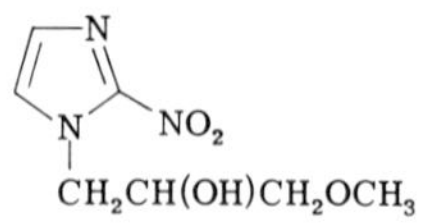

4

5

Misonidazole (**5**), a powerful hypoxic-cell sensitizer, has a nitro group in the molecule. We decided to use the nitro group as the electron acceptors. Thus our design was accomplished: The target molecules are N^1,N^{10}-bis(4-nitrobenzoyl)spermidine (FNT-1)[1] (**6**) and N^1,N^{14}-bis(4-nitrobenzoyl)spermine (FNT-2)[1] (**7**). The Kyoto group (Nagao *et al.*, 1980a) developed a new method for synthesis of amide *via* aminolysis of 3-acyl-1,3-thiazolidine-2-thione (ATT) (**8**) and applied it to the synthesis of macrolactams (Nagao *et al.*, 1980b). Total syntheses of macrocyclic spermidine alkaloids, codonocarpine (Nagao *et al.*, 1980c), *dl*-lunarine, and *dl*-lunaridine (Nagao *et al.*, 1981) were also published.

Thus, syntheses of FNT-1 (**6**) and FNT-2 (**7**) were carried out efficiently as follows. A solution of spermidine (**2**) (0.22 g) in methylene chloride (25 ml) was added to a solution of 3-(4-nitrobenzoyl)-1,3-thiazolidine-2-thione (**8a**) (0.8 g, mp 166–167°C), prepared by usual treatment of 1,3-thiazolidine-2-thione thallium(I) salt and *p*-nitrobenzoyl chloride, in methylene chloride (25 ml). After being stirred at room temperature (r.t.) for 1 h under an atmosphere of nitrogen, the reaction mixture was washed with 2% sodium hydroxide solution (100 ml) to remove the 1,3-thiazolidine-2-thione (TT) released. The TT-free solution was washed with brine, dried over anhydrous sodium sulfate, and evaporated *in vacuo* to leave crude

---

[1] FNT-1 and FNT-2 were named according to the initial letters of E. Fujita, Y. Nagao, and S. Takao, at Kyoto University.

crystals. Recrystallization was carried out from ethanol to afford pure yellow needles (0.65 g, mp 126–127°C, 98% yield). Hydrochloride (**6**) was obtained as yellow needles, mp 167–168°C (from ethanol).

Similar methods were used to prepare FNT-2 (**7**) (mp 255–258°C, decomposition) in good yield (Nagao *et al.*, 1983).

2 + 2 × (structure **8a**) $\xrightarrow[\substack{CH_2Cl_2 \\ 98.0\%}]{r.t.}$ Free base $\xrightarrow[\substack{EtOH \\ r.t. \\ 71.4\%}]{HCl}$ FNT-1 (**6**)

1 + 2 × 8a $\xrightarrow[\substack{CH_2Cl_2 \\ 79.3\%}]{r.t.}$ Free base $\xrightarrow[\substack{EtOH \\ r.t. \\ 79.0\%}]{HCl}$ FNT-2 (**7**)

These two compounds (FNT-1 and FNT-2) were shown to have more effective radiosensitizing abilities than misonidazole (**5**) to hypoxic cells. Especially FNT-1 (**6**) was shown to have an activity 1.5 times greater than that of misonidazole, as the result of *in vitro* tests (see Section II). Although detailed mechanisms of their activity remain to be determined, consideration led to the design of these molecules, and our postulations were supported, in principle, by the biological tests.

II. Activity

Hypoxic cells, which are present in almost all tumor tissues, represent a problem in radiotherapy treatment for cancer, as these cells respond poorly to radiotherapy and to chemotherapy. Therefore, in the radiotherapeutic control of malignant tumor, it is desirable to obtain a hypoxic-cell radiosensitizer that is highly effective and minimally toxic. Misonidazole, a derivative of 2-nitroimidazole, is reportedly the most effective radiosensitizer of hypoxic cells. However, its neurotoxic effects limit the clinical application at doses sufficient to give optimum sensitization. Because the nitro group is assumed to be responsible for radiosensitizing ability (Shibata *et al.*, 1981), we tested a series of compounds that contain nitro group in their molecule. Among them, two compounds named FNT-1 and FNT-2 (see Section I) were found to have marked radiosensitizing effect to hypoxic HeLa cells.

III. Materials and Methods

A. Compounds

Two compounds (FNT-1 and FNT-2) were synthesized and supplied to us (Tokai group) by the Kyoto group.

B. Cells

We used HeLa S3 cells grown on the surface of plastic flasks (NUNC, Roskilde, Denmark) in Eagle's minimum essential medium (MEM, Nissui Seiyaku, Tokyo), supplemented with 10% calf serum (Flow Lab., Rockville, Maryland). These cells were incubated at 37°C in a CO_2 incubator at 100% humidity. A solution of 0.1% trypsin (Difco Lab., Detroit, Michigan) containing 0.02% EDTA was used to detach the cells for subculture.

IV. Radiation Experiments

The exponentially growing cells used in all experiments were suspended in plastic tubes (Falcon Plastics, Los Angeles, California) containing 0.5 ml of MEM ($4–5 \times 10^5$ cells/ml). The compounds were dissolved in MEM and added to the cell suspension before hypoxic treatment. To obtain hypoxic conditions, the tubes were stoppered with tightly fitting rubber diaphragms; these were punctured with two injection needles (18- and 22-gauge) connected via a three-way stopcock to a hypoxic system. Hypoxia was produced by flushing the medium for 1 h with 95% nitrogen and 5% carbon dioxide gas containing less than 5 ppm oxygen (Nippon Sanso Co., Ltd., Oyama) through one injection needle, under gentle shaking. Thereafter, both needles were removed and the tubes were irradiated (Ohizumi et al., 1980). Irradiation with ^{60}Co γ rays was at a dose rate of 2.34 Gy/min in a Mix-Dp phantom with a six-tube capacity. The absorbed dose was calibrated by using an ionization chamber (AE-130LS, Applied Engineering, Inc., Tokyo) and a TLD dosimeter (Harshow Chemical Co. Ltd., Cleveland). After irradiation, cell samples were centrifuged, resuspended, and diluted. For each test, cells were plated at different densities in 60-mm diameter plastic dishes (Corning Glass Works, New York) containing 5 ml of MEM supplemented with 10% calf serum, and incubated at 37°C for 10 to 12 days. The colonies thus formed were fixed with methanol, stained with Giemsa (Merck, Darmstadt, Federal Republic of Germany), and counted.

V. Radiosensitizing Effects

Figures 1 and 2 show the survival curves for drug-treated or untreated HeLa S3 cells irradiated in the presence and absence of oxygen. The enhancement ratios were obtained from the D_0 ratio in the absence and presence of the radiosensitizer. The abbreviation D_0 describes the slope of the exponential portion of the survival curve, after the initial shoulder, and it is the dose required to reduce the surviving fraction of the cells to 37%. In our system, the D_0 value was 5.87 Gy for hypoxic cells and 1.72 Gy for aerobic cells. In the case of FNT-1, an increase in the concentration brought about a progressive increase in the sensitization of hypoxic cells. Cell killing was nil when cells were exposed to 0.1 mM FNT-2; however, when the concentration was increased to 1 mM, there was a similar sensitizing effect to that seen with 0.3 mM FNT-1.

Calculated enhancement ratios (ER) of FNT-1 and FNT-2 at tested concentrations are shown in Table I. The ERs for different concentrations of misonidazole are also presented for comparison. These results proved that, at 1 mM drug concentration, FNT-1 has about 1.5 times greater sensitizing effect than misonidazole.

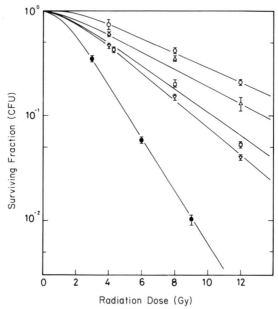

Fig. 1. Radiosensitizing effect of FNT-1 on hypoxic cells. Hypoxic (○). Hypoxic + 0.1 mM FNT-1 (△). Hypoxic + 0.5 mM FNT-1 (□). Hypoxic + 1 mM FNT-1 (▽). Aerobic (●).

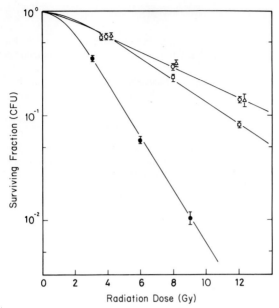

Fig. 2. Radiosensitizing effect of FNT-2 on hypoxic cells. Hypoxic (○). Hypoxic + 0.1 m*M* FNT-2 (△). Hypoxic + 1 m*M* FNT-2 (□). Aerobic (●).

These results were obtained in *in vitro* experiments; therefore, the toxicity of FNT-1 and FNT-2 to the cells and further *in vivo* investigations of these compounds are under way to determine possible safe and effective clinical application.

TABLE I

Enhancement Ratios (ER) of FNT-1,
FNT-2, and Misonidazole

Compound	Concentration (m*M*)	ER
FNT-1	0.1	1.18
	0.5	1.65
	1.0	2.10
FNT-2	1.0	1.45
Misonidazole	0.1	1.05
	0.5	1.12
	1.0	1.32

References

Becker, M. M., and Dervan, P. B. (1979). Molecular recognition of nucleic acid by small molecules. Binding affinity and structure specificity of bis(methidium) spermine. *J. Am. Chem. Soc.* **101**, 3644–3666.

Nagao, Y., Seno, K., Kawabata, K., Miyasaka, T., Takao, S., and Fujita, E. (1980a). Monitored aminolysis of 3-acylthiazolidine-2-thione: a new convenient synthesis of amide. *Tetrahedron Lett.* **21**, 841–844.

Nagao, Y., Seno, K., Miyasaka, T., and Fujita, E. (1980b). Monitored aminolysis of 3-acylthiazolidine-2-thione: a new synthesis of macrocyclic amides. *Chem. Lett.* No. 2 159–162.

Nagao, Y., Seno, K., and Fujita, E. (1980c). Total synthesis of a macrocyclic spermidine alkaloid, codonocarpine. *Tetrahedron Lett.* **21**, 4931–4934.

Nagao, Y., Takao, S., Miyasaka, T., and Fujita, E. (1981). Total synthesis of macrocyclic spermidine alkaloids, dl-lunarine and dl-lunaridine. *J. Chem. Soc. Chem. Commun.* No. 6, 286–287.

Nagao, Y., Takao, S., Fujita, E., Murayama, C., Mori, T., Asao, T., and Suzue, T. (1983). Development of new hypoxic cell sensitizers: amides of nitrobenzoic acid with spermidine and spermine. *Experientia* **39**, 1116–1118.

Ohizumi, Y., Shibata, C., and Mori, T. (1980). Effect of hypoxia on the cytotoxicity of misonidazole in HeLa S3 cells in vitro. *Gann* **71**, 319.

Shibata, C., Hori, H., Inayama, S., and Mori, T. (1981). Radiosensitizing effect of 2,4-dinitroimidazole-1-ethanol and its cytotoxicity in HeLa S3 cells. *Strahlentherapie* **157**, 481–485.

9 Anoxic-Cell Radiosensitization Induced by Heterocyclic Compounds

Eiichi Kano
Susumu Tsubouchi
Takashi Kondo
Michi Inui
Shinji Yoshikawa

Department of Experimental Radiology and Health Physics
Fukui Medical University, School of Medicine
Fukui 910-11, Japan

Masayo Furukawa

Department of Anatomy
School of Medicine, Osaka City University
Osaka 545, Japan

I. Introduction

The anoxic cell compartment of *in vivo* solid tumors limits to some extent the effects of therapeutic radiation (Gray *et al.*, 1953). The development of anoxic-cell radiosensitizers, as represented by the imidazole derivatives, has been given considerable attention (Adams and Cooke, 1969). Hyperbaric oxygen was also considered for this purpose. Misonidazole, one of the imidazole derivatives, has a radiosensitization effect on anoxic cell killing. However, clinical application was not feasible because the drug proved to be toxic to the central nervous system. The extent of neurotoxicity of the imidazole derivatives correlates with the lipophilicity of the drugs (Brown and Workman, 1980). If the hydrophilicity of the drug could be increased to the extent that the toxicity to the central nervous system would be diminished, then the effect of anoxic-cell radiosensitization of the drug in unit drug amount/body weight or body surface could be maintained.

We assayed a series of compounds, *o*-, *m*-, and *p*-nitrophenyl-tetrazoles, for their possible anoxic-cell radiosensitization effects. The differential effects were observed among the three isomers by cell survival assays in colony formations of Chinese hamster V-79 strain of cells, *in vitro*.

II. Materials and Methods

In order to assess the effect of drugs on cell survival after irradiation, colony-forming assays *in vitro* and murine lethal toxicity assay *in vivo* were carried out.

A. *In Vitro* Assays

1. *Cells*

Chinese hamster V-79 cells were colonially cloned and used throughout the present series of experiments. Cells were cultured stationarily in a CO_2 incubator.

2. *Culture Media*

The cells were maintained in growth medium MLN-15, 1 liter of which contained 730 ml of Eagle's MEM, 20 ml of 2.5 w/v% lactalbumin hydrolysate solution (Difco Laboratories, Detroit, Michigan), 100 ml of NCTC 135 solution (Difco), 150 ml of inactivated bovine serum, and antibiotics. Numerals following the abbreviation MLN- represent the serum volume percentages.

3. *Drugs*

The *o*-, *m*-, and *p*-nitrophenyltetrazoles, with a molecular weight of 191, were synthesized by the authors using a procedure developed by

Herbst *et al.* (1952). The structural formulas for the three isomers are shown here.

o-Nitrophenyltetrazole   *m*-Nitrophenyltetrazole   *p*-Nitrophenyltetrazole

Half-wave reduction potentials of the three isomers and misonidazole, in 500 μM and at pH values ranging from 7.11 to 7.35, were measured with a polarograph, Shimadzu RP-2 versus saturated calomel electrode (SCE), instead of the one-electron reduction potentials, E_7^1 (Table I).

Cells were treated with the drugs in the final concentration of 5 mM in MEM, for graded periods.

4. X-Ray Generator, Dosimeter, and Their Conditions

Physical parameters of X irradiation by a generator, Model KXC-17 Toshiba, were 140 kVp, 5 mA, 2-mm Al filter, at an exposure rate of 0.3 Gy/min, measured by a Radocon II dosimeter, Model 555 of Victoreen.

5. Anoxic Chamber System

The principle of the anoxic chamber system is schematically illustrated in Fig. 1. Medium in the culture plate (1), on which cells had been attached, was siphoned off, and the culture plate was placed in the chamber (2). The chamber was closed airtightly. Nitrogen gas, which was humidified to saturation by being blown into water in an airtight flask (5), was passed into this chamber for graded periods and at graded flow rates. The graded amounts of drug solution from the reservoir (6), into which N$_2$ gas humidified to saturation had been passed, were measured by syringe (4) and poured onto the plate (1). The N$_2$ gas was allowed to flow for graded periods and at graded flow rates. Thereafter, all the connection ducts and a valve (3) were tightly closed. The thus deoxygenated chamber was disconnected from the entire anoxic chamber unit. The isolated chamber containing the plate was irradiated with graded doses of X rays. To measure the dose rate of X rays in the chamber, a Radocon sensor was inserted into the chamber through a hole on the side wall of the chamber. The hole was closed airtightly except when the dose of X rays was being measured intracellularly.

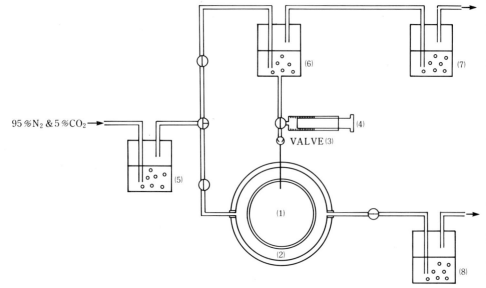

Fig. 1. Schematic illustration of the anoxic chamber system. Cells adhering to the culture plate (1) were refed with 3 ml MEM prior to the deoxygenation and the succeeding X irradiation. The culture plate(s) was placed in the chamber (2). The chamber was closed airtightly, and N_2 gas humidified to saturation (5) was allowed to flow into the chamber (2). Deoxygenated drug solution (6) was measured by syringe (4) and poured onto the cells (1). Nitrogen gas was further allowed to flow prior to X irradiation. The container was disconnected by the tight closing of a valve (3) and ducts. The isolated chamber containing culture plate(s) with cells was then exposed to X rays. The N_2 gas was exhausted through cups (7 and 8).

6. Culture Conditions

1. The cells were seeded in appropriate numbers per plastic plate to yield the pertinent number of colonies, as the surviving fractions. About 100 surviving colonies for the plate, 6 cm in diameter, were suitable for colony formation in the present culture system.

2. The plates were incubated overnight in water-saturated air with 5% CO_2 at 37°C by CO_2 incubator, prior to the X irradiation.

3. The control cell growth was monitored before and during the experiments on the successive day to that of the cell seeding.

4. After the various treatments, the cells attached to the plates were rinsed with MEM-0, fed with 6 ml of fresh MLN-15 per plate, and incubated for colony formation of the surviving cells.

7. *Experimental Procedures*

After an overnight incubation, medium on the plates was siphoned off. The plates were exposed to N_2 gas humidified to saturation, supplemented with 5% (v/v) of CO_2 gas, for 10 min at the flow rate of 1000 ml/min; then 3 ml of the deoxygenated drug solutions were added and the humidified N_2 and CO_2 gas mixture allowed to flow for another 30 min at the flow rate of 1000 ml/min. To the control plates were added 3 ml of MEM and incubation carried out in air humidified to saturation with 5% (v/v) of CO_2 gas for 40 min.

The pretreated and control groups of plates were then X irradiated.

8. *Survival Criterion*

After the final treatments, the cells on the plates were incubated for 6 to 8 days to obtain colonies of a macroscopic size and composed of 50 cells or more. The colonies were stained with methylene blue solution for half an hour at 37°C, and the number of colonies per plate was counted. The uncorrected cell surviving fraction from each treatment was routinely estimated as the ratio, the mean number of colonies formed per plate divided by the number of inoculated cells per plate. The estimated fractions were then corrected for the surviving fraction of the untreated control, plating efficiency. Three or more replicate plates were used for each survival point in an experiment, and the replicate experiments were done two to four times, depending on the consistency of the results obtained. The multiplicity of the cells was estimated during the experiments, which was just a little more than unity.

B. *In Vivo* Assays

1. *Mice*

The conventional male ICR/JCC mice 8 weeks of age were fed in isolated cages.

2. *Drugs*

p-Nitrophenyltetrazole was dissolved in 1 *N* NaOH, and the solution was neutralized with 0.1 *N* $NaHCO_3$ to a final concentration of 5 mg/ml and given ip, in graded doses ranging from 200 to 1200 mg/kg body weight.

3. *Experimental Procedures*

These so-treated mice were observed for 30 days, and histology-related autopsies were done on mice that died.

III. Results

The half-wave reduction potentials of the three isomers (*o*-, *m*-, and *p*-nitrophenyltetrazole) and misonidazole are shown in Table I.

A. Anoxic-Cell Radiosensitization Effects of *o*-, *m*-, and *p*-Nitrophenyltetrazoles *in Vitro*

Chinese hamster V-79 cells in plastic plates, from which culture medium had been siphoned off beforehand, were deoxygenated for 10 min. One of the three isomers in 5 mM in deoxygenated MEM was poured onto the plates and further deoxygenated for 30 min prior to the X irradiation with graded doses. After the X irradiation, the plates were oxygenated in air, and the medium containing the drug was siphoned off. The plates were then rinsed and incubated for colony formation. As shown in Fig. 2, the radiosensitization effect was observed in the form of steepening of the slopes on the exponentially regressing areas of the dose–survival curves. The slope of *p*-nitrophenyltetrazole under the deoxygenated conditions was parallel to that of the untreated control under aerated conditions.

Parameters of the survival curves are tabulated in Table II. All three isomers showed anoxic-cell radiosensitization effects with enhancement ratios in D_0 values ranging between 1.91 and 2.41. Among the three iso-

TABLE I

Half-Wave Reduction Potentials of Tetrazoles

Drugs	Concentration (μM)	pH	HWRP vs. SCE[a] (mV)
o-Nitrophenyltetrazole	500	7.32	480
m-Nitrophenyltetrazole	500	7.31	432
p-Nitrophenyltetrazole	500	7.11	450
Misonidazole	500	7.35	352

[a] Half-wave reduction potentials versus saturated calomel electrode by polarography. See text.

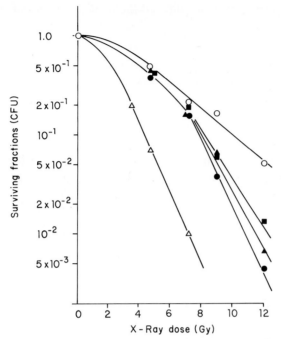

Fig. 2. Radiation dose–survival curves of V-79 cells in air and N_2 gas. CFU, colony-forming units. ($\triangle$) Control in air. ($\bigcirc$) Control in N_2. ($\blacksquare$) o-Nitrophenyltetrazole. ($\blacktriangle$) m-Nitrophenyltetrazole. ($\bullet$) p-Nitrophenyltetrazole.

TABLE II

Anoxic-Cell Radiosensitizing Effects of Nitrophenyltetrazoles[a]

Atmosphere	Drug	D_0 (Gy)	D_q (Gy)	Enhancement ratio (D_0)
Air	None	1.25	1.60	—
N_2	None	3.25	2.45	—
N_2	o-Nitrophenyltetrazole	1.70	4.10	1.91
N_2	m-Nitrophenyltetrazole	1.60	4.50	2.03
N_2	p-Nitrophenyltetrazole	1.35	4.85	2.41

[a] Cells were treated for 30 min under aerated and deoxygenated conditions. Enhancement ratios in D_0 were calculated in a D_0 of the deoxygenated, without drug treatment, divided by D_0 of the deoxygenated, with drug treatment.

mers, *p*-nitrophenyltetrazole showed the highest enhancement ratio in a D_0 of 2.41.

B. Toxicity of *p*-Nitrophenyltetrazole to Aerated and Deoxygenated Cells *in Vitro*

We determined the acute lethal cytotoxicity of *p*-nitrophenyltetrazole, which showed the highest enhancement ratio. Deoxygenated and aerated cells were treated with this drug in 5 m*M* concentration for graded periods, and the treatment time–survival relationships are shown in Fig. 3. Lethal cytotoxicities differed between aerated and deoxygenated cells. The survival curves of the cells showed exponential regressions with the treatment periods. Slopes of the curves for aerated and deoxygenated cells were 324 and 138 min, respectively. *p*-Nitrophenyltetrazole had a more lethal cytotoxicity on the deoxygenated cells.

C. Acute Lethal Toxicity of *p*-Nitrophenyltetrazole in ICR/JCC Male Mice

All the mice given this drug in doses below 500 mg/kg body weight survived for the 30-day observation period. Some mice treated with over 500 mg/kg body weight died; thus the LD_{50} for murine acute death seemed to be about 600 mg/kg. Autopsy revealed that the liver and kidney were most sensitive to this drug. Livers of the acutely dying mice and kidneys of the survivors revealed evidence of degeneration (Table III).

IV. Discussion

Misonidazole, a derivative of imidazoles that has a high lipophilicity and therefore a high partition coefficient, is toxic to the central nervous system.

Brown *et al.* (Brown and Workman, 1980, Brown et al., 1982) screened a series of 2-nitroimidazoles with a variety of side chains at the 1 position for partition coefficient, E_7^1, acute LD_{50}, and an anoxic-cell radiosensitization effect. Among the derivatives obtained, SR-2508 (1-$CH_2CONHCH_2CH_2OH$-2-nitroimidazole), of low partition coefficient, low brain : plasma drug concentration ratio, and high tumor : plasma drug concentration ratio, showed a high anoxic-cell radiosensitization effect.

Adams *et al.* (1980) synthesized a series of 1- or 5-substituted 2-nitroimidazoles and determined the chemical properties and anoxic-cell ra-

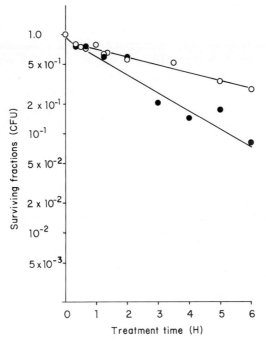

Fig. 3. Treatment time–survival curves of V-79 cells. (○) Aerated cell with *p*-Nitrophenyltetrazole. (●) Deoxygenated cell with *p*-Nitrophenyltetrazole.

TABLE III

Acute Lethal Toxicity of
p-Nitrophenyltetrazole in Mice[a]

Dose amount (mg/kg body weight)	Survivors	
	Ratio	%
0	5/5	100
200	4/4	100
250	4/4	100
300	10/10	100
350	5/5	100
400	10/10	100
450	1/1	(100)[b]
500	6/6	100
600	4/5	80
700	2/5	40
1000	4/5	80
1200	0/1	(0)[b]

[a] See text for experimental details (Section II,B) and conclusions (Section III,C).
[b] Figures in parentheses indicate that only one mouse was treated with this dose of the drug.

diosensitization effects. They concluded that the radiosensitization efficacy was greater than that which would be predicted on the basis of reduction potential achieved with nitroimidazoles substituted with a group carrying basic functions. The anoxic-cell radiosensitization effects of 5-sulfonyl-4-nitro-imidazoles (Adams *et al.*, 1981) were superior to those of nitro compounds previously assayed by these same investigators (Adams *et al.*, 1979).

We determined the chemical properties of *o*-, *m*-, and *p*-nitrophenyltetrazoles and observed the anoxic-cell radiosensitization effects of these compounds. Among the three isomers, *p*-nitrophenyltetrazole was the most effective, as represented in the slope D_0, on the radiation dose–survival curve of deoxygenated V-79 cells. The acute toxicity of $LD_{50/30}$ days in mice occurred in a dose of 600 mg/kg. The present drug concentration *in vitro* was 5 mM (i.e., 955 mg/liter medium). This means that the initial drug concentration in the serum was higher *in vivo* than *in vitro*. Some of the tetrazole derivatives may prove to be effective anoxic-cell radiosensitizers.

References

Adams, G. E., and Cooke, M. S. (1969). Electron-affinic sensitization. I. A structural basis for chemical radiosensitizers in bacteria. *Int. J. Radiat. Biol.* **15,** 457–471.

Adams, G. E., Clarke, E. D., Flockhart, I. R., Jacobs, R. S., Seimi, D. S., Stratford, I. J., Wardman, P., and Watts, M. E. (1979). Structure-activity relationships in the development of hypoxic cell radiosensitizers. I. Sensitization efficiency. *Int. J. Radiat. Biol.* **35,** 133–150.

Adams, G. E., Ahmed, I., Clarke, E. D., O'Neill, P., Parrick, J., Stratford, I. J., Wallace, R. G., Wardman, P., and Watts, M. E. (1980). Structure-activity relationships in the development of hypoxic cell radiosensitizers. III. Effects of basic substituents in nitroimidazole sidechains. *Int. J. Radiat. Biol.* **38,** 613–626.

Adams, G. E., Fielden, E. M., Hardy, C., Millar, B. C., Stratford, I. J., and Williamson, C. (1981). Radiosensitization of hypoxic mammalian cells *in vitro* by some 5-substituted-4-nitroimidazoles. *Int. J. Radiat. Biol.* **40,** 153–161.

Brown, D. M., Parker, E., and Brown, J. M. (1982). Structure-activity relationships of 1-substituted 2-nitroimidazoles: effect of partition coefficient and side-chain hydroxyl groups on radiosensitization *in vitro*. *Radiat. Res.* **90,** 98–108.

Brown, J. M., and Workman, P. (1980). Partition coefficient as a guide to the development of radiosensitizers which are less toxic than misonidazole. *Radiat. Res.* **82,** 171–190.

Gray, L. H., Conger, A. D., Ebert, M., Hornsey, S., and Scott, O. C. A. (1953). The concentration of oxygen dissolved in tissues at the time of irradiation as a factor in radiotherapy. *Br. J. Radiol.* **26,** 638–648.

Herbst, R. M., Roberts, C. W., Givens, H. F., and Harvill, E. K. (1952). The synthesis of nitro- and amino-phenyltetrazoles. *J. Org. Chem.* **17,** 262–271.

10 Electron-Affinic Agents: Development of the Optimum Radiosensitizer and Chemosensitizer for Clinical Application

J. Martin Brown

Division of Radiobiology Research
Department of Radiology
Stanford University School of Medicine
Stanford, California

I. Are Hypoxic Cells Important in Radiotherapy?

Since the early 1920s it has been known that tissues irradiated in the absence of oxygen are 2.5 to 3.0 times more resistant to the damaging effects of ionizing radiation. The possibility that this might present a problem in radiotherapy was soon appreciated (Crabtree and Cramer, 1933), but it was not until the pioneering work of Gray and colleagues

(Gray *et al.*, 1953; Thomlinson and Gray, 1955) that this problem was considered to involve serious limitations in the cure rates in radiotherapy. Thomlinson and Gray (1955) showed that the histological structure of human bronchogenic carcinoma fitted a model in which necrosis occurred as a result of the utilization of oxygen through respiring tumor tissue. Specifically, they showed that the distance from the blood vessels in the normal tissue stroma to necrosis in the tumor tissue was typically 100–150 μm, through the healthy tumor tissue. They suggested that viable hypoxic tumor cells might be present in a thin rim around the necrotic areas, that is, at a distance of 100 to 150 μm from the blood vessels. This is the classic model of hypoxia in tumors and is illustrated in Fig. 1. These hypoxic cells have been termed *chronically hypoxic cells* to distinguish them from cells made hypoxic (*acutely hypoxic cells*) by a mechanism involving the temporary occlusion of a blood vessel or momentary slowing of blood flow in such a vessel (Brown, 1979; Sutherland and Franko, 1980).

However likely these models are, they do not demonstrate the presence of viable, radiobiologically resistant hypoxic cells in tumors. One of the most common ways of doing this is to obtain a survival curve of the tumor cells irradiated *in situ,* under normal air-breathing conditions. The presence of hypoxic cells in the tumor is demonstrated by the finding that the

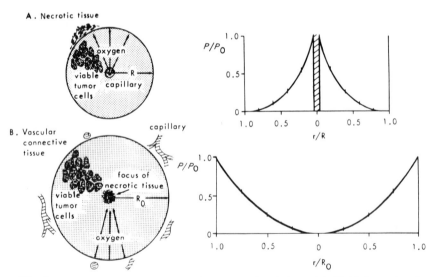

Fig. 1. The classical model of hypoxia in tumors (chronic hypoxia). Viable hypoxic cells are assumed to result from limitation of diffusion of oxygen through respiring tissue and are often adjacent to necrotic areas. The oxygen diffusion can be outward from an isolated capillary (A) or inward from blood vessels at the periphery of a cylinder of tumor cells (B). From Tannock (1972) by permission of the author and publisher. For detailed definitions of P/P_0, r/R, and r/R_0, see Tannock (1972).

resistant portion of the survival curve of the cells from tumors irradiated in air-breathing animals is parallel to that obtained from the cells in tumors irradiated when all of the cells have been made artificially anoxic. This curve of 100% hypoxic cells can be easily obtained by clamping the tumor or killing the animal prior to irradiation. The proportion of hypoxic cells in the tumor can be calculated from the distance between the two parallel lines. Actual survival curves have been obtained for different animal tumors, and almost all have shown the presence of hypoxic cells, as demonstrated by the parallel nature of the survival curves obtained from tumors in air-breathing mice and tumors in dead mice. Figure 2 shows six such examples taken from a review by Tannock (1972).

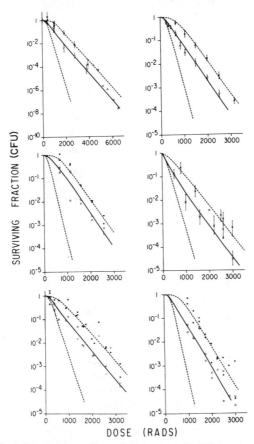

Fig. 2. Published data on the cell survival curves of solid tumors. (○) Results from animals breathing air. (●) Irradiation under hypoxic conditions. (----) Response of fully hypoxic and fully aerobic cells. (○——○) Assumed values for the proportion of well-oxygenated cells and D_0 and n values. From Tannock (1972) by permission of the author and publisher. See Tannock (1972) for the original references.

The question of whether human tumors also contain hypoxic cells cannot be answered as directly. However, evidence for the presence of hypoxic cells in human tumors was obtained from trials using hyperbaric oxygen (HBO) with radiotherapy. Table I shows the results of one such trial, a cooperative study by the British Medical Research Council (MRC), in which stage III carcinoma of the cervix was treated using conventional fractionated radiotherapy, with or without hyperbaric oxygen. Two points are worthy of note. First, with treatments in air, 6 fractions are clearly inferior to conventional daily treatments of 25 to 30 fractions. Second, treatment of tumors with HBO increases the local control rate and 5-year survival of the patients—dramatically so for the 6-fraction treatments but also for the conventional daily treatments. It should be noted, however, that there was an increased morbidity rate for the HBO treatments, so it cannot be concluded that use of HBO increased the therapeutic ratio. However, two important conclusions can be drawn: (1) Hypoxic cells are present and limit the control rate of these tumors, even in conventional daily fractionation; and (2) the use of the hypoxic-cell sensitizer, oxygen, dramatically increases 5-year survival when less than an optimum regimen (6 fractions) is used. This could be extremely important when using chemical hypoxic-cell sensitizers in situations where treatment involves only a few doses of radiation.

However, high-pressure oxygen is expensive and difficult to use. What is needed is a chemical sensitizer that acts in the same way as oxygen but can reach the hypoxic tumor cells and sensitize them to radiation. In 1974, such a group of chemicals, the *nitroimidazoles*, was discovered by Adams and co-workers (Asquith *et al.*, 1974). Misonidazole (MIS) is the best

TABLE I

MRC Hyperbaric Oxygen Trial, Carcinoma of the Cervix Uteri: Stage III[a]

	HBO (%)	Air (%)	Comments
5-year survival			
6 Fractions Portsmouth (37 pts)	42	17	In air, results
6 Fractions Oxford (23 pts)	46	8	were poor
25 Fractions Glasgow (127 pts)	50	37	Combined
30 Fractions Mt Vernon (56 pts)	39	28	$p < .05$
Local control 5 years			
Glasgow	87	60	Highly significant
Mt. Vernon	76	50	differences
Severe morbidity			
Bowel	12	4	

[a] Data extracted from Watson *et al.* (1978).

known of these radiosensitizers, and it is a highly effective radiosensitizer of a wide spectrum of animal tumors (Denekamp et al., 1980). It also appears to be active against human malignancies (Thomlinson et al., 1976; Ash et al., 1979). It is clear, however, that the neurological side effects of MIS are severe, thus limiting the drug levels and hence the degree of radiosensitization that can be achieved (Dische et al., 1977; Urtasun et al., 1978; Wasserman et al., 1979). In fact, with conventional daily fractionation, the doses of MIS are limited to the extent that tumor concentrations of the drug at the time of radiation are only approximately 20 μg/g. Such a concentration would be expected to increase the radiosensitivity of hypoxic tumor cells by only a factor of 1.1 to 1.3. This is unlikely to result in a detectable increase in local control rate, considering that reoxygenation will probably occur between radiation fractions (Kallman, 1972). It would be ideal to have a radiosensitizer that could be used with each fraction in a conventional radiotherapy regimen, at a concentration that gave an enhancement ratio for the hypoxic cells of 2.5 or greater. Such a drug would either be approximately 10 times less neurotoxic than MIS with the same radiosensitizing efficiency (so that an approximately 10 times larger dose could be delivered) or have a 10 times greater radiosensitizing efficiency with the same toxicity as MIS.

In 1978, an extensive program was designed to look for ways of achieving this 10-fold gain over MIS. Four specific possibilities were given attention (Section II).

II.   Improvement on Misonidazole

A.   A More Effective Radiosensitizer of Comparable Toxicity

The finding that electron affinity is an excellent predictor for radiosensitizing efficiency (Adams et al., 1979) has enabled synthesis of compounds with a greater radiosensitizing efficacy than MIS, on a rational basis. One promising series of compounds are the 5-substituted methyl-2-nitroimidazoles, which are more electron affinic than MIS because of the presence of electron-attracting substituents at the 5 position in the nitroimidazole ring. Methods of testing these compounds involve in vitro and in vivo radiosensitizing experiments using Chinese hamster ovary (CHO) cells in vitro and EMT-6 tumors in vivo, assessment of tumor and plasma drug levels using reverse-phase high-performance liquid chromatography (HPLC), and toxicity testing. All of the assays involved and procedures used have been described in detail elsewhere (Brown *et al.*, 1981).

Figure 3 shows data on the enhancement ratio as a function of drug concentration of two of these compounds, SR-2537 and SR-2553, which are more electron affinic than MIS. As expected from their higher electron affinity, each of these compounds is a more effective radiosensitizer than MIS by a factor of approximately 10. In other words, the same degree of radiosensitization is achieved with a 10-fold lower concentration than with MIS. Because each of these two compounds had an acute LD_{50} in mice, and this was comparable to that of MIS (5–10 mmol/kg), it would appear that both would be strong candidates as radiosensitizers superior to MIS.

We thus compared the radiosensitization produced in EMT-6 tumors irradiated *in vivo* with a fixed dose of 1750 rads given at varying times after either ip or iv administrations of 2 mmol/kg SR-2537 or SR-2553. In each experiment we also ran comparable groups given the same molar dose of MIS. The results obtained from this experiment were disappointing: Far from showing a more effective radiosensitization than MIS, each compound showed significantly less radiosensitization of the hypoxic cells in the tumor. However, we also found that tumor concentrations of these drugs were considerably lower than those obtained with MIS, and also that the elimination half-lives were very short (Brown *et al.*, 1982a).

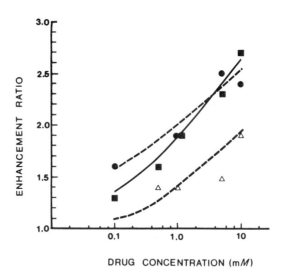

Fig. 3. Sensitizer enhancement ratio as a function of drug concentration after a 1-h exposure of the drugs to hypoxic HA-1 cells at 22°C. (●) SR-2537 ($E_{1/2} = -0.25$), (■) SR-2553 ($E_{1/2} = -0.23$), (△) MIS ($E_{1/2} = -0.35$).

In order to overcome this perceived problem of low tumor concentrations (probably caused by the rapid elimination of these compounds), multiple iv administrations of the drugs were given. Mice of the BALB/c strain bearing intradermal EMT-6 tumors were given an initial iv administration of 1 mmol/kg with subsequent injections of 0.5 mmol/kg every 10 min. Misonidazole (1 mmol/kg ip) was injected initially, with additional injections of 0.5 mmol/kg every 30 min. As can be seen from Fig. 4, these schedules were successful in maintaining tumor concentrations of SR-2537 and MIS of approximately 0.5 mM. However, even under these conditions (Fig. 4B) SR-2537 was inferior to MIS, despite achieving equal tumor concentrations. This is precisely the reverse of the situation *in vitro* (Fig. 3), in which SR-2537 was significantly more effective than MIS in

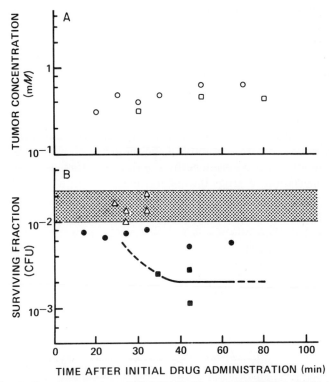

Fig. 4. (A) The concentration of SR-2537 (● ○) and MIS (■ □) in EMT-6 tumors at various times after multiple injections of each drug. (B) The surviving fraction of the cells in EMT-6 tumors after a dose of 1750 rads given to the tumor at different times after the initial injection of 1 mmol/kg of either SR-2537 or MIS. The shaded area shows the range of surviving fraction for saline-injected mice (△) also irradiated with 1750 rads. From Brown *et al*. (1982a).

radiosensitizing hypoxic cells. We obtained similar disappointing results with several other compounds with radiosensitizing effect 5 to 10 times greater than that of MIS *in vitro*.

It would thus appear that 2-nitroimidazoles of 5 to 10 times greater radiosensitizing efficacy than MIS (because of their increased electron affinity) are not able to radiosensitize hypoxic cells as well as does MIS *in vivo*. The reasons for this poor sensitization are not yet clear but presumably are the result of an inability of these drugs to reach the hypoxic regions of tumors and subsequently diffuse intact across the cell membrane into these hypoxic cells. This could be attributable to an increased reactivity of these compounds because of their higher electron affinity. Thus there was no improvement on the radiosensitizing ability of MIS by the required factor of 5 to 10 simply by changing the electron affinity of the 2-nitroimidazole ring.

B. A Less Toxic Radiosensitizer of Comparable Radiosensitizing Efficiency

Figure 5 shows the rationale used to develop a compound of lower toxicity but equal radiosensitizing efficiency to MIS. From the work of Adams *et al.* (1979) it is known that the extent of radiosensitization is dependent on the electron affinity of the molecule. For nitroimidazoles, the electron affinity is determined by the ring structure. It is also known that the penetration of drugs into neural tissues (i.e., across the blood–brain and blood–nerve barriers) depends on their lipid solubility or *li-*

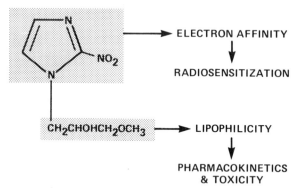

Fig. 5. The structural formula of MIS showing that the nitroimidazole ring largely determines the electron affinity of the molecule, whereas the aliphatic side chain at the 1 position primarily governs its lipophilicity.

pophilicity (Soloway *et al.*, 1960; Binns, 1964). This lipophilicity is largely governed by aliphatic side chain at the 1 position of the ring. In addition to affecting the penetration of drugs into neural tissues, however, lipophilicity also governs other aspects of the pharmacokinetics, in particular the elimination half-life of the drugs from the plasma. This suggests a second way in which toxicity could be reduced without affecting the degree of radiosensitization. Because the extent of radiosensitization depends only on concentration of the drug in the hypoxic cells at the time of radiation— whereas the toxicity is likely to be a function of the area under the curve of drug concentration versus time (Mellet, 1974)—it follows that a drug with a shorter plasma half-life could be less toxic than one with a longer half-life without being a less efficient radiosensitizer.

Studies were done under the working hypothesis that neurotoxicity may be a function of lipophilicity, and a range of 2-nitroimidazoles of similar electron affinity but differing in lipophilicity (measured by the octanol–water partition coefficient P), by a factor of 100 were synthesized. For each of these compounds, plasma, tumor, and brain levels were assessed in mice and in dogs, after a single injection. Figure 6 shows

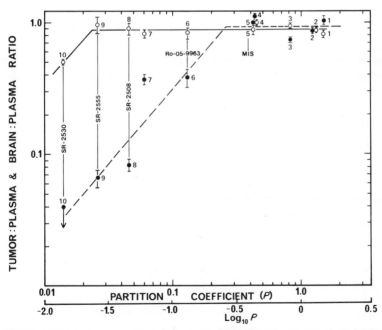

Fig. 6. The mean values (± 1 SE) of the tumor : plasma ratio ($\bigcirc$) and the brain : plasma ratio ($\bullet$) for a series of ten 2-nitroimidazoles of similar electron affinity. [Brown and Workman (1980).

the results of this study in mice. Similar results have been obtained in dogs (White *et al.*, 1980).

It can be seen from Fig. 6 that the tumor : plasma ratio is largely independent of the partition coefficient over almost the entire range studied from P values of 0.026 to 1.5. However, the brain : plasma ratio showed a marked dependency on lipophilicity at partition coefficients below approximately 0.4. These results suggest that compounds of low lipophilicity might be less neurotoxic than MIS.

With regard to the ability of these 2-nitroimidazoles to sensitize hypoxic cells, tests were done both with tumors *in vivo* and with hypoxic cells *in vitro*. For the EMT-6 tumor transplanted intradermally in BALB/c mice, all the compounds with a partition coefficient of 0.04 and higher gave equivalent levels of radiosensitization. However, below partition coefficients of 0.04 there is clearly less radiosensitization for equimolar injected doses. This is shown, for example, by the comparison between the 2-nitroimidazole amide SR-2508 (side chain = $CH_2CONHCH_2$-CH_2OH; $P = 0.046$) and the similar 2-nitroimidazole SR-2555 [side chain = $CH_2CON(CH_2CH_2OH)_2$; $P = 0.026$]. Figure 7 shows the results of this comparison for equimolar injected doses. Even though both drugs given iv showed similar peak tumor levels and similar half-lives, the extent of radiosensitization produced by SR-2555 was less than that produced by SR-2508. In other experiments, the extent of radiosensitization produced by MIS and SR-2508 was the same (Brown *et al.*, 1981). The results obtained with hypoxic CHO cells *in vitro* were similar. All compounds with partition coefficients of 0.04 and above showed the same extent of radiosensitization, whereas when the partition coefficient falls below this level, the compounds become increasingly inactive as radiosensitizers *in vitro* (Brown *et al.*, 1982b). This shows that the loss of radiosensitization *in vivo* for the compounds of low lipophilicity is not due to their ability to diffuse through the tumor to the hypoxic cells but rather to their inability to penetrate these hypoxic cells. This idea was recently confirmed by measuring the intracellular concentrations of 2-nitroimidazoles, as a function of their lipophilicity (Brown *et al.*, 1983).

The neurotoxicity of a selected number of these compounds was also studied using performance on an accelerating rotarod as a measure of neurotoxicity. Table II shows the results of drug toxicity testing for the four 2-nitroimidazoles MIS, desmethylmisonidazole (DESMIS), SR-2508, and SR-2555. It can be seen that as the partition coefficient is reduced, the toxicity of the compounds is also reduced both in acute toxicity to a single dose and in the neurotoxicity following repeated daily injections, as determined by the rotarod technique. From these data, the relative toxicities (on a molar basis) of MIS, DESMIS, SR-2508, and SR-2555 are

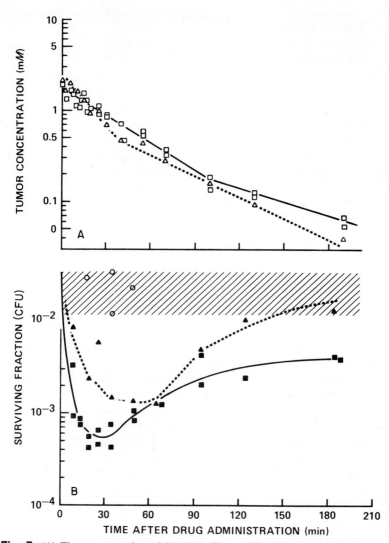

Fig. 7. (A) The concentration of SR-2508 (□) and SR-2555 (△) in EMT-6 tumors at various times after an iv administration of 2 mmol/kg of each drug. (B) The surviving fraction of the cells of the same EMT-6 tumors as in (A) after a radiation dose of 20 Gy given at different times after an iv administration of 2 mmol/kg of either SR-2508 (■) or SR-2555 (▲). (○) Saline controls. From Brown *et al.* (1981).

TABLE II

Comparative Toxicities of Four 2-Nitroimidazoles to BALB/c Mice[a]

Compound	P^b	Acute $LD_{50/2d}$ (with 95% C.L.)		Daily dose to give neuropathy[c]	
		mg/g	mmol/kg	mg/g	mmol/kg
MIS	0.43	1.7 (1.5–1.9)	8.5 (7.5–9.5)	0.6	3.0
DESMIS	0.13	3.4 (3.2–3.6)	18.2 (16.9–19.3)	1.3	7.0
SR-2508	0.046	4.9 (4.3–5.6)	22.9 (20.1–25.7)	>2.0	>9.3
SR-2555	0.026	8.9 (7.9–10.0)	34.5 (30.6–38.4)	>3.0	>11.6

[a] From Brown et al. (1981).

[b] The octanol–water partition coefficient.

[c] Defined as 50% reduction in rotarod retention time 4–5 weeks after the start of daily (5 days/week) drug injections.

$1:2.3:>3.1:>3.9$ for the neurotoxicity assay. Conroy et al. (1982) also compared these four drugs using the same assay as well as one based on ototoxicity. They obtained similar results for both assays with the ratios of doses to give equivalent toxicities of $1:1.8:5:10$ for MIS, DESMIS, SR-2508, and SR-2555, respectively.

All the data on the radiosensitizing effectiveness and on the neurotoxicity (as judged both by peripheral nerve concentration in the dog and on the rotarod assay in the mouse) were pooled to produce the overall "therapeutic index" shown in Fig. 8. It can be seen that SR-2508 is close to the ideal compound for 2-nitroimidazoles with electron affinity similar to MIS, and phase I clinical testing of this compound is now underway in the United States. From these mouse and dog experiments, the tumor concentrations of SR-2508 of at least 7–8 times those for MIS will be achievable clinically, with the same degree of neurotoxicity. Using the toxicity data of Conroy et al. (1982), this value becomes approximately 10. Early results of the clinical phase I testing have confirmed that SR-2508 is less toxic than MIS.

C. Enhancement of the Efficacy but Not the Toxicity of MIS by Removal of Competing SH

The rationale for this possibility is shown in Fig. 9, which illustrates the oxygen-fixation hypothesis developed by Alper (1956) and Howard-Flanders (1960) to explain the oxygen effect, and its later extension by Willson

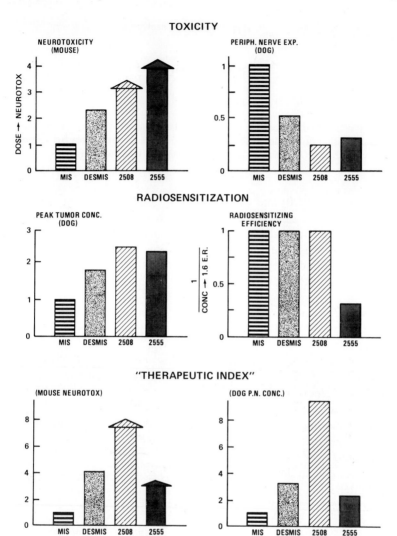

Fig. 8. The derivation of a "therapeutic index" for three 2-nitroimidazoles that are less lipophilic than MIS (cf. MIS = 1). This index is based on two estimates of drug toxicity: the rotarod assay in mice and the peripheral nerve concentrations in dogs (White *et al.*, 1980). It is also based on the peak tumor concentration of each drug after an equimolar iv injection in dogs (White *et al.*, 1980) and on the radiosensitizing efficiency of each drug for hypoxic cells *in vitro* (Brown *et al.*, 1982b). These are multiplied together in the appropriate way to give the "therapeutic index," which is essentially the equivalent tumor concentration of MIS, for each of the drugs, to produce the same level of neurotoxicity as MIS.

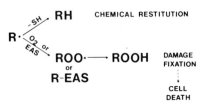

Fig. 9. Illustration of the oxygen-fixation hypothesis, showing the competition between chemical restitution of the target (DNA) radical R· by H donation from SH and damage fixation by binding of O_2 or an electron-affinic sensitizer (EAS) to the radical.

and Emmerson (1970) and Chapman *et al.* (1973) to include the mechanism for the sensitization of hypoxic cells by electron-affinic sensitizers. Although there is still debate that the damage-fixation hypothesis is the mechanism of sensitization by electron-affinic agents (Adams and Jameson, 1980), the finding that the predictions of this hypothesis were borne out in the present case is at least partial support for the validity of the hypothesis.

The prediction of the model shown in Fig. 9 of relevance in the present situation is that because chemical restitution and damage fixation are competitive processes, the rates of each will be modifiable by changing the concentrations of the restituting or fixing species. Thus, it is likely that there will be a greater radiosensitization of hypoxic cells by a given concentration of electron-affinic sensitizer (EAS) if the endogenous concentration of hydrogen-donating SH compounds is reduced. The principal hydrogen-donating species in the cell are the non-protein-bound sulfhydryls, of which the tripeptide glutathione (GSH) constitutes more than 95%, in most species of mammalian cells.

Use was made of diethyl maleate (DEM), which is a specific depleter of intracellular GSH at nontoxic concentrations. Concentrations of diethyl maleate can be used that deplete intracellular GSH levels to less than 1% of control values without producing any cellular toxicity (Bump *et al.*, 1982a). Figure 10 shows data on CHO cells treated for 1 h under aerobic conditions with various concentrations of diethyl maleate prior to irradiation, under either hypoxic or aerobic conditions. It can be seen that GSH depletion produced a dose-modifying sensitization of the hypoxic cells without altering radiosensitivity of the aerobic cells. This is as would be expected from the competitive reaction of the oxygen-fixation hypothesis shown in Fig. 9. There is a residual oxygen-enhancement ratio of approximately 1.5 at GSH levels of less than 1%; thus there may be other hydrogen-donating species in the cell in addition to GSH or the competitive oxygen-fixation hypothesis cannot account for the entire oxygen effect.

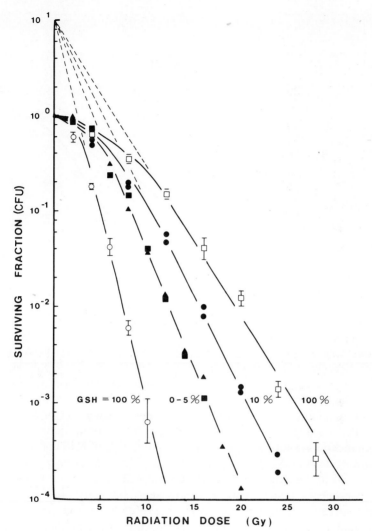

Fig. 10. Cell survival curves of CHO cells (Toronto line) irradiated in suspension with various doses of X ray with or without a 1-h pretreatment of the cells with various concentrations of DEM. The measured GSH levels as a percentage of control levels are shown. Not shown are the DEM-pretreated air controls, which showed no radiosensitization; that is, they fall on the GSH = 100% air control. ($\bigcirc$) Air control, GSH = 100%. ($\square$) N_2 Control, GSH = 100%. ($\bullet$) N_2, 7×10^{-5} M DEM, GSH = 10%. ($\blacktriangle$) N_2, 2×10^{-4} M DEM, GSH = 1–5%. ($\blacksquare$) N_2, 1×10^{-3} M DEM, GSH = 0% (Y. C. Taylor, unpublished).

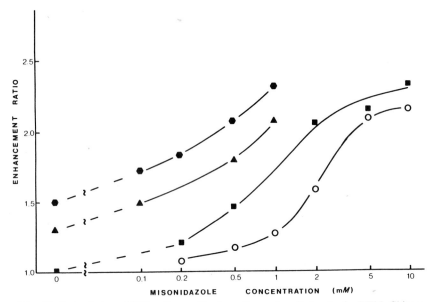

Fig. 11. Potentiation of MIS radiosensitization of hypoxic cells *in vitro* by DEM. Chinese hamster ovary (HA-1) cells were incubated at 25°C for 1 h with DEM (■, 2.5×10^{-5} M; ▲, 5×10^{-5} M; ●, 2×10^{-4} M) in tissue culture plates under 5% CO_2 in N_2. Misonidazole was added concurrently with DEM. Cells were irradiated under hypoxic conditions at 25°C. (○) Controls. Data shown are averages from two to four experiments. Data from Bump *et al.* (1982a).

The effect of GSH depletion on the radiosensitization produced by different concentrations of MIS was also given attention. Figure 11 shows the enhancement ratio of hypoxic cells as a function of MIS concentration for control cells and for cells pretreated for 1 h with varying concentrations of DEM, which depleted intracellular GSH levels to 30, 10, and <5% of controls, respectively. It can be seen that cells with GSH levels lower than normal require less MIS to produce a given sensitizer-enhancement ratio. For example, the cells with 10% GSH levels require approximately one-tenth the concentration of MIS to produce an enhancement ratio of 1.5 to 2.0. This could be extremely useful if the GSH levels can be depleted in tumors without enhancing the neurotoxicity.

Figure 12 shows data on GSH levels for mouse EMT-6 tumors, as a function of time after injecting the tumor-bearing mice with varying doses of DEM. These data clearly show that GSH levels can be substantially reduced in tumors at nontoxic doses of DEM (LD_{50} = 1200 mg/kg).

From these data on the intracellular concentrations of GSH in tumors and from the previous *in vitro* data (Figs. 10 and 11), it would seem that

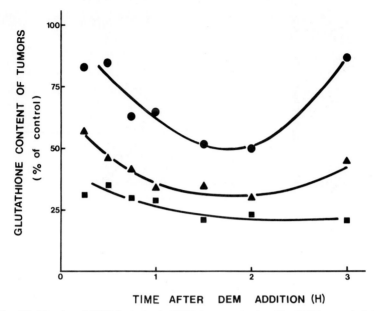

TIME AFTER DEM ADDITION (H)

Fig. 12. Kinetics of GSH depletion in EMT-6 tumors *in vivo*. The DEM was administered ip in peanut oil in dosages as follows (mg/kg): ●, 300; ▲, 500; ■, 720. Tumors were removed at the indicated times, homogenized in 10% trichloroacetic acid, and GSH assayed enzymatically by the method of Tietze (1969). Data from Bump *et al.* (1982b).

the tumors can probably be sensitized to irradiation by nontoxic levels of DEM alone and that the maximum sensitization would occur approximately 90 min after the injection. This was confirmed along with findings that radiosensitization over and above that produced by GSH depletion can be achieved at MIS concentrations low enough to produce no radiosensitization of their own. These data are shown in Fig. 13. In this case, EMT-6 tumors were irradiated in saline-injected mice, in mice treated with a low dose of MIS (25 mg/kg), or in mice treated with DEM (720 mg/kg) plus this same low dose of MIS. In these doubly injected mice, the MIS was given 45 min after the DEM injection, and the mice were irradiated 45 min later (i.e., 90 min after the DEM injection). The enhancement ratio of the hypoxic cells to the DEM alone was 1.3, that of the MIS alone 1.0, and that of the combination 2.0. From previous data it is known that a MIS dose of approximately 10 times that given (i.e., 250 mg/kg) is required to produce an enhancement ratio as large as 2.0.

Thus a large enhancement ratio of the hypoxic cells can be produced at small clinically achievable doses of MIS. However, it remains to be seen whether significant reductions in the GSH content of human tumors can

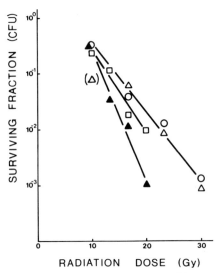

Fig. 13. The cell survival of EMT-6 cells irradiated as solid tumors in BALB/c mice and assayed *in vitro*. The mice were given DEM (ip in peanut oil) 90 min before irradiation and 45 min prior to MIS injection. (△) MIS, 25 mg/kg; (□) DEM, 720 mg/kg; (▲) MIS + DEM. From Bump *et al.* (1982a).

be obtained at clinically achievable doses of DEM. It is also important to determine whether generalized GSH depletion would enhance the systemic toxicity of MIS or other electron-affinic agents. It is also feasible that less toxic substances capable of depleting GSH *in vivo* can be formulated. This is now an area of active interest.

D. Reduction or Elimination of the Neurotoxicity of MIS

It has been suggested that the neurotoxicity of MIS and other nitroimidazoles might be the result of depletion of pyridoxal by the nitro-reduction product of MIS, aminomisonidazole (amino-MIS) (Eifel *et al.*, 1983). This suggestion was based on the observation that a number of clinically useful amines and hydrazines such as isoniazid, cycloserine, hydralazine, ethionamide, and penicillamine are neurotoxic, and the so-induced morphological changes in central and peripheral nerves are similar to those seen with MIS. Because the toxicity of these drugs is related to the depletion of pyridoxal and pyridoxal phosphate by binding of the amino group to the aldehyde group of pyridoxal to form a Schiff's base (Dakshinamurti, 1977), it was logical to assume that this might also be the mechanism involved in MIS neurotoxicity. Pyridoxal (vitamin B_6) is a critical cofactor in many enzyme reactions including the decarboxylation of glutamate to form γ-aminobutyric acid (GABA), an inhibitory neurotransmitter required in central afferent systems. The depletion of pyridoxal nutritionally or by the drugs just listed can cause a neuropathy and seizures that are completely reversed (or prevented) by administration of adequate doses (equimolar concentrations) of pyridoxine.

Because the compounds just listed deplete pyridoxal by reaction of their amino groups, it is therefore reasonable to assume that the reactive species of MIS is not MIS itself but the final reduction of the nitro group, amino-MIS (NH_2-MIS). If this were the case, NH_2-MIS would be more toxic than MIS itself, and this was shown by Born *et al.* (1980), who found it to be eight times more toxic than MIS itself. This final reduction product was shown to occur *in vivo* by Chin and Rauth (1981). These investigators noted the presence of reduced MIS products in mouse G.I. tract, liver, and brain after administration of MIS.

To test the hypothesis that pyridoxal depletion might be responsible for the toxicity of MIS, we injected mice daily with the drug, with and without a simultaneous injection of pyridoxine. The mice were monitored regularly for weight and for signs of neurological deficiency using two indices of neurotoxicity: foot splay (the distance apart of the rear feet when a mouse is raised gently by the tail) and a positive tail–body angle (TBA) on holding a mouse vertically by the tail. The first sign of such toxicity was invariably the loss of the mouse's ability to lift its body above a vertical position when holding it by the tail (loss of TBA). Figure 14 shows the data from an experiment in which mice were given daily (7 days/week) ip administrations of MIS (580 mg/kg) with or without simultaneous ip injections of pyridoxine (200 mg/kg). In the mice treated with MIS alone, there was a considerable weight loss and they died much earlier than did mice treated with the same dose of MIS plus pyridoxine. Also shown on these graphs are the points at which the first sign of neurotoxicity was noted (a large diamond), and the mean times (with SE limits) to the development of this first sign of neurotoxicity were 15.1 (13.7–16.7) and >38.0 (>33.8–>43.5) days for the MIS and MIS plus pyridoxine groups, respectively. About twice as many injections of MIS were tolerated by the mice also given pyridoxine.

These data show that the simultaneous administration of pyridoxine reduces the toxicity of MIS in mice. However, this could have occurred by altering the pharmacokinetics of MIS so as to reduce the radiosensitization produced. However, there was no effect of simultaneous pyridoxine administration on the pharmacokinetics of MIS or any effect of multiply daily injections of pyridoxine on the subsequent elimination half-life

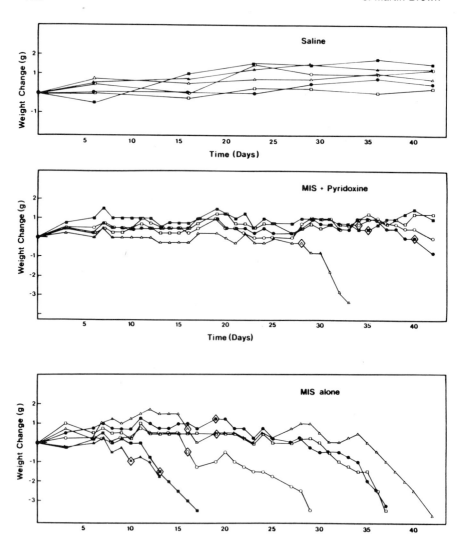

Fig. 14. The monitoring of body weight (grams) of female BALB/c mice during daily ip administrations of either saline or MIS alone (580 mg/kg), or MIS plus pyridoxine (200 mg/kg) given simultaneously. Data points represent the change in weight of individual animals compared to their weight prior to injection. (◇) The day the drug-injected mice demonstrated loss of TBA, as described in the text. (P. J. Eifel, D. M. Brown, W. W. Lee, and J. M. Brown, unpublished).

and peak plasma level of MIS subsequently injected. We also tested the radiosensitization produced by MIS with or without pyridoxine in EMT-6 tumors irradiated *in vivo*. As predicted from the pharmacokinetic data, there were no changes in the radiosensitization produced by MIS by the simultaneous administration of pyridoxine (Eifel *et al.*, 1983).

If pyridoxal depletion proves to be an important mechanism in the development of the neurotoxicity of MIS and other nitroimidazole sensitizers in humans, pyridoxine or pyridoxal administration may allow for administration of more effective doses of these radiosensitizing drugs.

It should also be noted that the four different methods suggested here for producing a superior radiosensitizer to MIS are essentially independent. In other words, these methods could be combined. For example, although it is likely that the drug SR-2508 can be given in doses 5 to 10 times greater than those currently being used with MIS, it still might be advantageous to enhance the radiosensitizing ability of any given dose of SR-2508 by simultaneous depletion of intracellular GSH levels. Thus, the prospects are bright for having within the next 4 to 5 years an ideal radiosensitizer, one that can be given to patients without producing any toxicity but that produces maximum radiosensitization of the hypoxic tumor cells. Once this becomes available, it can be determined under what conditions, if any, hypoxic cells are a limitation to the local control rates that can be achieved with conventional fractionated radiotherapy.

III. Electron-Affinic Agents as Chemosensitizers

A. Is There a Therapeutic Gain?

In addition to their radiosensitizing ability, it has been shown that MIS and other 2-nitroimidazoles are capable of sensitizing tumors in mice to a variety of alkylating agents including cyclophosphamide, melphalan, and the nitrosoureas (Rose *et al.*, 1980; Clement *et al.*, 1980; Tannock, 1980; Martin *et al.*, 1981; Law *et al.*, 1981; Twentyman, 1981; Siemann, 1981; Mulcahy *et al.*, 1981). Although most of these investigators found that the cytotoxicity of the alkylating agents to the normal tissues is enhanced by MIS, almost all concluded that the enhancement of the tumor response is greater than that of normal tissues, and thus there is a therapeutic gain (McNally, 1982).

A major question not resolved by any of these studies is whether the differential enhancement of the cytotoxicity of alkylating agents to tumor cells would occur at clinically realistic dose levels of MIS. Most workers gave doses of MIS of 600 to 1000 mg/kg, which produce plasma levels 5–10 times higher than can be achieved in humans. In studies in which doses of MIS approaching clinical levels were used, there was little or no chemosensitization. However, one must bear in mind that the plasma half-life of MIS in the mouse is 10 times shorter than that in humans, and it is therefore possible that prolonged exposure of tumor cells to MIS, even at relatively low doses, might increase the chemosensitizing effect.

An attempt to answer this question was made by simulating in the mouse the prolonged low levels of MIS that can be tolerated in humans in order to determine whether useful sensitization of the cytotoxic effect of cyclophosphamide, melphalan, and the nitrosourea CCNU on tumor cells might be achieved by MIS in the clinic (Brown and Hirst, 1982; Hirst and Brown, 1982).

In these studies, there was a significant chemosensitization for tumors under conditions in which the pharmacokinetics of MIS in humans has been simulated in the mouse. Figures 15 and 16 show data for cyclophosphamide (CY) and for melphalan (L-PAM). Figures 15A and 16A and B show the response of RIF-1 sarcoma to increasing doses of the alkylating agents given either with or without MIS. Figures 15B and 16C show the plasma concentrations of MIS achieved in the same animals as used for the tumor response. These plasma levels were obtained by giving multiple small injections of MIS every half hour. The plasma concentrations obtained closely simulate those reported for humans by Urtasun *et al.* (1977) following a single oral 7-g administration of MIS. In each case, the dose of alkylating agents was given at 4 h after the start of this prolonged exposure to MIS. As can be seen, the tumor is rendered more sensitive to the alkylating agent by a dose-modification factor (DMF) of approximately 2.0. In parallel experiments in our laboratory, the response of the bone marrow stem cells (CFU-S) and white blood cells to these alkylating agents was measured with or without a prolonged MIS exposure. For each of these two dose-limiting normal tissue end points, no sensitization to the chemotherapeutic agent was produced by MIS.

Similar experiments were done with CCNU using the KHT tumor and bone marrow stem cells and spermatogonia as the normal tissues (Hirst and Brown, 1982). Here too there was a significant enhancement of the tumor response with no enhancement of the two normal tissue end points. Thus the enhancement ratios for the tumors (measured either as surviving fraction or as regrowth delay) represent therapeutic gains.

The use of MIS in combination with several chemotherapeutic agents suggests that a tumor response essentially equivalent to doubling the dose of the chemotherapeutic agents may be obtained and with no additional increase in normal tissue toxicity.

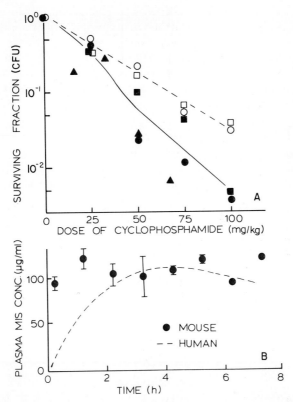

Fig. 15. Effects of prior treatment with saline (○, □), a large single dose of 750 mg/kg MIS (▲), or prolonged exposure to low-level (15 mg/kg) MIS (●, ■) on the survival of RIF-1 tumor cells exposed to a range of CY doses. The different symbols show the results of two independent experiments. Lines were drawn by eye through the saline and the multiple MIS points (A). (B) Plasma levels achieved with multiple MIS injections in one of these experiments (●). The dashed line repesents a typical human exposure after the oral administration of 7 g MIS (Urtasun *et al.*, 1977). From Brown and Hirst (1982).

B. Is There a Better Chemosensitizer than MIS?

Although the results just given augur well for the clinical use of MIS with chemotherapeutic agents, there are data that MIS may not be the most effective chemosensitizer. Indeed, evidence has been presented by Workman and Twentyman (1982) indicating that nitroimidazoles more lipophilic than MIS are more efficient than MIS at enhancing the *in vivo* tumor cell killing by CCNU. These authors investigated a series of nitroimidazoles with similar electron affinities but with widely differing octanol–water partition coefficients (*P*), and showed that the amount of

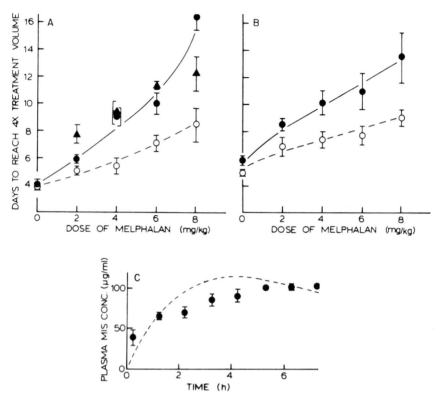

Fig. 16. (A, B) Effects, in two separate experiments, of different doses of L-PAM, with
(●) or without (○) prolonged low-level MIS exposure, on the time to reach four times
treatment volume. Also shown is the enhancement of L-PAM cytotoxicity produced by a
large single dose of MIS (750 mg/kg) given 30 min prior to L-PAM injection (▲). Error bars
represent ±1 SE. The plasma levels of MIS in one of these experiments (A) are shown in
(C). The dashed line represents a typical human drug profile after a single 7-g oral administration of MIS (Urtasun *et al.*, 1977). From Brown and Hirst (1982).

enhancement achieved by the series exhibits a parabolic dependence on
log P, with a peak value close to that for benznidazole (Ro-07-1051; $P =$
8.5). These experiments raised the possibility that there may be one or
several other nitroimidazoles that can enhance tumor response to a much
greater extent than MIS.

However, before these data can be extrapolated, there are at least three
important questions that must be addressed. It has to be determined (1)
whether the greater enhancement of CCNU cytotoxicity by benznidazole
is also seen in dose-limiting normal tissues, (2) whether benznidazole can
continue to show its effect when administered at clinically relevant dose

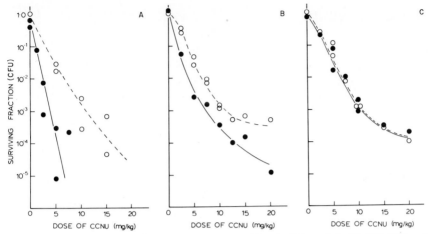

Fig. 17. Effects of large single doses of (A) benznidazole (520 mg/kg), (B) MIS (750 mg/kg), or (C) SR-2508 (800 mg/kg) in combination with CCNU on the survival of KHT tumor cells treated *in vivo* and assayed *in vitro*. (○) Saline + CCNU. Data from two to three experiments were pooled in each case. From Hirst *et al.* (1983a).

levels, and (3) whether benznidazole is effective against tumors other than the KHT used in the study of Workman and Twentyman (1982).

The ability of three nitroimidazoles of widely different lipophilicities (benznidazole, MIS, and SR-2508) to enhance the cytotoxicity of CCNU was assessed, and the responses of two mouse tumors (the KHT sarcoma and the SCC VII/St carcinoma) and two normal tissues (bone marrow stem cells and spermatogonia) were evaluated after single and multiple doses of these nitroimidazoles designed to simulate the human pharmacokinetics (Hirst *et al.*, 1983a).

Figure 17 shows data for the three nitroimidazoles of equal electron affinity. These compounds were given in large single parenteral doses to mice bearing the KHT tumor and treated immediately with various doses of CCNU. As also found by Workman and Twentyman (1982), lipophilicity influences significantly the ability of nitroimidazoles to sensitize to CCNU, the most lipophilic and effective compound being benznidazole. The least lipophilic, SR-2508, was essentially ineffective at enhancing the response of the KHT tumor to CCNU. The same evidence was found with the less CCNU-responsive tumor, the SCC-VII/St carcinoma. However, when the response of the two normal tissues to CCNU in combination with one of these three nitroimidazoles was examined, a similar enhancement of both of these normal tissue end points was evident. This is shown in the case of bone marrow in Fig. 18. There is a substantial enhancement

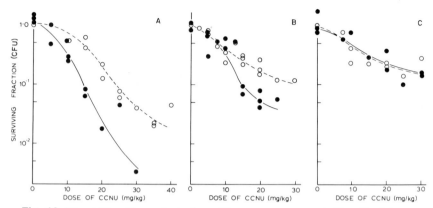

Fig. 18. The ability of large single doses (●, same amounts as in Fig. 17) of the three sensitizers: (A) benznidazole, (B) MIS, or (C) SR-2508 to enhance the killing of bone marrow stem cells by a range of CCNU doses. (○) Saline + CCNU. From Hirst *et al.* (1983a).

of the normal tissue toxicity seen with a large single dose of benznidazole preceding the administration of CCNU. There was also an enhancement of the effect of MIS but only at CCNU doses over 10 mg/kg. Thus, for these large single doses of nitroimidazoles (irrelevant to the clinical situation), there is no apparent therapeutic gain in using a nitroimidazole as lipophilic as benznidazole.

As to the low multiple doses of nitroimidazoles designed to simulate the human pharmacokinetics of these drugs, Fig. 19 shows the results obtained for this schedule with the three nitroimidazoles used with the KHT tumor. The mean sensitizer level in the blood for the 4 h prior to CCNU injection was 50–70 μg/ml for benznidazole, 50–100 μg/ml for MIS, and 50–70 μg/ml for SR-2508. As can be seen in this figure, a similar but greater enhancement of the CCNU response was seen with benznidazole, and little or no enhancement was seen with SR-2508. Again, however, as shown in Fig. 20, there was a large enhancement by benznidazole of the response of the bone marrow to CCNU toxicity, resulting in apparently little or no improvement in the therapeutic gain compared to MIS.

Table III gives a summary of the enhancement ratios obtained for the two different mouse tumors and two different normal tissues for the large single doses of sensitizer and the prolonged low-level exposures to sensitizers used. There was no improvement in the therapeutic gain factor in changing from MIS to benznidazole in using large single doses of sensitizer, and there was a loss of the therapeutic gain when using the more clinically relevant low-level exposures to the sensitizers.

Although the mechanism of enhancement of CCNU cytotoxicity by nitroimidazoles is poorly understood, it may not be coincidental that the

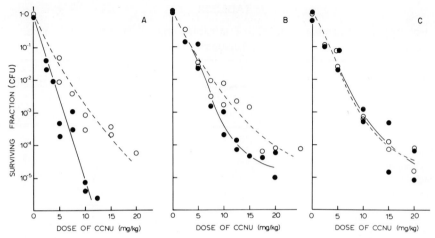

Fig. 19. Effects of prolonged exposure (●; for benznidazole, 14 mg/kg per dose; for MIS and SR-2508, 0.6 mmol/kg for first dose and 0.15 mmol/kg for second to fifteenth dose) to the three sensitizers, (A–C) as in Fig. 18, on cell killing in the KHT tumor by a range of CCNU doses. (○) Saline + CCNU. Data from two to three experiments were pooled. From Hirst *et al.* (1983a).

more lipophilic compounds have a greater effect against CCNU, which is itself lipophilic. This clearly raises the possibility—particularly in that the response of normal tissues increases in parallel to that of the tumors—that the enhancement of cytotoxicity by benznidazole is largely the result

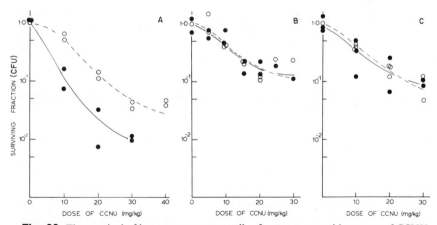

Fig. 20. The survival of bone marrow stem cells after treatment with a range of CCNU doses, in combination with saline (○) or prolonged low-level exposure (●, 15 mg/kg per dose) to the three sensitizers: (A–C) as in Fig. 18. Data from two to three experiments were pooled. From Hirst *et al.* (1983a).

TABLE III

Relative Effectiveness of the Nitroimidazoles against Tumors and Normal Tissues[a]

Nitroimidazole	Enhancement ratio[b]				
	KHT Tumor	SCC VII/St Tumor	Bone marrow	Testis	TGF[c]
	Large single doses of sensitizer				
Benznidazole	2.7	1.8	1.9	>4.0	1.5
(2 mmol/kg)		2.0	1.7	3.3	
MIS	1.5	1.7	1.0	1.6	1.4
(3.75 mmol/kg)	1.9	1.6	1.5	1.5	
SR-2508	1.0	1.0	1.0	1.0	1.0
(3.75 mmol/kg)	1.0	1.0	1.0	1.0	
	Prolonged low-level exposure to sensitizers				
Benznidazole	1.8	—	2.0	>4.0	1.0
	2.1	—	2.1	2.6	
MIS	1.3	—	1.0	1.0	1.4
	1.6	<1.3	1.0	1.0	
SR-2058	1.0	1.0	1.0	1.4	1.0
	1.0	1.0	1.0	1.0	

[a] From Hirst *et al.* (1983a).

[b] Enhancement ratios were calculated at two dose levels of CCNU alone: 10 mg/kg (upper value), 20 mg/kg (lower value).

[c] Therapeutic gain factors (TGF) were calculated by dividing the mean of the two enhancement ratios for the KHT tumor by the mean of the two enhancement ratios for the dose-limiting normal tissue (bone marrow). Similar values could be calculated for other combinations of tumor and normal tissue system.

of altered pharmacokinetics of CCNU. Thus, more hydrophilic chemotherapeutic agents might be expected to interact differently with nitroimidazoles. As can be seen from Figs. 18 and 20, SR-2508 was ineffective in enhancing CCNU toxicity in tumors when administered either in a large single dose or in the form of a prolonged low-level exposure.

However, it has been shown (Law *et al.*, 1981) that a large single dose of SR-2508 will enhance cyclophosphamide toxicity almost as effectively as MIS. In subsequent experiments with prolonged exposures to low levels to SR-2508, there was an evident enhancement of cyclophosphamide cytotoxicity similar to that achieved with comparable levels of MIS (Hirst *et al.*, 1983b). Thus, the ability to enhance cyclophosphamide toxicity extends to more hydrophilic nitroimidazoles than it does for

CCNU enhancement. The optimum drug for the enhancement of chemotherapeutic response may be different for each chemotherapeutic agent.

C. Mechanisms of Chemosensitization

A major stumbling block in the development of the optimum chemosensitizer for clinical use is our lack of knowledge of the mechanism of chemosensitization. However, it is reasonable to assume that the enhancement of tumor cytotoxicity seen *in vivo* is at least in part the result of the same mechanism that produces a similar effect *in vitro*. Such an *in vitro* effect was originally shown by Stratford *et al*. (1980), who found that cells incubated under hypoxic conditions with MIS were subsequently more sensitive to killing by a variety of chemotherapeutic drugs. This effect does not occur unless the cells are incubated under hypoxic conditions with MIS, a finding that implicates the anaerobic metabolism of MIS in the mechanism (Brown, 1982). This requirement of hypoxia for the phenomenon of chemosensitization could well explain the preferential effect on tumors compared to normal tissues, because it is primarily tumors that contain hypoxic cells. Working from the hypothesis that the preferential sensitization by MIS and other nitroimidazoles of tumors *in vivo* is at least partly a reflection of the same mechanism giving rise to chemosensitization *in vitro,* the possible mechanisms for the enhancement of cytotoxicity of a model bifunctional alkylating agent, melphalan (L-PAM), by MIS were studied using CHO cells *in vitro* (Taylor *et al.,* 1982).

Hypoxic (but not aerobic) treatment of CHO cells with MIS at 37°C for 2 h increases the sensitivity of these cells to subsequent killing by L-PAM by a DMF of approximately 4 (Taylor *et al.*, 1982). Although toxicity occurs with prolonged exposure to MIS under these conditions, this chemosensitization is apparent in the absence of toxicity and does not require the presence of MIS or hypoxia during the subsequent challenge with L-PAM.

Three likely mechanisms for this chemosensitization are

1. *Depletion of the intracellular protector glutathione (GSH):* A 2-h hypoxic pretreatment of CHO cells with MIS depletes GSH levels to approximately 10% of control levels. Because GSH can "intercept" alkylating agents before they reach the DNA, this could result in the chemosensitization. This 90% depletion of glutathione was simulated using diethyl maleate (DEM), and there was an enhancement to subsequent L-PAM treatment by a DMF of 1.4. Because a DMF of 4.0 was seen after

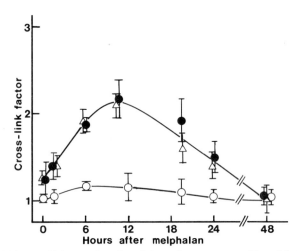

Fig. 21. DNA cross-links as a function of time after treatment with melphalan (L-PAM). Control (○) and MIS-pretreated (●, 5 mM, 2 h) cells were exposed to 1.5 μg/ml L-PAM for 1 h, after which they were left in drug-free growth medium for up to 48 h. (△) Control cells exposed to 6 μg/ml L-PAM for 1 h. Samples were removed at various times for assay by alkaline elution. (Y. C. Taylor, J. W. Evans, and J. M. Brown, unpublished).

pretreatment with MIS, GSH depletion by MIS can therefore account for only approximately 15% of the subsequent sensitization to L-PAM.

2. *Increased intracellular uptake of L-PAM:* The binding of ^{14}C-labeled L-PAM to cellular macromolecules with and without MIS pretreatment was examined. There was an increase by a DMF of 1.4 with the MIS pretreatment. However, cells pretreated with DEM to produce a 90% GSH depletion also have a 40% increase in binding (i.e., DMF for binding = 1.4). Thus the increased binding of L-PAM to cellular macromolecules in MIS-pretreated cells is entirely accounted for by GSH depletion and does not relate to the large sensitization. Hence there is no evidence for a direct effect of MIS on the intracellular uptake of L-PAM.

3. *Increased efficiency of DNA interstrand cross-link formation:* This possibility was investigated by using the alkaline elution assay developed by Kohn *et al.* (1976), and the number of DNA interstrand cross-links for any dose of L-PAM was increased by a factor of 4 following hypoxic preincubation with MIS (Y. C. Taylor, J. W. Evans, and J. M. Brown, unpublished). These data are shown in Figs. 21 and 22. Figure 21 shows the development of cross-links in the L-PAM–treated cells as a function of time following the 1-h treatment by L-PAM. As has been found by others, DNA cross-links do not develop immediately but increase gradually to a maximum at 6 to 12 h after treatment with L-PAM. The total

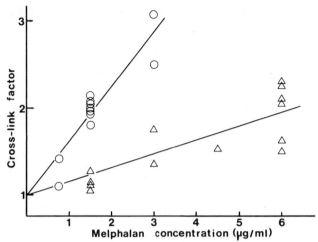

Fig. 22. Dose–response curve for L-PAM–induced DNA cross-links in control (△) and MIS-pretreated (○, 5 mM, 2 h) cells. Cross-link factors were calculated from alkaline elution data from cells assayed 6–12 h after L-PAM treatment, the time at which cross-linking is at a maximum (Fig. 21). The ratio of the slope of the two lines fitted by least-squares regression is 3.9, essentially identical to the DMF for the enhancement of cell killing by MIS pretreatment of the cells. (Y. C. Taylor, J. W. Evans, and J. M. Brown, unpublished).

number of cross links and their development and decay in L-PAM–treated cells preincubated with MIS can be precisely matched by a four-fold greater dose of L-PAM alone. This factor of 4 is also seen in a summary of experiments showing the peak number of cross-links (i.e., measured at 12 h after L-PAM) in cells treated with L-PAM with or without MIS (Fig. 22). If allowance is made for a DMF of 1.4 resulting from GSH depletion, then a given L-PAM molecule bound to DNA has a threefold greater chance of forming a lethal DNA interstrand cross-link if the cell has been pretreated with MIS. This may be the result of an interference with the enzymatic excision of the monoadduct before it becomes a cross-link.

As a further test of the specificity of the enhancement of cross-link formation by MIS, experiments were done in which the hypoxic treatment with MIS was performed immediately after the 1-h incubation of cells under aerobic conditions with L-PAM. The rationale of this experiment was that because cross-links can take up to 12 h to be produced, and if MIS is enhancing this cross-link production, then significant sensitization should be produced even with MIS given after L-PAM. Under these conditions, the sensitization would be somewhat less than with the pretreatment, because the effect of the removal of intracellular GSH would

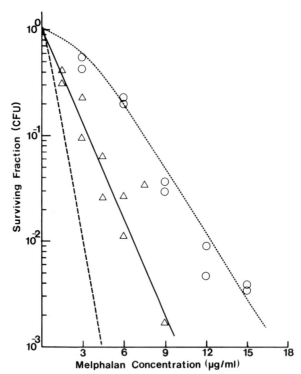

Fig. 23. Enhancement of L-PAM toxicity by *posttreatment* incubation with MIS under hypoxic conditions (△). Chinese hamster ovary cells were exposed to various concentrations of L-PAM for 1 h, the L-PAM removed, and then the cells incubated for an additional 2 h under hypoxic conditions with or without 5 m*M* MIS. The dashed lines show the survival curves obtained in other experiments for MIS-pretreated (longer dashes) and control (○·····○) cells. (Y. C. Taylor, J. W. Evans, and J. M. Brown, unpublished).

not be present when the MIS was given after L-PAM. Figure 23 shows the results of this experiment. Incubation of the cells under hypoxic conditions with MIS after L-PAM treatment also significantly sensitizes the cells, and this clearly rules out any influences of MIS on the uptake, metabolism, or distribution of L-PAM.

Assuming that the chemosensitizing effect of MIS is indeed due to enhanced cross-link formation, the chemosensitization will be limited to those agents that produce their major effect by cross-linking the DNA. This certainly applies to bifunctional alkylating agents such as cyclophosphamide, melphalan, chlorambucil, and nitrogen mustard, and also to the nitrosoureas. In fact, the effects of most of these compounds are enhanced by MIS *in vivo*. The situation with *cis*-platinum is more complicated, in that although chemosensitization has been shown *in vitro* (Stratford *et al.*, 1980), no chemosensitization has been found *in vivo* (J. M. Brown, unpublished).

IV. Summary

A. Radiosensitization

Experience with high-pressure oxygen in combination with radiotherapy has shown that, for some tumors at least, the presence of hypoxic cells is a limiting factor, even with conventional daily fractionation. Thus, hypoxic-cell radiosensitizers, of which MIS is the prototype drug, may play a role in improving the cure rate of some tumors when combined with daily fractionation or with low-dose radiation.

However, the toxicity of MIS limits the dose that can be given with conventional daily radiotherapy to only one-fifth to one-tenth of that required to produce maximum radiosensitization of the hypoxic cells. In this chapter an attempt has been made to summarize the different approaches taken to overcome this problem and to develop drugs that would improve on MIS. These approaches can be broken down into four pathways:

1. *A more effective radiosensitizer of comparable toxicity:* Although it is relatively simple to synthesize drugs of greater radiosensitizing efficiency *in vitro* than MIS by increasing their electron affinity, this does not translate into a similar increase in radiosensitizing efficiency *in vivo*. Although several drugs that are more efficient radiosensitizers than MIS were tested *in vitro,* with achievement of adequate tumor concentrations, a more effective radiosensitization than that produced by MIS was not evident *in vivo*.

2. *A less toxic radiosensitizer of comparable radiosensitizing efficiency:* Because the dose-limiting toxicity of MIS is neurotoxicity, such a drug might be one that is selectively excluded from neural tissues. A way to achieve this is to reduce the lipid solubility (lipophilicity) of the compound while still retaining its electron affinity, thus reducing the concentration of drug in the neural tissues (brain, peripheral nerves) without affecting the tumor concentration. However, if the reduction in lipophilicity is too great, the drug ceases to radiosensitize effectively, both *in vitro* and *in vivo*, as a result of its inability to penetrate the cell membrane and enter the cell. It would appear that a lipophilicity given by an octanol–water partition coefficient of approximately 0.04 is optimum (cf. MIS = 0.43), with the 2-nitroimidazole amide SR-2508 being the most promising

in this series. Tumor levels of this drug of up to 10 times greater than those obtainable with MIS should be attainable clinically and with no increase in neurotoxicity. This compound is presently in phase I clinical testing in the United States, under the auspices of the Radiotherapy Oncology Group, and has already proved itself less toxic than MIS.

3. *Enhancement of the efficacy but not the toxicity of MIS by removal of competing SH:* Because it is likely that MIS acts by fixing target radical damage in competition with restitution of the radical by H donation from intracellular glutathione (GSH), it follows that a given concentration of MIS will produce greater radiosensitization if the intracellular level of GSH is depleted. The compound diethyl maleate (DEM) was used to test this hypothesis both *in vitro* and *in vivo*. With this drug, tumor levels of GSH can be reduced by 80 to 90% at nontoxic doses, and the radiosensitizing efficiency of MIS is increased by 5- to 10-fold. Whether or not this is an effective approach for clinical use must await further testing.

4. *Reduction or elimination of the neurotoxicity of MIS:* There is evidence that the neurotoxicity of MIS is the result of depletion of pyridoxal phosphate (vitamin B_6), an essential coenzyme in the formation of the inhibitory neurotransmitter, γ-aminobutyric acid (GABA). This depletion, and hence the neurotoxicity, can be largely prevented by simultaneous administration of pyridoxine with MIS.

Because most of these approaches are independent, they could be combined to overcome the systemic toxicity of electron-affinic sensitizers. With this choice, optimum doses of an electron-affinic agent will eventually be delivered with conventional radiation fractionation.

B. Chemosensitization

In addition to being effective radiosensitizers, MIS and other 2-nitroimidazoles have been found to sensitize tumors in mice to a variety of alkylating agents including cyclophosphamide, melphalan, and the nitrosoureas. This effect can be achieved at clinical levels of MIS, and moreover at these clinically simulated levels, the chemosensitizing effect of MIS is restricted entirely to the tumors, with *no* sensitizing effect on several normal tissues studied. Thus the combined use of MIS and chemotherapeutic agents shows promise.

Work is under way to determine if more effective compounds can be formulated. Although drugs that are more lipophilic than MIS do sensitize tumors to the nitrosourea CCNU with greater efficacy, this does not appear to translate into an improved therapeutic gain, because there is a concomitant increase in the sensitization produced in normal tissues. For other chemotherapeutic agents there appears to be much less (if any) influence of the lipophilicity of the 2-nitroimidazole on the chemosensitizing ability.

However, rational design of a new chemosensitizing drug must await knowledge of the mechanism involved. There is new evidence that the principle mechanism for the sensitization to L-PAM by MIS *in vitro* is a specific enhancement of DNA interstrand cross-link formation. Further knowledge of the mechanics of this occurrence should aid in synthesizing effective compounds.

Acknowledgments

My sincere gratitude is extended to colleagues Drs. E. A. Bump, P. J. Eifel, D. G. Hirst, and Y. C. Taylor for helpful discussions and for permission to quote unpublished data. This work was supported by Research Grants CA-15201 and CA-25990, and Research Contract CM-87207, from the U.S. National Cancer Institute, DHHS.

References

Adams, G. E., and Jameson, D. G. (1980). Time effects in molecular radiation biology. *Radiat. Environ. Biophys.* **17,** 95–113.

Adams, G. E., Clarke, E. D., Flockhart, I. R., Jacobs, R. S., Sehmi, D. S., Stratford, I. J., Wardman, P., Watts, M. E., Parrick, J., Wallace, R. G., and Smithen, C. E. (1979). Structure-activity relationships in the development of hypoxic cell radiosensitizers. I. Sensitization efficiency. *Int. J. Radiat. Biol.* **35,** 133–150.

Alper, T. (1956). The modification of damage caused by primary ionization of biological targets. *Radiat. Res.* **5,** 573–586.

Ash, D. V., Peckham, M. J., and Steel, G. G. (1979). The quantitative response of human tumours to radiation and misonidazole. *Br. J. Cancer* **40,** 883–889.

Asquith, J. C., Watts, M. E., Patel, K., Smithen, C. E., and Adams, G. E. (1974). Electron affinic sensitization. V. Radiosensitization of hypoxic bacteria and mammalian cells *in vitro* by some nitroimidazoles and nitropyrazoles. *Radiat. Res.* **60,** 108–118.

Binns, T. B. (ed.) (1964). "Absorption and Distribution of Drugs." Livingstone, Edinburgh.

Born, J. L., Hadley, W. M., Anderson, S. L., and Yuhas, J. M. (1980). *In* "Radiation Sensitizers: Their Use in the Clinical Management of Cancer" (L. W. Brady, ed.), pp. 79–82. Masson, New York.

Brown, D. M., Yu, N. Y., Brown, J. M., and Lee, W. W. (1982a). *In vitro* and *in vivo* radiosensitization by 2-nitroimidazoles more electron-affinic than misonidazole. *Int. J. Radiat. Oncol. Biol. Phys.* **8,** 435–438.

Brown, D. M., Parker, E. T., and Brown, J. M. (1982b). Structure-activity relationships of 1-substituted-2-nitroimidazoles: effect of partition coefficient and side chain hydroxyl groups on radiosensitization *in vitro*. *Radiat. Res.* **90,** 98–108.

Brown, D. M., Gonzales-Mendez, R., and Brown, J. M. (1983). Factors influencing intracellular uptake and radiosensitization by 2-nitroimidazoles *in vitro*. *Radiat. Res.* **93,** 492–505.

Brown, J. M. (1979). Evidence for acutely hypoxic cells in mouse tumours, and a possible mechanism of reoxygenation. *Br. J. Radiol.* **52**, 650–656.

Brown, J. M. (1982). The mechanisms of cytotoxicity and chemosensitization by misonidazole and other nitroimidazoles. *Int. J. Radiat. Oncol. Biol. Phys.* **8**, 675–682.

Brown, J. M., and Hirst, D. G. (1982). Effect of clinical levels of misonidazole on the response of tumour and normal tissues in the mouse to alkylating agents. *Br. J. Cancer* **45**, 700–708.

Brown, J. M., and Workman, P. (1980). Partition coefficient as a guide to the development of radiosensitizers which are less toxic than misonidazole. *Radiat. Res.* **82**, 171–190.

Brown, J. M., Yu, N. Y., Brown, D. M., and Lee, W. W. (1981). SR-2508: a 2-nitroimidazole amide which should be superior to misonidazole as a radiosensitizer for clinical use. *Int. J. Radiat. Oncol. Biol. Phys.* **7**, 695–703.

Bump, E. A., Yu, N. Y., and Brown, J. M. (1982a). The use of drugs which deplete intracellular glutathione in hypoxic cell radiosensitization. *Int. J. Radiat. Oncol. Biol. Phys.* **8**, 439–442.

Bump, E. A., Yu, N. Y., Taylor, Y. C., Brown, J. M., Travis, E. L., and Boyd, M. R. (1982b). Radiosensitization and chemosensitization by diethylmaleate. *Proc. Conf. Radio-protectors Anticarcinogens 1st.*

Chapman, J. D., Greenstock, C. L., Reuvers, A. P., McDonald, E., and Dunlop, I. (1973). Radiation chemical studies with nitrofurazone as related to its mechanism of radiosensitization. *Radiat. Res.* **53**, 190–203.

Chin, J. B., and Rauth, A. M. (1981). The metabolism and pharmacokinetics of the hypoxic cell radiosensitizer and cytotoxic agent, misonidazole, in C3H mice. *Radiat. Res.* **86**, 341–357.

Clement, J. J., Gorman, M. S., Wodinsky, I., Catane, R., and Johnson, R. K. (1980). Enhancement of antitumor activity of alkylating agents by the radiation sensitizer misonidazole. *Cancer Res.* **40**, 4165.

Conroy, P. J., McNeill, T. H., Passalacqua, W., Merritt, J., Reich, K. R., and Walker, S. (1982). Nitroimidazole neurotoxicity: are mouse studies predictive? *Int. J. Radiat. Oncol. Biol. Phys.* **8**, 799–803.

Crabtree, H. G., and Cramer, W. (1933). The action of radium on cancer cells. II. Some factors determining the susceptibility of cancer cells to radium. *Proc. R. Soc. London Ser. B* **113**, 238–250.

Dakshinamurti, K. (1977). *In* "Nutrition and the Brain" (R. J. Wurtman and J. J. Wurtman, eds.), Vol. 1, pp. 289–306. Raven, New York.

Denekamp, J., Hirst, D. G., Stewart, F. A., and Terry, N. H. A. (1980). Is tumour radiosensitization by misonidazole a general phenomenon? *Br. J. Cancer* **41**, 1–9.

Dische, S., Saunders, M. I., Lee, M. E., Adams, G. E., and Flockhart, I. R. (1977). Clinical testing of the radiosensitizer Ro-07-0582. Experience with multiple doses. *Br. J. Cancer* **35**, 567–579.

Eifel, P. J., Brown, D. M., Lee, W. W., and Brown, J. M. (1983). Misonidazole neurotoxicity in mice decreased by administration with pyridoxine. *Int. J. Radiat. Oncol. Biol. Phys.* (In press).

Gray, L. H., Conger, A. D., Ebert, M., Hornsey, S., and Scott, O. C. A. (1953). The concentration of oxygen dissolved in tissues at the time of irradiation as a factor in radiotherapy. *Br. J. Radiol.* **26**, 638–648.

Hirst, D. G., and Brown, J. M. (1982). The therapeutic potential of misonidazole enhancement of alkylating agent cytotoxicity. *Int. J. Radiat. Oncol. Biol. Phys.* **8**, 639–642.

Hirst, D. G., Brown, J. M., and Hazelhurst, J. L. (1983a). Effect of partition coefficient on the ability of nitroimidazoles to enhance the cytotoxicity of 1-(2-chloroethyl)-3-cyclo-hexyl-1-nitrosourea. *Cancer Res.* **43**, 1961–1965.

Hirst, D. G., Hazelhurst, J. L., and Brown, J. M. (1983b). Sensitization of normal and malignant tissues to cyclophosphamide by nitroimidazoles with different partition coefficients. *Br. J. Cancer,* (In press).

Howard-Flanders, P. (1960). Effect of oxygen on the radiosensitivity of bacteriophage in the presence of sulphydryl compounds. *Nature (London)* **186**, 485–487.

Kallman, R. F. (1972). The phenomenon of reoxygenation and its implications for fraction-ated radiotherapy. *Radiology (Easton, Pa.)* **105**, 135–142.

Kohn, K. W., Erickson, L. C., Ewig, R. A. G., and Friedman, C. A. (1976). Fractionation of DNA from mammalian cells by alkaline elution. *Biochemistry* **15**, 4629–4637.

Law, M. P., Hirst, D. G., and Brown, J. M. (1981). The enhancing effect of misonidazole on the response of the RIF-1 tumour to cyclophosphamide. *Br. J. Cancer* **44**, 208.

Martin, W. M. C., McNally, N. J., and DeRonde, J. (1981). The potentiation of cyclophos-phamide cytotoxicity by misonidazole. *Br. J. Cancer* **43**, 756.

McNally, N. J. (1982). Enhancement of chemotherapy agents. *Int. J. Radiat. Oncol. Biol. Phys.* **8**, 593–598.

Mellet, L. B. (1974). The constancy of the product of concentration and time. *In* "Antineo-plastic and Immuno-Suppressive Agents" (A. C. Sartorelli and D. G. Johns, eds.), pp. 330–340. Springer-Verlag, Berlin.

Mulcahy, R. T., Siemann, D. W., and Sutherland, R. M. (1981). *In vivo* response of KHT sarcomas to combined chemotherapy with misonidazole and BCNU. *Br. J. Cancer* **43**, 93.

Rose, C. M., Millar, J. L., Peacock, J. H., Phelps, T. A., and Stephens, T. (1980). Differen-tial enhancement of melphalan cytotoxicity in tumor and normal tissue by misonidazole. *In* "Radiation Sensitizers: Their Use in the Clinical Management of Cancer" (L. W. Brady, ed.), p. 405. Manor, New York.

Siemann, D. W. (1981). The *in vivo* combination of the nitroimidazole misonidazole and the chemotherapeutic agent CCNU. *Br. J. Cancer* **43**, 367.

Soloway, A. H., Whitman, B., and Messer, J. R. (1960). Penetration of brain and brain tumor by aromatic compounds as a function of molecular substituents. *J. Pharmacol. Exp. Ther.* **129**, 310–314.

Stratford, I. J., Adams, G. E., Horsman, M. R., Kandaiya, S., Rajaratnam, S., Smith, E., and Williamson, C. (1980). The interaction of misonidazole with radiation, chemothera-peutic agents or heat. A preliminary report. *Cancer Clin. Trials* **3**, 231.

Sutherland, R. M., and Franko, A. J. (1980). On the nature of the radiobiologically hypoxic fraction in tumors. *Int. J. Radiat. Oncol. Biol. Phys.* **6**, 117–120.

Tannock, I. F. (1972). Oxygen diffusion and the distribution of cellular radiosensitivity in tumours. *Br. J. Radiol.* **45**, 515–524.

Tannock, I. F. (1980). The *in vivo* interaction of anti-cancer drugs with misonidazole or metronidazole: cyclophosphamide and BCNU. *Br. J. Cancer* **42**, 871.

Taylor, Y. C., Bump, E. A., and Brown, J. M. (1982). Studies of the mechanism of chemo-sensitization by misonidazole *in vitro*. *Int. J. Radiat. Oncol. Biol. Phys.* **8**, 705–708.

Thomlinson, R. H., and Gray, L. H. (1955). The histological structure of some human lung cancers and the possible implications for radiotherapy. *Br. J. Cancer* **9**, 539–549.

Thomlinson, R. H., Dische, S., and Gray, A. J. (1976). Clinical testing of the radiosensitizer Ro-07-0582. III. Response of tumours. *Clin. Radiol.* **27**, 167–174.

Tietze, F. (1969). Enzymatic method for quantitative determination of nanogram amounts of total and oxidized glutathione: applications to mammalian blood and other tissues. *Anal. Biochem.* **27**, 502–522.

Twentyman, P. R. (1981). Modification of tumour and host response to cyclophosphamide by misonidazole and WR-2721. *Br. J. Cancer* **43,** 745.

Urtasun, R. C., Band, P., Chapman, J. D., Rabin, H. R., Wilson, A. F., and Fryer, C. G. (1977). Clinical phase 1 study of the hypoxic cell radiosensitizer Ro-07-0582, a 2-nitroimidazole derivative. *Radiology (Easton, Pa.)* **122,** 801.

Urtasun, R. C., Chapman, J. D., Feldstein, M. L., Band, R. P., Rabin, H. R., Wilson, A. F., Marynowski, B., Starreveld, E., and Shnitka, T. (1978). Peripheral neuropathy related to misonidazole: incidence and pathology. *Br. J. Cancer* **37** (Suppl. III), 271–275.

Wasserman, T. H., Phillips, T. L., Johnson, R. J., Gomer, C. J., Lawrence, G. A., Sadee, W., Marques, R. A., Levin, V. A., and Van Raalte, G. (1979). Initial United States clinical and pharmacologic evaluation of misonidazole (Ro-07-0582), an hypoxic cell radiosensitizer. *Int. J. Radiat. Oncol. Biol. Phys.* **5,** 775–786.

Watson, E. R., Halnan, K. E., Dische, S., Saunders, M. I., Cade, I. S., McEwan, J. B., Wiernik, F., Perrins, D. J. D., and Sutherland, I. (1978). Hyperbaric oxygen and radiotherapy: a Medical Research Council trial in carcinoma of the cervix. *Br. J. Radiol.* **51,** 879–887.

White, R. A. S., Workman, P., and Brown, J. M. (1980). The pharmacokinetics, tumor and neural tissue penetrating properties in the dog of SR-2508 and SR-2555—hydrophilic radiosensitizers potentially less toxic than misonidazole. *Radiat. Res.* **84,** 542–561.

Willson, R. L., and Emmerson, P. T. (1970). Reaction of triacetone-N-oxyl with radiation-induced radicals from DNA and from deoxyribonucleotides in aqueous solution. *In* "Radiation Protection and Sensitization" (H. L. Morison and M. Quintiliani, eds.), pp. 72–79. Taylor & Francis, London.

Workman, P., and Twentyman, P. R. (1982). Enhancement by electron-affinic agents of the therapeutic effects of cytotoxic agents against the KHT tumor: structure activity relationships. *Int. J. Radiat. Oncol. Biol. Phys.* **8,** 623–626.

11 Clinical Results of Misonidazole in Combination with Radiation

Koji Ono
Mitsuyuki Abe

Department of Radiology
Faculty of Medicine, Kyoto University
Kyoto 606, Japan

I. Introduction

Hypoxic cells in tumors have been considered responsible for the failure after radiotherapy. Radiation therapy under conditions of hyperbaric oxygen or mixed gas of 95% O_2 + 5% CO_2 was attempted, but results were not satisfactory (Abe *et al.*, 1977; Glassburn *et al.*, 1977). The oxygen seems to be totally utilized before it can reach the hypoxic-cell region.

Electron-affinic chemicals that sensitize hypoxic cells but not oxic ones, and are biochemically stable in tumors have been developed (Adams *et al.*, 1971; Chapman *et al.*, 1972; Foster and Willson, 1973; Asquith *et al.*, 1974; Begg *et al.*, 1974; Sheldon *et al.*, 1974; Sheldon and Smith, 1975; Ono *et al.*, 1978). Misonidazole (MISO), 2-nitroimidazole, is a most promising drug now being clinically applied (Dische *et al.*, 1976, 1977; Gray *et al.*, 1976; Wasserman *et al.*, 1979; Kogelnik, 1980; Onoyama *et al.*, 1981). The clinical results of MISO and its efficacy and safety are discussed herein.

Modification of Radiosensitivity in Cancer Treatment
Copyright © 1984 by Academic Press Japan, Inc.
All rights of reproduction in any form reserved.
ISBN 0-12-676020-9

$$CH_2CH(OH)CH_2OCH_3$$

Misonidazole

II. Materials and Methods

Open clinical trials of MISO in Kyoto University Hospital, Japan, were initiated in March 1979 and closed in June 1980. A total of 89 patients with advanced relatively radioresistant cancers were entered into this trial. The sites of disease and the numbers of patients are listed in Table I. Most of the patients had a relatively radioresistant malignancy, including carcinomas of the lung and esophagus, and locally advanced head and neck tumors. The adverse reactions to MISO were analyzed for all patients enrolled in this study, and radiosensitizing effects of the drug were estimated for patients with carcinomas of the lung and esophagus, and head and neck tumors.

The combination of MISO and radiation fractionation is described next. Radiation of 4 Gy twice weekly combined with 1.0 or 1.5 g/m^2 of MISO was given mainly to patients with lung cancer. Uneven fractionation radiotherapy combined with 1.0 or 1.5 g/m^2 of MISO once weekly was given to patients with esophageal and/or lung cancers. All patients with head and neck tumors and some patients with lung cancer were treated by conventional fractionation radiotherapy combined with 0.5 g/body of MISO, five times weekly. Several patients with uterine cancer were given

TABLE I

Type of Disease and No. of Patients
Treated by Radiation + MISO

Primary site	No. patients	% Total
Lung	30	34
Esophagus	14	16
Head and neck	14	16
Uterus	13	14
Brain	8	9
Others	10	11
	89	100

a high-dose intracavitary radiotherapy combined with 2.0 or 2.5 g/m^2 of MISO.

Radiosensitizing effects of MISO were evaluated by the tumor response in all patients, and the effects on survival time were analyzed in patients with lung cancer. Tumor response was classified into three categories: CR (complete response), PR (partial response), and NR (no response). Partial response means a decrease of >50% in tumor size and no response a decrease of <50%. The 50% tumor regression dose (TRD_{50})—that is, the dose necessary to reduce the tumor size to 50% of the initial—was calculated for measurable tumors.

III. Results: Radiosensitizing Effects of MISO in Radiotherapy

A.   Effects of MISO on Head and Neck Tumors

The distribution of the tumor size indicated by T classification in patients treated by MISO plus radiation and those treated by radiation alone is given in Table II. The proportion of T3 and T4 cases was relatively greater in the MISO-treated group than in the control. Anatomical sites of the tumors in both groups are shown in Table III. All but one were treated by conventional fractionation radiotherapy of 2 Gy five times weekly in combination with a daily dose of 0.5 g/body of MISO. One patient was treated with uneven fractionation radiotherapy combined with 1.0 g/m^2 of MISO once weekly. Cumulative radiation doses ranging from 40 to 70 Gy were delivered.

Ten patients with T3 or T4 tumor in the MISO-treated group and 12 with the corresponding tumor in the control group were examined to evaluate the radiosensitizing effects of MISO. One patient with T4 maxil-

TABLE II

Distribution of Tumor Size (T Classification) in Patients with Head and Neck Tumors

Treatment group	Tumor size classification				Total patients
	T1	T2	T3	T4	
MISO	1	2	5	6	14
Control	0	9	8	4	21
	1	11	13	10	35

TABLE III

Anatomical Sites of Head and Neck
Tumors

	Treatment group	
Anatomical site	MISO	Control
Paranasal sinus	3	3
Nasopharynx	1	4
Mesopharynx	0	6
Hypopharynx	2	0
Mouth floor	1	1
Tongue	2	3
Larynx	3	2
Gingiva	2	2
	14	21

lary cancer treated with BrdU-infusion radiotherapy was excluded from the analysis. The proportion of CR, PR, and NR in both groups is demonstrated in Table IV. Complete response was obtained in 70% of all patients in the MISO group, while the response was only 33.3% in the control group. All patients in the MISO group achieved CR or PR. Clinical courses of patients with CR, in both groups, are presented in Fig. 1. Local recurrence several months after radiotherapy was seen in four of seven MISO-treated patients and in two of four control patients.

Case No. 65: A 53-Year-Old Woman with Nasopharyngeal Cancer

Biopsy revealed a well-differentiated squamous cell carcinoma. At the start of radiation therapy, the nasopharyngeal region was completely occupied by the tumor, and the base of the skull was destroyed (Fig. 2A). Lymph node metastasis in the neck region was nil. Radiation with 2 Gy combined with 0.5 g/body of MISO was delivered five times weekly. After a cumulative dose of 70 Gy the tumor disappeared, and the patient is well with no evidence of recurrence or metastasis for 2 years (Fig. 2B).

B. Effects of MISO on Esophageal Cancer

Fourteen patients with esophageal cancer were treated by radiation in combination with MISO, and 43 patients were treated by radiation alone. The distribution of morphological types of esophageal cancer is given in

TABLE IV

Distribution of Tumor Response in
Patients with Head and Neck Tumors

	Treatment group[a]	
Tumor response	MISO	Control
CR	7 (70)	4 (34)
PR	3 (30)	7 (58)
NR	0 (0)	1 (8)
	10 (100)	12 (100)

[a] Percentage of total given in parentheses.

Table V. Most patients in both groups had a spiral form of cancer about 5 to 10 cm in length on the X ray. In eight patients, 1.0 or 1.5 g/m^2 of MISO was given once weekly in combination with an uneven fractionation radiotherapy. In six patients, 0.5 g/body of MISO and 2 Gy of radiation were delivered five times weekly. In the control group, irradiation was delivered five fractions weekly with an absorbed dose of 2 Gy/fraction.

The tumor regression curve in the MISO-treated group was compared with that of the control, and the TRD_{50} values in both groups were calculated from the curves (Fig. 3). In the MISO-treated group, TRD_{50} decreased by a factor of 1.3, as compared with that of the control. No

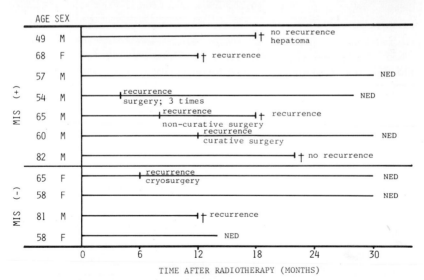

Fig. 1. Clinical course of patients with a complete response.

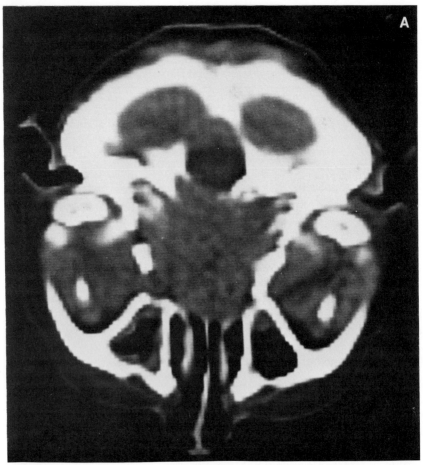

Fig. 2. A 53-year-old woman with nasopharyngeal cancer. (A) CT film before radiation therapy. (B) CT film 2 years after radiation therapy in combination with MISO.

TABLE V

Distribution of Morphological Types of
Esophageal Cancer

Type classification	Treatment group	
	MISO	Control
Polypoid	2	4
Serrated	2	7
Spiral	10	30
Funneled	0	2
	14	43

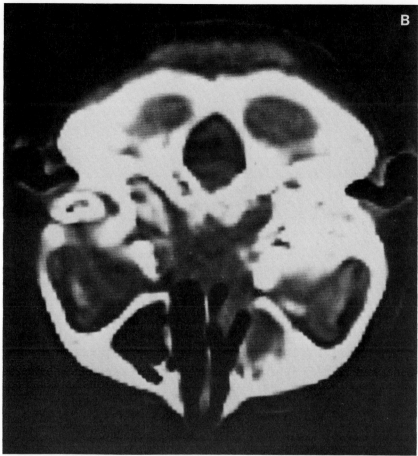

Fig. 2. (Cont.)

significant difference in the dose-modifying factors (DMF) of MISO was observed with changes in the drug dose and radiation fractionation schedules.

Case No. 54: An 83-Year-Old Woman with Esophageal Cancer

A tumor about 15 cm in length was evident on X-ray films (Fig. 4A). Radiation (2 Gy) from a ^{60}Co unit five times weekly was delivered to the lesion through parallel opposing fields of 17×8 cm. Misonidazole (0.5 g/ body) was given po 4 h before each irradiation. The tumor response to this combined radiation therapy was dramatic. There were no tumors on the

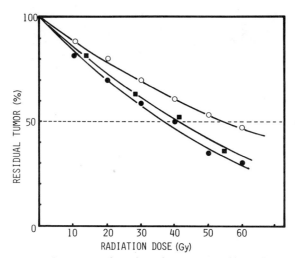

Fig. 3. Tumor regression curves of esophageal cancer treated by radiation in combination with MISO, and with radiation alone. (○) Conventional fractionation, $n = 43$. (■) Uneven fractionation + MISO, $n = 8$. (●) Conventional fractionation + MISO, $n = 6$.

X-ray film after an accumulated dose of 26 Gy (Fig. 4B). About 1 month after the completion of radiation therapy with 60 Gy, she died of pneumonia. Histopathological examination at necropsy revealed total lack of cancer cells in the field that had been irradiated.

C. Effects of MISO on Lung Cancer

Misonidazole was given to 30 patients on radiation therapy, 15 of whom received 4 Gy of radiation and 1.0 or 1.5 g/m² of MISO twice weekly. Misonidazole (0.5 g/body) and radiation (2 Gy) were delivered five times weekly, in 10 of the 30 patients. The remaining five patients were given an uneven fractionation radiotherapy in combination with 1.0 or 1.5 g/m² of MISO, once weekly. In the control group, all patients were treated with 4 Gy of radiation twice weekly.

Distributions of the histology and the disease stage are presented in Tables VI and VII, respectively.

Tumor regression rate was calculated from the changes in the tumor size, computed as the product of maximum length × maximum width, as measured on the X-ray films. The tumor regression rate was expressed as a percentage of that over the initial tumor size. Figure 5 shows the tumor regression curves. No difference in the tumor regression rate was observed between patients treated with 1.0 g/m² of MISO twice weekly and

TABLE VI

Distribution of Histology in Patients with Lung Cancer

Histology	No. patients	% Total
Squamous cell carcinoma	15	50
Adenocarcinoma	4	13
Small cell carcinoma	6	20
Large cell carcinoma	4	13
Undifferentiated cell carcinoma	1	4
	30	100

the control. The 50% tumor regression dose (TRD_{50}) was 41.5 Gy for patients given 1.5 g/m^2 of MISO twice weekly, compared to 55.5 Gy for the control. Therefore, the DMF of MISO was estimated to be 1.3 when the patients were given 1.5 g/m^2 of the drug.

Figure 6 demonstrates the survival curves in cases of MISO plus radiation and radiation alone. The 2-year survival rate of patients treated with MISO plus radiation was better than that of patients treated with radiation alone. The survival rate in patients treated by conventional or uneven fractionation radiotherapy in combination with MISO was better than that of the control group, whereas in patients treated with 4 Gy of radiation combined with 1.0 or 1.5 g/m^2 of MISO twice weekly, the figure was diminished. Patients in this group died within 6 months after the treatment.

Case No. 26:   *A 56-Year-Old Woman with Lung Cancer*

A tumor of about 8 × 8.5 cm was seen on X-ray films of the right lung (Fig. 7A). Squamous cell carcinoma of the lung was evident in the bron-

TABLE VII

Distribution of Disease Stage in Patients with Lung Cancer

Stage	No. patients	% Total
I	3	10
II	10	33
III	14	47
IV	3	10
	30	100

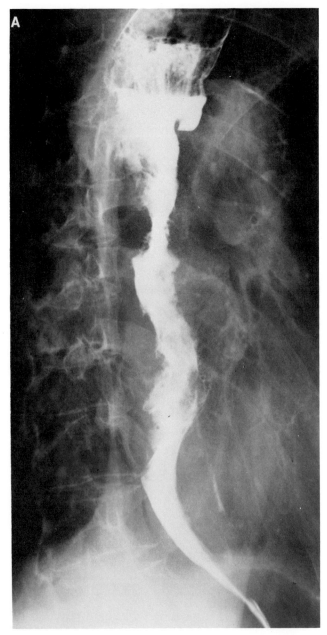

Fig. 4. An 83-year-old woman with esophageal cancer. (A) Esophagogram before radiation therapy. (B) Esophagogram after an accumulated dose of 26 Gy of radiation plus MISO.

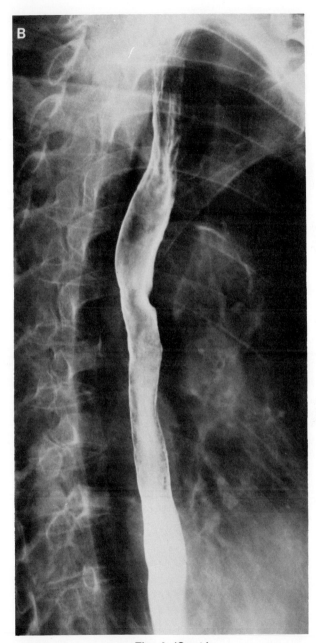

Fig. 4. (Cont.)

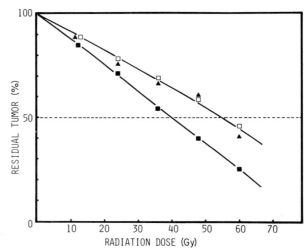

Fig. 5. Tumor regression curves of lung cancer treated by radiation (4 Gy twice weekly) in combination with MISO (▲, 1.0 g/m², $n = 7$; ■, 1.5 g/m², $n = 8$) and radiation alone (□, 4 Gy twice weekly, $n = 13$).

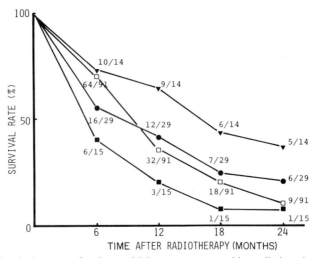

Fig. 6. Survival curves of patients with lung cancer treated by radiation plus MISO and radiation alone. (▼) Conventional fractionation + MISO 0.5 g/body; uneven fractionation + MISO 1.0 or 1.5 g/m². (●) MISO group (total). (□) Conventional fractionation (historical). (■) 4 Gy + MISO 1.0 or 1.5 g/m² twice weekly.

choscopic biopsy. She was treated by uneven fractionation radiotherapy: 5 Gy once weekly followed by 1 Gy four times weekly. She was given 1.0 g/m^2 of MISO po 4 h before irradiation with 6 Gy. After a cumulative dose of 60 Gy, the tumor disappeared, with radiation-induced pulmonary fibrosis (Fig. 7B). One year thereafter, an inoperable large tumor was found in the transverse colon and was diagnosed by biopsy to be the primary tumor. This tumor was treated by radiation combined with hyperthermia, but there was no response and she died. There were no recurrences in the lung.

D.   Adverse Effects of MISO

Adverse reactions regarded as side effects of MISO treatment during and after radiotherapy were 16 in 13 patients: 2 gastrointestinal disorders, 12 neurological symptoms, and 2 fever (Fig. 8). Skin rash never occurred in our clinical trials.

Gastrointestinal disorders such as nausea and vomiting were observed in two patients who received 2.5 g/m^2 of MISO once weekly combined with high-dose intracavitary radiotherapy for the treatment of uterine cancer. These side effects disappeared after the cessation of the drug administration. Elevation of temperature over 38°C attributed to the drug occurred in two patients with lung cancer.

Side effects such as peripheral sensory neuropathy, ototoxicity, and/or CNS disorders occurred in nine patients. These adverse effects were found in 50% of patients who received 4 Gy twice weekly combined with 1.5 g/m^2 of MISO and amounting to a total dose of over 9 g/m^2. One patient had an ototoxicity at an accumulated dose of 9 g/m^2 of MISO, and in one patient ototoxicity and peripheral neuropathy developed. The patient who received 13.5 g/m^2 of MISO exhibited symptoms of vertigo, excitation, and hallucination combined with peripheral neuropathy. The CNS disorders disappeared in a few days after the cessation of the drug administration and followed by steroid hormone treatment. In 39 patients treated with 0.5 g of MISO five times weekly, 3 had peripheral neuropathy and 1 patient exhibited peripheral neuropathy and a severe CNS disorder. A semicomatose state continued for several days and improvement was gradual. This patient had advanced uterine cancer, and right hydronephrosis was evident at the start of radiation therapy combined with MISO. Despite radiation therapy, bilateral hydronephrosis occurred and the BUN level was high. Disturbances related to excretion of MISO from the kidney probably led to an accumulation of the drug and hence to the development of neurological complications.

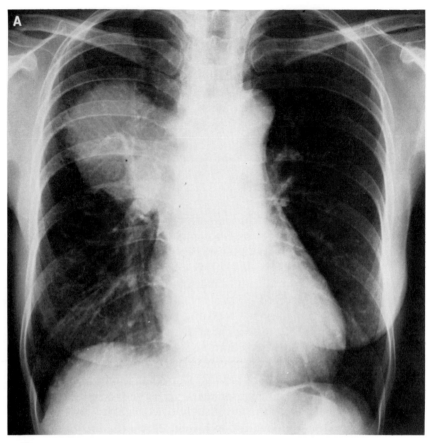

Fig. 7. A 56-year-old woman with lung cancer. (A) Chest radiogram before radiation therapy. (B) Chest radiogram after an accumulated dose of 60 Gy of radiation plus MISO.

IV. Discussion and Conclusion

Although the phase I study was designed to determine the toxicity and pharmacology, radiosensitizing effects of MISO on the tumor response and the effects on the survival were also analyzed in patients with lung cancer. Radiosensitizing effects of MISO were also observed in the phase I study in the United Kingdom (Thomlinson *et al.*, 1976) and in the United States (Phillips *et al.*, 1981). In the Radiation Therapy Oncology Group (RTOG) study, five patients with multiple lesions were treated: four with bilateral cervical metastases and one with bilateral pulmonary metastases. One side was treated by radiation plus MISO and the other by

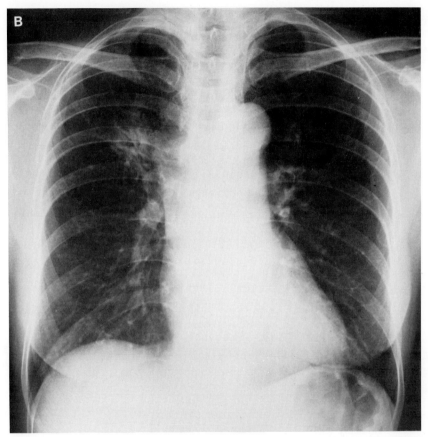

Fig. 7. (Cont.)

radiation after urinary excretion of MISO. The tumor response of the two sides was compared, and better response was observed in the side treated by radiation plus MISO (Phillips *et al.*, 1981). In the United Kingdom, a patient with multiple skin nodules related to squamous cell carcinoma of the uterine cervix was treated in the phase I study. The enhancement ratio was estimated to be 1.2 from the examination of the regression and regrowth of these skin nodules (Thomlinson *et al.*, 1976). In these two trials, patients were treated with high-dose fractionation radiotherapy combined with a large dose of MISO. In our clinical trial, the enhancement ratio of 1.3 was estimated from TRD_{50} analysis in patients with esophageal and lung cancers. Although the average serum level of MISO in patients treated with 0.5 g/body five times weekly was less than 0.1 mM, the relatively large enhancement ratio of 1.3 was obtained in patients with

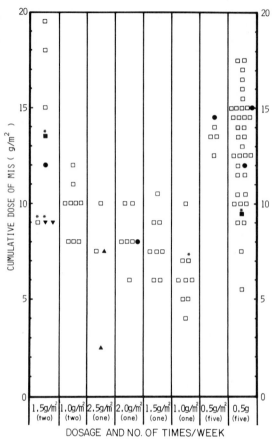

Fig. 8. Adverse reactions to MISO and drug dose. (□) No reactions; (⊡) fever >38°C; (●) peripheral neuropathy (PN); (▼) ototoxicity; (▾) ototoxicity + PN; (■) CNS disorders; (▮) CNS disorders + PN; (▲) G.I. disorders.

esophageal cancer. It has been demonstrated in *in vitro* systems that preincubation of cells in MISO results in the removal of endogenous thiols (Hall and Biaglow, 1977; Hall *et al.*, 1982). Therefore, prolonged exposure of cells to this drug prior to irradiation might account for the relatively large enhancement ratio.

The cause of early death and the poor rates of survival in patients treated with 4 Gy of radiation combined with 1.0 or 1.5 g/m² of MISO twice weekly is not clear; however, the severe radiation pneumonitis that occurred in these patients may be one reason.

Adverse reactions regarded as side effects of MISO treatment during and after radiotherapy occurred in 13 patients (14.6%). This rate is low compared with other reported data (Phillips *et al.*, 1982). The serum level of MISO was relatively low in our study. Thirty-nine patients (43.8%) were treated with radiation in combination with 0.5 g/body of MISO five times weekly, and the serum level of MISO was estimated to be less than 0.1 mM (Onoyama *et al.*, 1981). The total dose delivered was less than 10 g/m^2 in 76% of total patients enrolled in this study.

Because severe neurological side effects occurred in one patient with bilateral hydronephrosis, renal function was considered to play a role in the occurrence of these side effects. Therefore, renal function tests should be done before administering MISO.

The phase III study on MISO is in progress.

References

Abe, M., Yabumoto, E., Nishidai, T., and Takahashi, M. (1977). Trials of new forms of radiotherapy for locally advanced bronchogenic carcinoma. Irradiation under 95% O$_2$ plus 5% CO$_2$ inhalation uneven fractionation irradiation and intraoperative irradiation. *Strahlentherapie* **153**, 149–158.

Adams, G. E., Asquith, J. C., Dewey, D. L., Foster, J. L., Michael, B. D., and Willson, R. L. (1971). Part II paranitroacetophenone. A radiosensitizer of anoxic bacterial and mammalian cells. *Int. J. Radiat. Biol.* **19**, 575–585.

Asquith, J. C., Watts, M. E., Patel, K., Smithen, C. E., and Adams, G. E. (1974). Electron affinic sensitization. V. Radiosensitization of hypoxic bacteria and mammalian cells *in vitro* by some nitroimidazoles and nitropyrazoles. *Radiat. Res.* **60**, 105–118.

Begg, A. C., Sheldon, O. W., and Foster, J. L. (1974). Demonstration of radiosensitization of hypoxic cells in solid tumors by metronidazole. *Br. J. Radiol.* **47**, 399–404.

Chapman, J. D., Reuvers, A. P., Borsa, J., Petkau, A., and McCalla, D. R. (1972). Nitro-furans as radiosensitizers of hypoxic mammalian cells. *Cancer Res.* **32**, 2616–2624.

Dische, S., Gray, A. J., and Zanelli, G. D. (1976). Clinical testing of the radiosensitizer Ro-07-0582. II. Radiosensitization of normal and hypoxic skin. *Clin. Radiol.* **27**, 159–166.

Dische, S., Saunders, M. I., and Lee, M. E. (1977). Clinical testing of the radiosensitizer Ro-07-0582: experience with multiple doses. *Br. J. Cancer* **35**, 567–569.

Foster, J. L., and Willson, R. L. (1973). Radiosensitization of anoxic cells by metronidazole. *Br. J. Radiol.* **46**, 234–235.

Glassburn, J. R., Brady, L. W., and Plenk, H. P. (1977). Hyperbaric oxygen in radiation therapy. *Cancer (Philadelphia)* **39**, 751–767.

Gray, A. J., Dische, S., Adams, G. E., Flockhart, I. R., and Foster, J. L. (1976). Clinical testing of the radiosensitizer Ro-07-0582. I. Dose tolerance, serum and tumor concentrations. *Clin. Radiol.* **27**, 151–157.

Hall, E. J., and Biaglow, J. (1977). Ro-07-0582 as a radiosensitizer and cytotoxic agent. *Int. J. Radiat. Oncol. Biol. Phys.* **2**, 521–530.

Hall, E. J., Astor, M., Biaglow, J., and Parham, J. C. (1982). The enhanced sensitivity to killing by X-rays after prolonged exposure to several nitroimidazoles. *Int. J. Radiat. Oncol. Biol. Phys.* **8**, 447–451.

Kogelnik, H. D. (1980). Clinical experience with misonidazole. High dose fractions versus low doses. *Cancer Clin. Trials* **3**, 179–186.

Ono, K., Nakajima, T., Hiraoka, M., Matsumiya, A., and Onoyama, Y. (1978). Radiosensitizing effect of misonidazole on mammary carcinoma of C3H mice. *Kawasaki Med. J.* **4,** 183–191.

Onoyama, Y., Nakajima, T., Umekawa, T., Nakajima, H., Taniguchi, S., and Yamashita, A. (1981). Clinical trial of the hypoxic cell radiosensitizer. *Gann no Rinsho* **27,** 1461–1466.

Phillips, T. L., Wasserman, T. H., Johnson, R. J., Levin, V. A., and Van Raalte, G. (1981). Final report on the United States phase I clinical trial of the hypoxic cell radiosensitizer, misonidazole (Ro-07-0582: NSC #261037). *Cancer (Philadelphia)* **48,** 1697–1704.

Phillips, T. L., Wasserman, T. D., Stetz, J., and Brady, L. W. (1982). Clinical trials of hypoxic cell sensitizers. *Int. J. Radiat. Oncol. Biol. Phys.* **8,** 327–334.

Sheldon, P. W., and Smith, A. M. (1975). Modest radiosensitization of solid tumors in C3H mice by the hypoxic cell radiosensitizer NDPP. *Br. J. Cancer* **31,** 81–88.

Sheldon, P. W., Foster, J. L., and Fowler, J. F. (1974). Radiosensitization of C3H mouse mammary tumors by a 2-nitro-imidazole drug. *Br. J. Cancer* **30,** 560–565.

Thomlinson, R. H., Dische, S., Gray, A. J., and Errington, L. M. (1976). Clinical testing of the radiosensitizer Ro-07-0582. III. Response of tumors. *Clin. Radiol.* **27,** 167–174.

Wasserman, T. H., Phillips, T. L., Johnson, R. J., Gomer, C. J., Lawrence, G. A., Sadee, W., Marques, R. A., Levin, V. A., and Van Raalte, G. (1979). Initial United States clinical and pharmacological evaluation of misonidazole (Ro-07-0582) an hypoxic cell radiosensitizer. *Int. J. Radiat. Oncol. Biol. Phys.* **5,** 775–786.

12 Clinical and Pharmacological Study of Misonidazole: With Special Reference to Pharmacokinesis and Toxicology in Japanese Patients

Yasuto Onoyama

Department of Radiology
Osaka City University Medical School
Osaka 545, Japan

I. Introduction

Hypoxic cells are more radioresistant to killing effects of low-LET radiation than are oxic cells by a factor of 2.5 to 3.0 (Gray, 1961). Radioresistance of these cells in solid tumors has been regarded as a limiting factor in the local control of human cancer by radiotherapy (Thomlinson and Gray, 1955). Attempts to improve the situation led to the use of hyperbaric oxygen, high-LET radiation, etc.; however a more promising and easier method involves the combined use of chemicals that can selec-

Modification of Radiosensitivity in Cancer Treatment

195

tively sensitize the hypoxic cells to conventional low-LET radiation yet have no effect on normal oxic cells. Adams and colleagues (Adams and Dewey, 1963; Adams and Cooke, 1969) found that electron-affinic compounds could sensitize hypoxic cells as oxygen does and that there was a close relationship between electron affinity and potency of drugs as a hypoxic-cell sensitizer. Various electron-affinic substances, such as triacetoamine N-oxyl (TAN) (Parker et al., 1969), p-nitroacetophenone (PNAP) (Adams et al., 1971), and p-nitro-3-dimethylaminopropiophenone hydrochloride (NDPP) (Adams et al., 1972), were studied, but there was no sensitizing effect in vivo, mainly because of the low water solubility, toxicity, etc. Finally in the early 1970s, nitroimidazole derivatives, especially 2-nitroimidazole (Ro-07-0582, misonidazole), were found to be excellent hypoxic-cell sensitizers in cultured mammalian cells and in some rodent tumors (Asquith et al., 1974; Sheldon et al., 1974; Hall et al., 1975; Denekamp and Harris, 1975; Moore et al., 1976; Adams et al., 1976; Ono et al., 1978). Results obtained in those studies led to the rapid introduction of these compounds into clinical trials in Canada, the United Kingdom, and then in the United States (Urtasun et al., 1977; Dische et al., 1977; Wasserman et al., 1979). In Japan, experimental studies of misonidazole were initiated in 1976 by the research group organized by Sugahara, and clinical trials to determine its safety and effect in the Japanese started in late 1978. Worldwide clinical trials are in progress to evaluate the efficacy of misonidazole for clinical cancer therapy.

Designs of clinical trials for radiosensitizers differ somewhat from those for anticancer drugs. The phase I study aims to establish the toxicity, maximum tolerance dose, and pharmacokinesis of the drug among the patients receiving radiotherapy for palliative purposes. The phase II studies are directed toward specific tumor sites and histologies, and generally involve a specific regimen of radiation and drug to establish the adequate combination of both modalities. The purpose of the phase III study is to determine the efficacy of the drug, taking the benefit of sensitization and unfavorable side effects into consideration. Therefore, large-scale controlled and randomized investigations are usually required. Misonidazole is the first sensitizer that has been evaluated by systematic large-scale clinical trials; however, the compound is not an ideal drug, mainly because of its toxicity, and it is regarded as the first-generation sensitizer for hypoxic cells. However, it seems to be worthwhile to clarify the processes of the clinical studies in order to facilitate further development of new sensitizers. The purpose of this chapter is to describe the clinical results obtained in the phase studies, which have been performed through the collaboration of various institutions. Special attention is directed to pharmacokinesis and toxicology in Japanese patients.

II. Pharmacokinetic and Toxicological Study

A phase I clinical study of misonidazole in Japan was initiated in March 1979 with seven institutions collaborating (Appendix 1), including ours, and closed in June 1980. The main purpose of the study was to determine the safe and tolerable dose regimen of the sensitizer and to study the pharmacokinetic properties in the Japanese.

A. Design of Phase I Study and Patient Population

The dose regimen in the trials was determined by collecting data available at that time from the clinical trials in the United Kingdom, Canada, and the United States (Foster *et al.*, 1975; Urtasun *et al.*, 1977; Dische *et al.*, 1977; Phillips *et al.*, 1978) and evaluating these data by discrimination analysis, which showed that neuropathy occurred in less than 15% of all the patients. The curves in Fig. 1 show the upper limit of the fractional

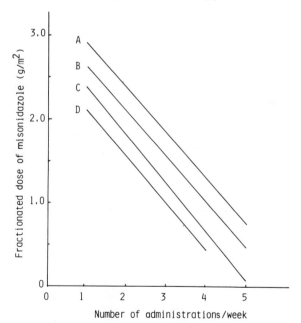

Fig. 1. Curves indicating fractional dose and weekly fractions, with which the incidence of neuropathy occurs at a rate of 15% in patients. By discrimination analysis of the collected data, a formula was derived, $Y = -0.499220X + (3.85220 - 0.11862 Z)$, where Y means single dose of misonidazole, X the fraction number per week, and Z the total dose, respectively.

TABLE I

Schedule of Misonidazole Administration[a]

Regimen	Doses/week	Single dose (g/m^2)	Maximal dose (g/m^2)
A	1	1.0	10.0
B	1	1.5	10.0
C	1	2.0	10.0
D	2	1.0	10.0
E	2	1.5	10.0
F	5	0.3	8.5
G	5	0.5	6.5

[a] Administration po 4–5 h prior to irradiation.

dose of misonidazole in relation to the total amount and weekly fractions that can be administered under the conditions previously mentioned. Seven regimens were adopted in our phase I study: 1.0, 1.5, and 2.0 g/m^2 once a week (with the maximum total dose up to 10.0 g/m^2), 1.0 and 1.5 g/m^2 twice a week (up to 10.0 g/m^2), and 0.3 and 0.5 g/m^2 five times a week (up to 8.5 and 6.5 g/m^2, respectively) (Table I). Misonidazole was given orally in the form of 100- or 500-mg capsules, 4–5 h before irradiation.

The patient population of our trial included those with advanced solid tumors who required radiotherapy but for whom control with radiation alone was ruled out. The following patients were excluded from the study: (1) patients over 70 years old, (2) systemically aggravated patients, (3) patients with cardiac, hepatic, renal, and hematological diseases, and (4) patients with neurological disorders, except those with brain tumors. A total of 106 patients were finally included in the clinical trial. All were adults with advanced malignancies of mixed primary sites and histologies, primary tumor in 78 cases, recurrent in 14, and metastatic in the remaining 14 (Table II). A single weekly dose was given to 22 patients, 29 two weekly doses, and 44 five weekly doses; 11 received doses other than the prescribed dose schedules (Table III). Drug administration was interrupted in some patients because of adverse reactions, so the mean total dose for all patients was 7.09 g/m^2 (Table III).

B. Pharmacokinesis of Misonidazole

The pharmacological studies involved measurements of variation of plasma levels according to time lapse, plasma levels at 4 to 5 h, accumula-

TABLE II

Distribution of Patients according to Drug Schedules and Tumor Sites

Tumor	No. of patients	Schedule of misonidazole[a]							
		A	B	C	D	E	F	G	Others
Brain	25	—	—	1	7	—	6	5	6
Head and neck	24	3	3	—	6	—	5	5	2
Lung and mediastinum	41	7	1	2	11	5	9	3	3
Esophagus	9	4	—	—	—	—	4	1	—
Uterus	3	—	—	—	—	—	3	—	—
Others	4	1	—	—	—	—	2	1	—
	106	15	4	3	24	5	29	15	11

[a] See Table I for description of dose schedules.

tion after consecutive administration, and urinary excretion. Frozen samples of plasma and urine were collected, and the concentrations of the sensitizer were measured by high-pressure liquid chromatography (HPLC) in the laboratory of Nippon Roche Co. Ltd.

Figure 2 shows plasma concentration curves of misonidazole and its desmethyl derivative after oral administration of various doses; the latter usually occupied around 5% of the concentration of misonidazole. Plasma levels reached the peak value at 2 h after administration with a mean half-life of 12 h, ranging from 10.3 to 13.1 h. Plasma concentrations at the time of irradiation (4–5 h after drug ingestion) had a linear relationship with the

TABLE III

Distribution of Patients according to Drug Schedules and Total Dose of Misonidazole

Total dose[a] (g/m²)	A	B	C	D	E	F	G	Others	Total
≦5.0	8	—	—	2	—	6	2	6	24
≦7.5	5	2	1	5	—	12	6	2	33
≦10.0	2	2	1	9	3	4	4	—	25
≦12.5	—	—	1	7	1	3	1	—	13
≦15.0	—	—	—	1	1	1	2	—	5
≦17.5	—	—	—	—	—	1	—	—	1
Body surface unknown	—	—	—	—	—	2	—	3	5
	15	4	3	24	5	29	15	11	106

[a] Mean total dose = 7.09 ± 0.32 g/m².

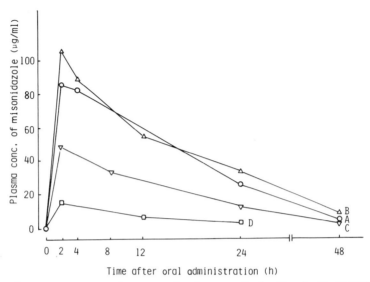

Fig. 2. Plasma concentration curves for the sum of misonidazole (Ro-07-0582) and desmethylmisonidazole (Ro-05-9963). $\triangle$, 2.0 g/m², $N = 1$; $\bigcirc$, 1.5 g/m², $N = 2$; $\triangledown$, 1.0 g/m², $N = 4$; $\square$, 0.3 g/m², $N = 7$.

dose of the drug administered (Fig. 3). Mean values for the sum of misonidazole and its metabolite were 23.4 μg/ml at a dose of 0.5 g/m², 43.6 μg/ml at 1.0 g/m², and 81.4 μg/ml at 2.0 g/m², respectively, in a total of 251 determinations (Table IV). Ingestion of food before taking the drug seemed to have some influence on the plasma level, such as delay of the peak and reduction of the area under the curve. Figure 4 shows accumulation of the drug among the patients who received five consecutive doses a week. Taking the concentration at 4 h on the first Monday as 100%, the plasma level tended to increase by 20 to 40% on Friday; however, it usually reverted to the original level after a 3-day interval.

Urinary excretion of the drug was measured in 10 patients. Total percentage excretion over 24 h of both misonidazole and its desmethyl derivative ranged from 6 to 12% of the oral dose (Table V). About one-third of the drug was excreted as the metabolite; in our series, however, the ratio of the metabolite tended to increase according to the given dose of misonidazole.

C. Adverse Reactions Observed in Phase I Study

Assessment of the side effects relating to misonidazole consisted of a thorough investigation with regard to subjective symptoms and objective

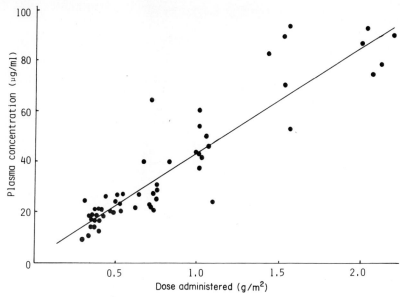

Fig. 3. Scattergram of plasma concentration (0582 + 9963) at 4 h after oral administration of misonidazole.

TABLE IV

Dosage of Misonidazole and Mean Plasma Level 4 h after Oral Administration[a]

Dosage (g/m²)	No. of doses	Mean plasma level (µg/ml)
0.3	129	15.51 ± 0.37[c]
0.5	34	23.41 ± 0.78
0.7	42	29.58 ± 1.67
1.0	23	43.60 ± 2.56
1.0[b]	2	46.14 ± 0.43
1.5	5	81.38 ± 5.02
1.5[b]	3	52.73 ± 1.80
2.0	12	81.40 ± 3.45
2.0[b]	1	90.30

[a] Plasma levels for misonidazole (Ro-07-0582) + desmethylmisonidazole (Ro-05-9963).
[b] After breakfast.
[c] Values given are ±SE.

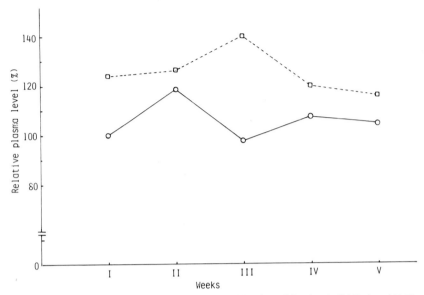

Fig. 4. Relative plasma concentrations of misonidazole on Monday (solid line) and Friday (dotted line) in two patients given five consecutive daily doses.

signs, as well as laboratory examinations including hematological and biochemical studies, during and after the misonidazole treatment.

Adverse reactions during radiotherapy combined with misonidazole included 60 symptoms in 33 patients, cumulatively, including 22 gastrointestinal disorders, 19 neurotoxicities, 4 skin rashes, elevation of serum transaminase, and 13 other reactions (Table VI). About two-thirds, or 38 symptoms, were regarded as side effects of misonidazole.

TABLE V

Urinary Excretion of Misonidazole and Desmethylmisonidazole
(0–24 h)

Dose (g/m²)	No. of patients	Excretion (% of dose)		
		0582	9963	0582 + 9963
0.3	4	4.2 (0.3–8.4)[a]	1.3 (0.2–1.8)	6.0 (0.5–10.1)
0.7	6	8.7 (3.0–16.2)	3.3 (1.7–3.5)	12.0 (5.5–22.7)

[a] Ranges are given in parentheses.

TABLE VI

Adverse Reactions to Misonidazole
among 106 Patients (Cumulative
Incidence in 33 Cases)

Symptoms	No. of patients[a]
Numbness	8 (5)
Paresthesia	2 (2)
Dizziness	2 (1)
Hallucination	1 (1)
Excitation	1 (1)
Lacrimation	1 (1)
Convulsion	1
Depression	1
Deafness and tinnitus	2 (2)
General malaise	4 (4)
Fever	6 (3)
Skin rash	4 (2)
Anorexia	8 (5)
Nausea	8 (7)
Vomiting	3 (1)
Epigastric discomfort	1 (1)
Constipation	1 (1)
Stomatitis	1 (1)
Leukopenia	2
GOT, GPT elevation	2
Blood pressure elevation	1
	60 (38)

[a] Numbers in parentheses refer to patients with symptoms thought to be due to misonidazole.

Gastrointestinal toxicities, such as nausea and vomiting, often occurred at the time of or after radiotherapy in 15 of 106 patients. It was difficult to interpret these symptoms because of the concomitant administration of radiotherapy, which did not specify radiation dose and portals in the phase I study. The incidence was dose related, in that the patients given higher doses had a higher incidence; however, misonidazole administration was interrupted in only two patients as a result of such side effects in our series, in which the maximal single dose was limited to 2.0 g/m^2.

Skin eruptions attributed to misonidazole treatment occurred in two patients. Maculopapular rashes appeared on the legs and trunk after the cumulative dose of 2.0 and 4.0 g/m^2, but disappeared spontaneously soon after withdrawal of the drug.

Serum transaminase was elevated in two patients after a dose of 3 and 8.5 g/m², respectively. Misonidazole was withdrawn in the former patient, but continued up to 10.0 g/m² in the latter. Transaminase levels reverted to normal ranges in both patients without any particular treatment at about 1 month after the cessation of the drug. Abnormal data in hematological examination were detected in several patients given the combined therapy; however, most abnormalities were related to the radiotherapy.

D. Neurotoxicity of Misonidazole

Neurotoxicity was the most important and dose-limiting side effect of misonidazole in the reports of phase I studies by other authors (Dische *et al.*, 1979; Phillips *et al.*, 1981). In our phase I study, neurological symptoms developed in 12 of 106 patients (11.3%) during or after the combined therapy. Symptoms in five of the patients were transient and disappeared in a few hours, or were not attributed to the drug. In seven patients, who exhibited symptoms that persisted for 24 h or longer, the neuropathy could be directly linked to misonidazole treatment (Table VII). Four had peripheral sensory neuropathy, two had ototoxicity, and one exhibited

TABLE VII

Patients Revealing Unequivocal Neuropathy[a]

Patient no.	Age	Sex	Tumor site	Drug schedule[b]	Cumulative dose at onset (g/m²)	Symptom
2–3	50	F	Epipharynx	D	10.6	Paresthesia of fingers and feet
3–15	68	M	Lung	E	7.5	Vertigo, excitation
3–16	45	F	Lung	E	12.3	Paresthesia of both legs
3–25	71	M	Lung	E	9.5	Hearing impairment
3–26	49	F	Lung	E	9.5	Hearing impairment
6–20	66	M	Lung	F	14.1	Paresthesia of left leg
7–7	53	F	Lung	C	4.1	Numbness of left fingers

[a] Patients with equivocal or transient symptoms not included.
[b] Refer to Tables I and III.

CNS symptoms, such as excitation, hallucination, and vertigo. Neurotoxicity occurred in 4 of 33 female patients and in 3 of 73 males, and all but one patient had a bronchogenic carcinoma. Cumulative dose at the onset of symptoms ranged from 4.1 to 14.1 g/m^2; however, it exceeded 7.5 g/m^2 with the exception of one patient. Most patients were given misonidazole according to a single or two weekly regimens with higher fractional dosage, with the exception of patient no. 6-20.

Incidence of neurotoxicity was analyzed in relation to total dose, fractional dosage, and number of fractions per week (Table VIII). In patients receiving a total dose of 10.0 g/m^2 or less, the incidence was 4 in 83 (4.8%), as compared to patients receiving more than 10.0 g/m^2 for whom the incidence was 3 in 18 (16.7%). A higher incidence (41.7%) was observed among 12 patients who received a higher fractional dose (>1.5 g/m^2). Of 75 patients receiving a total dose under 10.0 g/m^2, neuropathy occurred solely in those given a single weekly dose of more than 2.0 g/m^2 or twice-weekly doses of 1.5 g/m^2 of misonidazole (Table IX). The incidence of neurotoxicity was mainly dependent on total dose in our patients, but it was also related to fractional dosage and number of fractions per week.

TABLE VIII

Incidence of Neuropathy, Cumulative Dose, and Drug Schedule of Misonidazole[a]

Cumulative dose at onset of neuropathy (g/m^2)	A	B	C	D	E	F	G	Others	Total	
≤5.0	0/9	0/1	1/1	0/2	—	0/6	0/2	0/6	1/27	4/83 (4.8%)
≤7.5	0/4	0/2	—	0/5	1/1	0/12	0/6	0/2	1/32	
≤10.0	0/2	0/1	0/1	0/9	2/3	0/4	0/4	—	2/24	
≤12.5	—	—	0/1	1/7	1/1	0/3	0/1	—	2/13	3/18 (16.7%)
≤15.0	—	—	—	0/1	—	1/2	0/2	—	1/5	
Body surface unknown	—	—	—	—	—	0/2	—	0/3	0/5	
	0/15	0/4	1/3	1/24	4/5	1/29	0/15	0/11	7/106	
	1/22 (4.5%)			5/29 (17.2%)		1/44 (2.3%)		0/11 (0%)	(6.6%)	

[a] For description of schedules A–G, see Table I.

TABLE IX

Incidence of Neuropathy according to Fractional
Dosage of Misonidazole

Total dose (g/m²)	Fractional dosage (g/m²)				
	$\leqq 0.5$	$\leqq 1.0$	$\leqq 1.5$	$\leqq 2.0$	>2.0
$\leqq 10.0$					
Once/week	—	0/11	0/5	1/4	0/1
Twice/week	—	0/12	1/6	2/2	—
Five times/week	0/32	0/2	—	—	—
	0/32	0/25	1/11	3/6	0/1
		1/68 (1.5%)		3/7 (42.9%)	
>10.0					
Once/week	—	—	—	—	0/1
Twice/week	—	0/2	2/7	—	—
Five times/week	1/6	0/2	—	—	—
	1/6	0/4	2/7	—	0/1
		3/17 (17.6%)		0/1	

E. Tolerable Dose of Misonidazole in the Japanese Patient

Although doses given in our phase I study were lower than those in the Radiation Therapy Oncology Group (RTOG) trial, results of our pharmacokinetic study with misonidazole were essentially similar to those reported by Phillips *et al.* (1981) except for the following: Slightly higher plasma concentrations at 4 h after oral administration—43 μg/ml with a dose of 1.0 g/m² and 81 μg/ml with 2.0 g/m² (Table IV)—were observed in the series in Japan, as compared with 30 and 76 μg/ml with the corresponding doses in the RTOG series. However, the difference may be at least partly attributable to the fact that misonidazole was given before breakfast in our series, whereas it was given after a light meal in the RTOG series. The average urinary excretion over 24 h in the RTOG series amounted to 30% of the administered drugs, about half of which was identified as desmethylmisonidazole. On the contrary, only 6–12% was excreted in the urine, and the ratio occupied by the desmethyl metabolite was in the range between 20 and 30% in our series (Table V). The cause of this difference is not clear, but it may be partly attributable to the lower dose (up to 0.7 g/m^2) in the Japanese as compared with over 1.0 g/m^2 in the RTOG series. The percentage excretion and the ratio of desmethyl derivative tend to increase with the administered dose (Table V).

Incidence of neurotoxicities was as high as 50% in the RTOG phase I study, in which misonidazole was given in total doses ranging from 3 to 21 g/m^2 up to 5 g/m^2 as a fractional dose (Phillips et al., 1981). On the basis of their study, the RTOG recommended total doses to 6.0 g/m^2 in 1 week, 10.5 g/m^2 in 2 or 3 weeks, and 12.0 g/m^2 in 6 weeks. Maximum dose and average dose in our phase I study were 15.3 g/m^2 and 7.1 g/m^2, respectively. The incidence was 6.6%, as far as the unequivocal cases were concerned, or 11.3% when the transient or equivocal cases were included (Table VIII). In addition to the total dose, the fractional dose and frequency of the drug influenced the incidence in our series. Permissible incidence of major side effects of sensitizer should be determined in view of the balance between beneficial and hazardous effect; however, an incidence over 10% seems to be unacceptable. Therefore, we considered that doses of 1.5 g/m^2 once a week, 1.0 g/m^2 twice a week, and 0.5 g/m^2 five times a week with a total dose of 10.0 g/m^2 are tolerable for the Japanese. If plasma concentrations achieved with these dose levels are compared with the enhancement ratios measured in cultured cells containing the same levels of misonidazole concentration (Adams et al., 1976), concentration achievable with 0.5 g/m^2 should allow for an enhancement ratio of 1.3 to 1.4; with 1.0 g/m^2 this ratio should be 1.5 to 1.6, and with 1.5 g/m^2, 1.6–1.7. The enhancement ratios to be obtained may be lower because tumor concentrations are usually 60–80% of plasma concentration; however, a certain sensitizing effect can be expected with these dose levels.

III. Efficacy Study

Large-scale randomized trials on patients with specific tumor sites and histologies are required for the clinical evaluation of the efficacy of radiosensitizers. Such a study on misonidazole is now under way in several countries including Japan. Because of the double-blind method used in our phase III studies, no definite conclusion is possible. Therefore, we will describe our clinical observations during the nonrandomized trials and outline our phase III studies.

A. Observations in Phase I and Pilot Studies

Although the phase I study was not designed to evaluate sensitizing effects, observations were made on the purpose of the tumor irradiated

TABLE X

Sensitizing Effect of Misonidazole Observed in Phase I Study

Tumor site	No. of patients	Enhancement		
		Positive	Negative	Uncertain
Brain	25	1	6	18
Head and neck	24	6	4	14
Lung and mediastinum	41	15	6	20
Esophagus	9	5	0	4
Uterus	3	1	0	2
Others	4	3	1	0
	106	31	17	58

under conditions of misonidazole treatment. Most of the patients in the phase I study were given palliative treatment for advanced malignancies; however, in about one-half of all patients (48), evaluations on the primary effect on the tumor could be made (Table X). There was a significant increase in tumor regression in about two-thirds of the patients, as compared with findings in similar patients not given misonidazole. Tumor response seemed to be better in the patients with head and neck, lung, and esophageal cancers. The drug did not appear to be so effective for patients with brain tumors.

The same trend was observed in 27 patients in the pilot study in Osaka City University. Table XI summarizes our findings on the sensitizing effect according to tumor sites and histologies. Beneficial effects of misonidazole were remarkable in those with squamous cell carcinoma and undifferentiated large cell carcinoma, but were less marked in those with adenocarcinoma and glioma.

B. Phase II Studies

The phase II study of radiosensitizers was designed in an attempt to establish a safe and effective regimen of both radiation and sensitizer for each site of tumors. Combined use of radiosensitizer may force change in fractionation of radiation therapy and cause an unexpected adverse effect of radiation itself. A number of phase II studies with 20 to 50 patients per treatment have been carried out in the United States, United Kingdom, and European countries. In Japan most investigators proceeded to phase III study after the completion of Phase I; therefore only a limited number of such studies have been completed in the Japanese.

TABLE XI

Sensitizing Effect of Misonidazole Observed in a Pilot Study at
Osaka City University

Tumor description	No. of patients	Enhancement	
		Positive	Negative
Site			
Brain	6	1	5
Head and neck	9	6	3
Lung	8	5	3
Esophagus	4	2	2
	27	14	13
Histology			
Squamous cell carcinoma	16	9	7
Adenocarcinoma	5	2	3
Large cell undifferentiated carcinoma	2	2	0
Glioma	4	1	3
	27	14	13

Attempts to estimate the enhancement ratio of misonidazole in clinical radiotherapy were made by Ono et al., (1982). They stated that the dose of radiation required to reduce the tumor size of esophageal cancer to 50% of the initial size decreased by a factor of 1.3 by combined use of misonidazole, as compared with the historical control. The same degree of sensitization to lung cancer was observed when a fractional dose of 1.5 g/m^2 was combined with irradiation (4 Gy) twice a week.

These results suggest the presence of sensitizing effects of misonidazole in clinical cancer therapy, however, there was no evidence of effects on long-term survival. Studies on the length of survival of the patients with glioblastoma showed no prolongation by radiotherapy in conjunction with misonidazole (H. Niibe, personal communication).

In the United States, the RTOG conducted a total of 17 phase II studies. Results of the study on lung cancer (Simpson et al., 1982), esophageal cancer (Ydrach et al., 1982), glioma (Carabell et al., 1981), brain metastases (Phillips et al., 1980), and head and neck tumors (Fazekas et al., 1981) are summarized in Table XII. Although better tumor responses were observed in some tumors, the results of most phase II studies were equivocal and controversial. In some tumors, such as esophageal cancer, unconventional fractionation schemes of irradiation resulting from misonidazole treatment resulted in poorer control rates in the RTOG study.

TABLE XII

Results of RTOG Phase II Studies of Misonidazole

Tumor	No. of patients entered	Treatment schedule			Criteria of evaluation	Effect[a]
		Drug and radiation	Doses/ week	No. of doses		
Lung	51	2.0–1.75 g/m²	2	6	Tumor regression	+
		6.0 Gy	2	6	Survival	+
Esophagus	46	1.0–1.25 g/m²	2–3	12	Tumor regression	−
		4.0 Gy	2–3	12	Survival	−
Glioma	54	2.5 g/m²	1	6	Survival	±
		4.0 + 1.5 Gy	1 + 3[b]	24		
		(Boost 9 Gy)				
Brain metastasis	40	2.0 g/m²	2	6	Tumor regression	+
		6.0 Gy	2	6	Survival	±
Head and neck	50	2.5–2.0 g/m²	1	25	Tumor regression	+
		(2.5 + 2.1 Gy)	2 + 3[c]		Survival	+
		+ 1.8 Gy				
		(Boost 10–20 Gy				
		at 5 wk)				

[a] (+) Better than, (±) equal to, (−) worse than historical control.

[b] 4.0 Gy on Monday with MISO, 1.5 Gy on Wednesday, Thursday, and Friday without MISO.

[c] On Monday, the patient received two sessions of radiotherapy (2.5 + 2.1 Gy), 1.8 Gy three other times a week.

Furthermore, the limited number of patients receiving a given treatment and the lack of an adequate control group in phase II studies do not allow for a definite evaluation of the sensitizing effect of misonidazole.

C.   Phase III Studies

Several large-scale randomized trials are in progress in the United States, United Kingdom, and Europe. The RTOG phase III studies involving about 2200 patients with head and neck tumors, lung cancer, glioma, brain metastases, liver metastases, and cervical cancer, were opened in 1979 and were scheduled to be completed by the end of 1984 (Wasserman *et al.*, 1981).

In Japan, phase III studies of misonidazole have been organized with the collaboration of the 34 institutions listed in Appendix 2. Six studies with one- or two-dose regimens were initiated in 1980 and were scheduled to close in early 1983 (Table XIII). Items evaluated in these studies are local tumor control, change in performance state, length of survival, and

TABLE XIII

Phase III Studies of Misonidazole in Japan

Site of disease	Date opened	Drug schedule			Patients needed	No. of patients entered[a]
		Dose (g/m²)	Doses/ week	No. of doses		
Lung cancer	10/80	0.5	5	20	200	137
		1.0	2	10	100	
Esophageal cancer	1/81	0.5	5	20	200	113
		1.0	2	10	100	
Brain tumor	2/81	0.5	5	20		
Glioblastoma					100	99
Metastases					100	
Head and neck tumors	2/81	0.5	5	20	200	77
T$_{2-4}$ or N$_3$		0.6	4	16		
Cervix, stage III, IVA	2/81	0.5	5	20	200	89
		0.6	4	76		

[a] July 31, 1982.

side effects of the drug. Strict double-blind methods were adopted to exclude subjective impressions of beneficial and unfavorable effects of the drug. Half the total number of patients were given a placebo with the same external appearance as true misonidazole. The key for randomization was kept by a controller outside the group study. Dose regimens evolved in the phase I study ($1.0 \, g/m^2$ twice a week and $0.5 \, g/m^2$ five times a week) were generally used.

Two drug schedules were used in the lung cancer study. The first arm is radiotherapy of 2 Gy 5 days a week combined with $0.5 \, g/m^2$ of misonidazole in each session, for 4 weeks. In the second arm, patients receive irradiation of a large fraction of 4 Gy twice a week with a fractional dose of $1.0 \, g/m^2$ of the sensitizer for 5 weeks. Boost radiotherapy without misonidazole is allowed in both arms, if necessary. Two arms for esophageal cancer adopt essentially the same regimen of the drug and radiation as that used for lung cancer. Patients with glioblastoma or brain metastases receive radiotherapy of 2 Gy 5 days a week for 4 weeks combined with $0.5 \, g/m^2$ of misonidazole, in each session. Boost irradiation through the reduced field up to a total dose factor of 100 follows the cessation of the sensitizer. The schedules for head and neck cancer are radiotherapy of 2 Gy 5 days or 2.5 Gy 4 days a week for 4 weeks plus misonidazole at a dose of 0.5 or $0.6 \, g/m^2$, followed by boost irradiation without the sensi-

TABLE XIV

Adverse Reactions among 514 Japanese Patients in Phase III Study[a]

| | Site of tumor | | | | | |
Reported toxicities	Lung ($n = 137$)	Esophagus ($n = 113$)	Brain ($n = 99$)	Head and neck ($n = 77$)	Cervix ($n = 89$)	Total (%) ($n = 514$)
Peripheral neuropathy	6	2	2	5	0	15 (2.9)
CNS symptoms	1	0	1	0	3	5 (0.9)
Ototoxicity	0	0	0	0	0	0
GI symptoms	1	1	0	3	1	6 (1.2)
Skin rash	2	2	0	6	4	14 (2.7)
Liver dysfunction	0	5	0	0	3	8 (1.6)
Marrow suppression	1	0	0	0	1	2 (0.4)
	11 (8.0%)	10 (8.8%)	3 (3.0%)	14 (18.2%)	12 (13.5%)	50 (9.7)

[a] About half the patients were given misonidazole.

tizer. Patients with advanced cervical cancer receive whole-pelvic irradiation in a dose of 2 Gy 5 days or 2.2 Gy 4 days a week for 4 weeks in conjunction with misonidazole in the same dose regimen as for head and neck cancer. External irradiation is followed by intracavitary radiotherapy but without the drug.

A total of 514 patients were included in the phase III studies until June 1982. Adverse reactions observed in the studies are summarized in Table XIV. Peripheral neuropathy was recorded in 15 patients, CNS symptoms in 5, and skin rash in 14. The incidence of adverse reactions varied markedly according to the site of tumors. The highest incidence of 18.2% was encountered in patients with head and neck cancer, followed by those with cervical cancer, esophageal cancer, lung cancer, and brain tumors, in that order. The true incidence of neurotoxicity is unknown, but it can be estimated at about 8%, recalling that half of all the patients received "true misonidazole" and that all of the neurological symptoms could be attributable to the sensitizer. The incidence is in good agreement with the result of our phase I study and shows that the dose regimen in the phase III studies in Japan were acceptable, at least so far as the safety of the drug was concerned. The efficacy of misonidazole in clinical cancer therapy cannot yet be evaluated, because studies are still proceeding.

IV. Conclusions

Hypoxic cells are resistant to the effect of ionizing radiation and play an important role in the determination of the dose of radiation required to control the tumor. Hyperbaric oxygen and high-LET radiation are reportedly beneficial in overcoming this situation; however, these methods are expensive and difficult to use routinely. Rationale for the combined use of hypoxic-cell sensitizers with low-LET radiation is that these chemicals can act in the same way as oxygen and sensitize selectively the hypoxic cells in tumors. Because hypoxic cells do not exist in most normal tissues, improvement of the therapeutic ratio can be expected theoretically as the result of combination of these chemicals.

Of many candidate substances that were tested experimentally, misonidazole is the first hypoxic-cell sensitizer evaluated by large-scale clinical trial and shows considerable promise for cancer radiotherapy. Thousands of patients the world over have been included in clinical trials of misonidazole. Since 1979 more than 500 patients have been treated with the sensitizer in Japan.

Our phase I study established the pharmacokinesis, toxicology, and safe total and fractional dose in the Japanese. Pharmacokinetic behavior of misonidazole in the Japanese was essentially similar to that reported by authors in the United States and United Kingdom (Dische *et al.*, 1979; Phillips *et al.*, 1981). Neurotoxicity is the major dose-limiting side effect of misonidazole, as was also found in other countries. A total dose of 10 g/m^2 divided into 10 fractions twice a week or 20 fractions five times a week can be administered with only minimal incidence of neurotoxicity in the Japanese; this was confirmed in a large-scale phase III study.

Concerning the sensitizing effect of misonidazole, we observed the acceleration of tumor regression in several tumors. However, it is clear from our small-scale trials that doubling or tripling of control rates will not be attained by the combination of doses of misonidazole used in our study. Statistical evaluation in a large number of patients is required for the assessment of its efficacy in cancer therapy.

Misonidazole is not the ideal sensitizer mainly because of its neurotoxicity, and it may rather be regarded as the first-generation drug for hypoxic cells. Ideally, a radiosensitizer approximately 10 times less toxic or 10 times more effective than misonidazole with the same degree of sensitization or toxicity is required. Relationships between chemical structures and sensitizing effect or toxicity of nitroimidazole derivatives have been somewhat clarified. The extent of the sensitizing effect depends on the electron affinity of the molecule, which is determined by the ring structure, whereas the penetration of drugs into neural tissues depends on their lipophilicity, which is largely governed by the aliphatic side chain at the 1 position of the ring (Adams *et al.*, 1979). A more electron-affinic sensitizer, 2,4-dinitroimidazole, is being studied experimentally (Maruyama *et al.*, 1982), and less lipophilic chemicals such as desmethyl misonidazole and SR compounds are about to be introduced in the clinical trials (Brown *et al.*, 1981). Drugs with a more favorable ratio between the sensitizing effect and toxicity will no doubt be synthesized in the near future. Therefore, experiences with misonidazole should serve in evaluating new sensitizers.

Acknowledgments

Gratitude is extended to the investigators in the institutions listed in the Appendixes for their cooperation and to Nippon Roche Co. Ltd. for the supply of misonidazole and technical assistance. This work was supported in part by Grant Nos. 501063 and 56010065 from the Japanese Ministry of Education, and Grant No. 55-5 from the Japanese Ministry of Health and Welfare.

Appendix 1

Medical Schools Participating in Phase I Study of Misonidazole

Gumma University
Kawasaki University of Medical Science
Kyoto University
Kyoto Prefectural University
Tokai University
Yamaguchi University

Appendix 2

Medical Schools and Institutions Participating in Phase III Study of Misonidazole

Aichi Prefectural Cancer Center
Asahikawa University of Medical Science
Cancer Institute Hospital
Dokkyo University

Gumma University
Hokkaido University
Kagoshima University
Kanagawa Prefectural Center for Adult Diseases
Keio University
Kobe University
Kyoto University
Kyushu University
Metropolitan Komagome Hospital
Mie University
Nagoya University
Nagasaki University
National Medical Center
Nippon University
Nishi-Saitama National Hospital
Osaka City University
Osaka Prefectural Center for Adult Diseases
Osaka Red Cross Hospital
Osaka University
Saitama Prefectural Cancer Center
Sapporo National Hospital
Shiga University of Medical Science
Shinshu University
Tokai University
Tokyo Jikeikai University of Medical Science
Tokyo Medical School
Tokyo Medical and Dental University
Tokyo Women's Medical College
Yamaguchi University
Yokohama City University

References

Adams, G. E., and Cooke, M. S. (1969). Electron-affinic sensitization. I. A structural basis for chemical radiosensitizers in bacteria. *Int. J. Radiat. Biol.* **15,** 457–471.

Adams, G. E., and Dewey, D. L. (1963). Hydrated electrons and radiobiological sensitization. *Biochem. Biophys. Res. Commun.* **12,** 473–477.

Adams, G. E., Asquith, J. C., Dewey, D. L., Foster, J. L., Michael, B. D., and Wilson, R. L. (1971). Electron-affinic sensitization. II. Paranitroacetophenone, a radiosensitizer for anoxic bacterial and mammalian cells. *Int. J. Radiat. Biol.* **19,** 575–585.

Adams, G. E., Asquith, J. C., Watts, M. E., and Smithen, C. E. (1972). Radiosensitization of hypoxic cells in vitro: a water-soluble derivative of paranitroacetophenone. *Nature New Biol.* **239,** 23–24.

Adams, G. E., Flockhart, I. R., Smithen, C. E., Stratford, I. J., Wardman, P., and Watts, M. E. (1976). Electron-affinic sensitization. VII. A correlation between structures, one-electron reduction potentials, and efficiencies of nitroinidazole as hypoxic cell radiosensitizers. *Radiat. Res.* **67,** 9–20.

Adams, G. E., Clarke, E. D., Flockhart, I. R., Jacobs, R. S., Sehmi, D. S., Stratford, I. J., Wardman, P., Watts, M. E., Parrick, J., Wallace, R. G., and Smithen, C. D. (1979). Structure-activity relationships in the development of hypoxic cell radiosensitizers. I. Sensitization efficiency. *Int. J. Radiat. Biol.* **35,** 133–150.

Asquith, J. C., Watts, M. E., Patel, K., Smithen, C. E., and Adams, G. E. (1974). Electron-affinic sensitization. V. Radiosensitization of hypoxic bacteria and mammalian cells in vitro by some nitroimidazoles and nitropyrazoles. *Radiat. Res.* **60,** 108–118.

Brown, J. M., Yu, N. Y., Brown, D. M., and Lee, W. W. (1981). SR-2508: a 2-nitroimidazole amide which should be superior to misonidazole as a radiosensitizer for clinical use. *Int. J. Radiat. Oncol. Biol. Phys.* **7,** 695–703.

Carabell, S. C., Bruno, L. A., Weinstein, A. S., Richter, M. P., Chang, C. H., Weler, C. B., and Goodman, R. L. (1981). Misonidazole and radiotherapy to treat malignant glioma: a phase II trial of the Radiation Therapy Oncology Group. *Int. J. Radiat. Oncol. Biol. Phys.* **7,** 71–77.

Denekamp, J., and Harris, S. R. (1975). Tests of two electron-affinic radiosensitizers in vivo using regrowth of an experimental carcinoma. *Radiat. Res.* **61,** 191–203.

Dische, S., Saunders, M. I., Lee, M. E., Adams, G. E., and Flockhart, I. R. (1977). Clinical testing of the radiosensitizer Ro-07-0582: experience with multiple doses. *Br. J. Cancer* **35,** 567–579.

Dische, S., Saunders, M. I., Flockhart, I. R., Lee, M. E., and Anderson, P. (1979). Misonidazole—a drug for trial in radiotherapy and oncology. *Int. J. Radiat. Oncol. Biol. Phys.* **5,** 851–860.

Fazekas, J. T., Goodman, R. L., and McLean, C. J. (1981). The value of adjuvant misonidazole in the definitive irradiation of advanced head and neck squamous cancer: an RTOG pilot study (#78–02). *Int. J. Radiat. Oncol. Biol. Phys.* **7,** 1703–1708.

Foster, J. L., Flockhart, I. R., Dische, S., Gray, A., Lenox-Smith, I., and Smithen, C. E. (1975). Serum concentration measurement in man of the radiosensitizer Ro-07-0582: some preliminary results. *Br. J. Cancer* **31,** 679–683.

Gray, H. L. (1961). Radiobiologic basis of oxygen as a modifying factor in radiation therapy. *Am. J. Roentgenol. Radium Ther.* **85,** 803–815.

Hall, E. J., Phil, D., and Roizin-Towle, L. (1975). Hypoxic sensitizers: radiobiological studies at the cellular level. *Radiology (Easton, Pa.)* **117,** 453–457.

Maruyama, C., Hori, H., Inayama, S., and Mori, T. (1982). A comparative study on the radiosensitizing effects and cytotoxic properties of misonidazole and 2,4-dinitroimidazole-1-ethanol in HeLa S3 cells. *Gann* **73,** 588–591.

Moore, B. A., Palcic, B., and Skarsgard, L. D. (1976). Radiosensitizing and toxic effects of 2-nitrimidazole Ro-07-0582 in hypoxic mammalian cells. *Radiat. Res.* **67,** 459–473.

Ono, K., Nakajima, T., Hiraoka, M., Matsumiya, A., and Onoyama, Y. (1978). Radiosensitizing effect of misonidazole on mammary carcinoma of C3H mice. *Kawasaki Med. J.* **4,** 183–191.

Ono, K., Takahashi, M., Hiraoka, M., Dodo, Y., Lee, S., Hamanaka, D., Nishidai, T., and Abe, M. (1982). Radiotherapy in combination with hypoxic cell sensitizer misonidazole. *J. Jpn. Soc. Cancer Ther.* **17,** 1130–1131.

Parker, L. Skarsgard, L. D., and Emmerson, P. T. (1969). Sensitization of anoxic mammalian cells to X ray by triacetoneamine N-oxyl. Survival and toxicity studies *in vitro*. *Radiat. Res.* **38,** 493–500.

Phillips, T. L., Wasserman, T. H., Johnson, R. J., Gomer, C. J., Lawrence, G. A., Levine, M. L., Sadee, W., Penta, J. S., and Rubin, D. J. (1978). The hypoxic cell sensitizer programma in the United States. *Br. J. Cancer* **37**, (*Suppl. III*), 276–280.

Phillips, T. L., Newall, J., Order, S. E., Rubin, P., Wara, W. M., and Wasserman, T. H. (1980). A phase II evaluation of misonidazole in patients with brain metastases. *Int. J. Radiat. Oncol. Biol. Phys.* **6**, 1391–1392.

Phillips, T. L., Wasserman, T. H., Johnson, R. J., Levin, V. A., and VanRaalte, G. (1981). Final report on the United States phase I clinical trial of the hypoxic cell radiosensitizer, misonidazole (Ro-07-0582, NSC #261037). *Cancer (Philadelphia)* **48**, 1697–1704.

Sheldon, P. W., Foster, J. L., and Fowler, J. F. (1974). Radiosensitization of C3H mouse mammary tumours by a 2-nitroimidazole drugs. *Br. J. Cancer* **30**, 560–565.

Simpson, J. R., Perez, C. A., Phillips, T. L., Concannon, J. P., and Carella, R. J. (1982). Large fraction radiotherapy plus misonidazole for treatment of advanced lung cancer: report of phase I/II trial. *Int. J. Radiat. Oncol. Biol. Phys.* **8**, 303–308.

Thomlinson, R. H., and Gray, L. H. (1955). The histological structure of some human lung cancers and the possible implication for radiotherapy. *Br. J. Cancer* **9**, 539–549.

Urtasun, P., Band, P., Chapman, J. D., Rubin, H. R., Wilson, A. F., and Fryer, C. (1977). Clinical phase I study of the hypoxic cell radiosensitizer Ro-07-0582, a 2-nitroimidazole derivate. *Radiology (Easton, Pa.)* **122**, 801–804.

Wasserman, T. H., Phillips, T. L., Johnson, R. J., Gomer, C. J., Lawrence, G. A., Sadee, W., Marques, R. A., Levine, V. A., and VanRaalte, G. (1979). Initial United States clinical and pharmacologic evaluation of misonidazole (Ro-07-0582), an hypoxic cell radiosensitizer. *Int. J. Radiat. Oncol. Biol. Phys.* **5**, 775–786.

Wasserman, T. H., Stetz, J., and Phillips, T. L. (1981). Radiation Therapy Oncology Group clinical trials with misonidazole. *Cancer (Philadelphia)* **47**, 2382–2390.

Ydrach, A. A., Marcial, V. A., Parson, J., Concannon, J., Asbell, S. O., and George, F. (1982). Misonidazole and unconventional radiation in advanced squamous cell carcinoma of the esophagus: a phase II study of the Radiation Therapy Oncology Group. *Int. J. Radiat. Oncol. Biol. Phys.* **8**, 357–359.

PART FOUR

Biological Sensitization

13 Potentially Lethal Damage Repair and Its Implication in Cancer Treatment

Shigekazu Nakatsugawa

Department of Experimental Radiology
Faculty of Medicine, Kyoto University
Kyoto 606, Japan

Modification of Radiosensitivity in Cancer Treatment

I. Introduction

The current definition of damage and repair of mammalian cells was formulated after assessing cell survival using colony formation techniques. These procedures enable quantitative studies, and certain kinetic aspects of radiation damage and its repair have been clarified. However, as in the case of sublethal damage (SLD) and potentially lethal damage (PLD) repair, identification of the damaged target and the repair processes have not been investigated in detail.

In the 1960s and 1970s the existence of SLD and PLD repair in experimental tumors *in vivo* and human or murine tumor cells *in vitro* was confirmed (Belli *et al.*, 1967; Suit and Urano, 1969; McNally, 1972; Little *et al.*, 1973; Hahn *et al.*, 1974b; Shipley *et al.*, 1975a), and the relevance of repair of radiation damage following therapy for cancers was suggested. The antitumor drug-induced PLD and its repair were observed in *in vitro* cell cultures and *in vivo* murine tumors (see Section IV,A). In 1977, Weichselbaum *et al.* reported that cells from an osteosarcoma patient, one of the most radioresistant malignancies, had an extraordinarily high capacity to repair PLD after X ray. In their later studies, it was suggested that nonradiocurable tumor cells generally may undergo more extensive PLD repair than do the radiocurable cancer cells. Thus, PLD repair may be one of the most important factors determining tumor responses to radio- or chemotherapy. As for molecular mechanisms of PLD repair after UV and X-ray exposure, the relevance of excision repair was suggested by Weichselbaum *et al.* in 1978. The relationship between PLD repair and mutation or transformation was also investigated.

In the 1980s, specific inhibitors of PLD repair were detected by Nakatsugawa and Sugahara, and Iliakis. In 1982, Nakatsugawa *et al.* showed that inhibitors of X-PLD repair may potentiate the anticancer effects of chemotherapeutic drugs, especially of alkylating agents. Weichselbaum *et al.* (1982b) suggested that even in cells of human melanoma and osteosarcoma, which are radioresistant malignancies, there was little capacity for SLD repair. Other authors suggested that the radioresistance represented by the shoulder might depend on PLD repair. Thus, the classical concept and definition of SLD and PLD repair may have to be revised.

II. Definitions

A. Definition of PLD: Fixation and Repair

Potentially lethal damage and the related repair are determined according to cell survival, using colony formation. For this reason, there have been interesting but complicated phenomena in radiation biology and oncology, since the first report by Phillips and Tolmach (1966). They observed that X-ray survival of HeLa S3 cells in the exponentially growing phase was enhanced by postirradiation treatment with cycloheximide, an inhibitor of protein synthesis, but that the cell killing was enhanced with hydroxyurea, an inhibitor of DNA synthesis. Thus, PLD was defined as radiation damage that is potentially lethal but that can be modified to a nonlethal state by proper postirradiation conditioning, or may remain (potentially) lethal. Here, proper postirradiation conditioning means exposing irradiated cells to conditions where they cannot enter the first semiconservative DNA synthesis after irradiation, for example chemical treatment, low temperature, or exhausted medium (Whitmore and Gulyas, 1967; Weiss and Tolmach, 1967; Belli and Shelton, 1969; Little, 1971; Winans et al., 1972; Little and Hahn, 1973; Horowitz et al., 1975).

To investigate PLD and its repair, exponentially growing cells have been used in combination with postirradiation treatments (log phase PLD repair). Hahn and Little (1972) developed density-inhibited or plateau phase culture cell systems, as a model of tumor *in vitro*. In this system, cells are irradiated in the plateau phase, held for indicated periods of time in the same phase with various nonnutrient buffer solutions or exhausted medium (postirradiation treatment), and then trypsinized, suspended, and replated onto petri dishes to form colonies. Thus, in both systems, irradiated cells are kept for some time under inappropriate conditions for cell cycle progression and then released to grow exponentially. In the latter systems, it was found that not only ionizing radiation but also UV or bleomycin can induce PLD (Takabe et al., 1974; Hahn et al., 1974a; Hahn, 1975, 1976; Braun and Hahn, 1975; Barranco et al., 1975; Barranco, 1976). Similarly even in experimental tumors, anticancer drugs as well as X rays have been found to cause PLD (Hahn et al., 1973a; Twentyman and Bleehen, 1974, 1975b; Law et al., 1981; Horsman et al., 1982). Each of the agents induces different types of damage as detected biochemically. However, these damages apparently include PLD because, using colony formation assay, increased cell survival after posttreatment conditioning was observed. It is also not clear what types of biological phenomena are responsible for PLD repair, although some DNA repair processes might be involved. In this sense, PLD repair should probably be termed PLD recovery.

B. Definition of SLD and Its Repair

Other radiation damage and its repair were also operationally defined by Elkind and Sutton (1959, 1960) and Elkind et al. (1967). This is called sublethal damage (SLD) repair, or the Elkind and Sutton type of repair. They observed that, during an interval between split doses of irradiation, cell survival increased. It was also found that the extent of the increase correlated with the magnitude of the shoulder. Hahn (1968) observed that the plateau phase of Chinese hamster cells with no "shoulder" cannot repair SLD. No other agent other than X ray has been found to induce SLD, except for some antitumor agents (Mauro and Elkind, 1968; Dewey and Kight, 1969; Barranco et al., 1975; Barranco, 1976). However, the data on chemically induced SLD repair are most difficult to elucidate, possibly because there is a residual amount of chemicals in the cells during the pulse treatment.

The relationship between PLD and SLD repair has not been determined, but it has been clarified that in the plateau phase of cell culture or in experimental tumors, the appearance is additive (Little, 1969; Dritschilo et al., 1976; Utsumi and Elkind, 1979). Studies on SLD repair using cells from a patient with ataxia telangiectasia (AT, deficient in repair of PLD in plateau phase, see Section III,A), may aid in redefining both PLD and SLD repairs. Repair of PLD may appear in the form of change of slope of the survival curve, whereas SLD repair has been regarded as the change of "shoulder." However, several reports have suggested that even the shoulder of the survival curve depends at least partly on PLD repair. Fixation of PLD by postirradiation anisotonic treatment revealed that if most of PLD were fixed, the shoulder of the survival curve would be reduced, depending on the degree of fixation (Pohlit and Heyder, 1981). Some investigators suggested that if the time of PLD repair (holding period) is lengthened, the shoulder of the survival curve would increase (Frankenberg and Frankenberg-Schwager, 1981). This suggests that the width of the shoulder does not always represent the cells' capacity to repair SLD. Thus the classical concepts on PLD repair and SLD repair will be changed.

III. Possible Molecular Events and Modification of PLD and Its Repair

A. Plateau Phase PLD Repair

Since the plateau phase PLD repair was developed by Hahn and Little (1972), this repair in mammalian cells has been regarded as similar to liquid-holding recovery (LHR) in bacteria. However, LHR in bacteria can be observed only after UV irradiation. The involvement of excision-type repair in LHR has been suggested (Roberts and Aldous, 1949; Alper and

Gillies, 1960; Ganesan and Smith, 1968). In yeast, LHR can be seen after either X or UV irradiation, and the relevance of recombination repair as well as that of excision repair was suggested (Patrick *et al.*, 1964; Patrick and Hayness, 1964; Parry and Parry, 1976; Jain *et al.*, 1977).

In 1977, Fornace and Little suggested that cross-linking between DNA and chromatin protein in mammalian cells may be induced by ionizing radiation as well as alkylating agents and that the cross-links may be removed during the incubation of cells at 37°C. In addition to cross-links, ionizing radiation has been known to induce base damage as well as strand breaks.

As for the plateau phase PLD, Weichselbaum *et al.* (1978) and Cox *et al.* (1981) reported that AT cells are deficient in the capacity to repair X-ray-induced PLD but proficient in repairing UV-induced PLD, and that cells from a patient with xeroderma pigmentosum (XP) cannot repair UV PLD but can repair X-ray PLD. They suggested that plateau phase PLD repair, both after UV and after X-ray, may be the excision-type repair. As for UV PLD, because XP (complementation group A) cells are known to be deficient in excision repair (long patch repair) after UV exposure, the involvement of excision-type repair (long patch repair) can be proposed. However, with regard to X-ray PLD, there seem to be problems with the proposed model. This is partly because in AT cells, there are more than two complementation groups (Inoue *et al.*, 1981; Jaspers and Bootzma, 1982; Murnane and Painter, 1982); one is considered to be deficient in excision repair (short patch repair) of ionizing radiation base damage (Paterson *et al.*, 1976, 1979; Inoue *et al.*, 1977). The hypersensitivity of AT cells of other complementation groups may be due to their unchanged rate of scheduled DNA synthesis after radiation exposure (Ford and Lavin, 1981; Painter, 1981).

In 1975, Terzaghi and Little reported that malignant transformation of mouse embryo-derived 10T1/2 cells increased for the first 2 h after irradiation and then decreased, in the plateau phase PLD repair system. They proposed a model of error-prone fast repair and error-free slow repair. However, in 1979, Suzuki *et al.* reported that X-ray-induced mutation in Chinese hamster cells decreases constantly during the postirradiation conditioning. M. Watanabe and O. Nikaido (personal communication) observed that X-ray-induced malignant transformation decreased for periods of PLD repair. Both suggest no involvement of error-prone repair in the plateau phase PLD repair. It was also reported by Nakatsugawa *et al.* in 1978 that the frequency of X-ray-induced sister chromatid exchanges in mammalian cells was reduced for the first 60 min of the holding period in the plateau phase, whereas cell survivals increased up to 10 h or more after irradiation. They also suggested that an error-free fast and slow

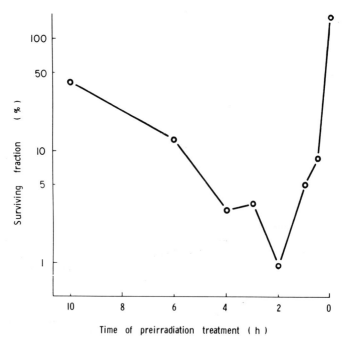

Fig. 1. Radiosensitizing effects of cordycepin (0.25 mM) given at the indicated time before 1000 rads of X irradiation. Chinese hamster *hai* cells in the stationary phase were trypsinized immediately after X-ray exposure and replated onto other dishes for colony formation (S. Nakatsugawa, unpublished).

repair may be involved in the plateau phase PLD repair. Pohlit and Heyder (1981) also suggested that there is a fast repair that is completed within 1 h after irradiation and a slow repair that is an unsaturated system with a time constant of several hours, determined by hypertonic postirradiation treatment. Using hyper- or hypotonic treatment immediately after irradiation, even in the plateau phase of Chinese hamster V-79 cells, as well as in the log phase, there is a fixation of PLD that is usually not expressed but is repaired even in cells explanted immediately after X-ray exposure, as reported by Raaphorst and Azzam (1981). They observed 1000-fold enhancement of cell killing by anisotonic treatment after 10 Gy of X irradiation, whereas a fourfold increase of surviving fractions took place during PLD repair. Similarly, as shown in Fig. 1, when cordycepin, a specific inhibitor of plateau phase PLD repair, is given 2 h before 1000 rads of X irradiation, more than 200-fold radiosensitization is achieved in the plateau phase of Chinese hamster cells. The almost complete diminution of the shoulder of the survival curve may be due to the inhibition of PLD repair (Fig. 2).

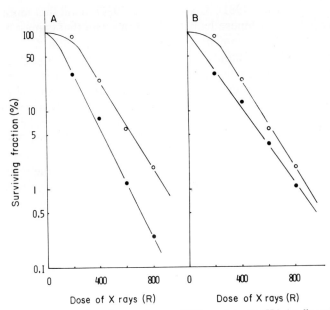

Fig. 2. Survival curves of stationary phases of Chinese hamster HA-1 cells replated after various doses of X irradiation. (A) ○, Cells treated with cordycepin (100 μg/ml) for 2 h before irradiation. ●, Cells X irradiated without cordycepin treatment. (B) ○, Cells treated with 3′-deoxyuridine (400 μg/ml) for 2 h before irradiation. ●, Cells not treated (S. Nakatsugawa, unpublished)

These data suggest that even the surviving fraction of cells explanted immediately after radiation may include large-scale PLD repair. Here, almost no cell cycle progression of the stationary-phase cells can be achieved during the holding period. Even after cells are released from the density-inhibited state, they must undergo a rather long lag period before the first DNA synthesis. Thus, during this lag before the first DNA replication after irradiation, excision-type repair (short patch repair, repair of cross-links or of base damage) must take place. After the first DNA synthesis, postreplicational repair may occur.

B. Log Phase PLD Repair

As for log phase PLD repair, there is little documentation of the existence of repair-deficient mutant cells. Radiosensitization of mammalian cells by postirradiation hyper- or hypotonic treatment—that is, fixation of PLD in exponentially growing cells as well as plateau phase of cells—has been reported (Utsumi and Elkind, 1979; Raaphorst and Dewey, 1979;

Raaphost and Azzam, 1981). Utsumi *et al.* (1981) found that mutant cells were selected from Chinese hamster V-79, a strain that cannot be sensitized by postirradiation tonicity change. They (H. Utsumi, C. K. Hill, E. Ben-Hur, and M. M. Elkind, personal communication) and Painter and Young (1982) also suggested that AT cells cannot be sensitized by anisotonic treatment. These data may indicate an involvement of not only DNA damage but also damage in membrane or chromatin structure in log phase PLD and its repair. The relevance of membrane damage repair, to repair of radiation damage, was suggested by Sato and co-workers (Sato and Kojima, 1971; Sato *et al.*, 1972; Sato and Nishizawa, 1975).

In the bacterial system, Yonei (1979, 1980) investigated the relationship between membrane fluidity and DNA damage repair, using repair-deficient mutant cells. These findings indicated a direct involvement or at least a close relevance of membrane function in damage repair. However, Nolan *et al.* (1981) found little or no involvement of membrane fluidity in PLD repair in mammalian cells. They studied the effect of membrane lipid perturbers such as butylated hydroxytoluene (BHT) on SLD and PLD repair at lower temperatures. Repair of PLD was not affected by membrane lipid perturbers in their system. As in the case of plateau phase PLD repair, studies on fixation of PLD in exponentially growing cells by anisotonic treatment suggest that most PLD may not be usually expressed or fixed at an isotonic condition, but rather repaired, resulting in 1.0 to 1.5 Gy of D_0 of the survival curve.

Damage to DNA in log phase PLD may be repaired by a repair process similar to that involved in plateau phase PLD repair—that is, excision-type repair (short patch) and postreplicational repair. Differences between log phase and plateau phase PLD repair may be due in part to the differences of their lag period before the first DNA replication after X irradiation. Similar factors may be involved in log phase and in plateau phase PLD repair. For example, H. Utsumi (personal communication) suggested that the log phase PLD repair-deficient cells are not sensitized by caffeine and cordycepin (3'-deoxyadenosine), whose inhibitory effects on plateau phase PLD repair were noted by Nakatsugawa and Sugahara in 1980. Caffeine and cordycepin reportedly sensitize cells in log phase to X ray, even when applied after irradiation (Robertson *et al.*, 1977a,b, 1978; Waldren and Rasco, 1978). As for the mechanism of radiosensitization by caffeine, increase in the level of DNA synthesis of irradiated cells may occur by induction of new replicon initiation rather than by inhibition of postreplication repair (Murnane *et al.*, 1981; Painter, 1980). As for the mechanisms of radiosensitization by cordycepin, Kada *et al.* (1982) reported that this drug inhibits DNA repair after γ irradiation, as determined by mutation induction in bacteria. However, there is little documentation of the detailed analysis of the mechanism of log phase and plateau phase PLD repair.

C. Repair of SLD

There are several reports on the chemical modification of log phase PLD repair (Phillips and Tolmach, 1966; Weiss and Tolmach, 1967; Djordjevic and Kim, 1969; Arlett, 1970). These workers studied the effects of postirradiation treatment of cells with inhibitors of macromolecules, DNA, RNA, or protein. However, there are discrepancies in the findings that are probably a result of the differences in experimental conditions. Some workers suggested that a reduction in the extrapolation number (n) can be obtained in the case of drugs. This adds support to the hypothesis that the shoulder of the survival curve depends partly on PLD repair.

However, Utsumi and Elkind (1979) suggested that log phase PLD might be independent of SLD repair, as an anisotonic treatment may affect log phase PLD repair as well as plateau phase PLD repair, but not SLD repair or UV sensitivity. There seem to be two agents that inhibit both SLD and PLD repairs in the plateau phase: actinomycin D and hyperthermia (Elkind et al., 1964; Elkind and Kano, 1970; Ben-Hur et al., 1974; Li et al., 1976; Dritschilo et al., 1979). Thus, there is apparently still much to learn of the relationship between SLD and PLD repair. Suzuki et al. found in 1979 that X-ray-induced mutation in mammalian cells was reduced when X-ray doses were split. They suggested that SLD repair might be error-free repair. However, studies on the molecular mechanisms of SLD repair using a repair-deficient mutant such as AT are required to support the proposed error-free repair model.

D. Repair of UV PLD

As for the molecular mechanisms in UV-PLD repair in the plateau phase, Weichselbaum et al. (1978) suggested that excision-type repair (long patch repair) may be involved in the increase of cell survival. McCormick and Maher (1981) suggested that the frequencies of UV-induced mutation in the plateau phase of mammalian cells can be reduced during the holding period. This also may support the idea that most of the UV-induced PLD may be repaired by excision-type repair (long patch type) during the relatively longer holding periods than that of X-ray-induced PLD, that is, 24–72 h of holding, which may correspond well with the time course of pyrimidine dimer excision.

It seems that the repair of UV-induced PLD in the log phase cells is much smaller than that in the plateau phase cells. The anisotonic treatment, much like cordycepin, does not affect UV sensitivity of log phase of cells (Utsumi and Elkind, 1979; S. Nakatsugawa, unpublished).

E. Chemical PLD Repair

5-Fluorouracil (5-FU) is not usually considered to cause DNA damage, but rather to inhibit deoxythymidilate (dTMP) synthetase, inhibit DNA synthesis, produce abnormal RNA, alter enzymes or proteins, or inhibit synthesis and utilization of uracil nucleotide (Madoc-Jones and Bruce, 1967; Balis, 1968; Hahn *et al.*, 1973a). Apparently there are no data suggesting DNA damage or its repair after 5-FU treatment. Bleomycin binds to DNA at the guanine or cytosine residue, induces DNA strand breaks, and inhibits DNA ligase. In the case of bleomycin-induced PLD repair (Hahn *et al.*, 1973a; Twentyman and Bleehen, 1973, 1974, 1975b; Twentyman, 1976a,b; Barranco *et al.*, 1975; Barranco, 1976), rejoining of DNA strand scissions may be involved in the repair processes. Alkylating agent-induced PLD may also be involved, as it is well known that these agents cause cross-linking between the different DNA strands, between guanine bases in the same strand, or between DNA and other molecules. Moreover, bifunctional alkylating agents as well as monofunctional alkylating agents are thought to induce adducts in DNA. Both monoadducts and cross-links may be repaired by base excision and nucleotide excision repair. However, it is not clear whether postreplicational repair (recombination) might be involved in the repair of alkylating agent-induced damage, although it does not seem likely (Cleaver, 1978; Hanawalt *et al.*, 1979). Among antitumor agents tested, only adriamycin and mitomycin C (Silvestrini *et al.*, 1963; Calendi *et al.*, 1965) does not seem to induce PLD (Hahn, 1976; T. Miyamoto, personal communication).

F. Summary

Specific inhibitors of PLD repair in plateau-phase cells after X irradiation, such as the nucleoside analogs, $3'$-deoxyadenosine ($3'$-dA), $3'$-deoxyguanosine ($3'$-dG), $2',3'$-dideoxythymidine, β-D-arabinofuranosyladenine and -cytosine, are now available (Table I) (Nakatsugawa and Sugahara, 1980; Nakatsugawa *et al.*, 1982a; Iliakis, 1980, 1981; O. Nikaido, personal communication). In the stationary phase of mammalian cells, it has been shown recently that the fidelity of DNA polymerases was less than that in exponentially growing cells (S. Linn, personal com-

TABLE I

Modifying Factors of X-Ray–Induced PLD Repair (Nakatsugawa's Model)

Altered or unaltered semiconservative DNA synthesis after X-exposure
   AT (ataxia telangiectasia), Caffeine, Aphidicolin, Cell cycle distribution at radiation exposure, Hyperthermia
Modulation of structure or stability of membrane or of chromatin
   Tonicity change, Hyperthermia
Alteration of intracellular nucleotide pool
   Chain terminators (3'-deoxyadenosine and -guanosine, 2',3'-dideoxythymidine, β-D-arabinofuranosyladenine and -cytosine), Hydroxyurea, Inhibitors of Poly(ADP-ribose) synthesis (Caffeine, 3-aminobenzamide, nicotinamide), Other base or nucleoside analogs
Modification of radiation damage (damage interaction)
   Actinomycin D, Adriamycin,
Energy metabolism alteration
   2-Deoxy-D-glucose
Defective excision repair
   AT, Inhibitors of Poly (ADP-ribose) synthesis
Inhibition of short patch repair replication [DNA polymerase β (α)]
   Chain terminators, Hyperthermia
Inhibition of ligation
   Chain terminators, Inhibitors of Poly (ADP-ribose) synthesis, Hyperthermia

---

munication). Therefore, it might be postulated that in stationary phase cells 3'-dA and 3'-dG, which are analogs of RNA precursors, might be incorporated into DNA, and through this mechanism, result in the inhibition of PLD repair. The aforementioned repair inhibitors are all terminators of DNA and RNA chain elongation. Some nucleosides and their analogs such as adenosine and formycin B, which are not chain terminators, have no effect on PLD repair (S. Nakatsugawa, unpublished data). The involvement of chain elongation in DNA repair might be limited to the repair replication and ligation steps.

Recently Cleaver (1983) and S. Linn, (personal communication) have suggested that both DNA polymerase α and β are involved in long patch repair replication after UV exposure. However, a specific inhibitor of α polymerase, aphidicolin does not inhibit repair of X-ray–induced PLD but rather enhances this repair (Iliakis et al., 1982; S. Nakatsugawa, unpublished data). The importance of short patch repair replication in the repair of X-ray–induced damage is not well known, but it may play a role in PLD repair. 3'-dA and 3'-dG do not affect UV sensitivity and SLD repair after X exposure, but these agents might inhibit chemically induced PLD repair as well as X-ray PLD repair (Nakatsugawa and Sugahara, 1980; Nakatsugawa et al., 1982a; Iliakis, 1980, 1981; Robertson et al. 1977b).

Therefore, these inhibitors may inhibit the short but not the long patch repair replication, as in the case UV-damage repair.

Another possibility is that the ligation step may be inhibited by these inhibitors. This has been suggested by the data of Bryant and Blocher (1982), which showed that 1-β-ara A inhibits the rejoining of DNA double-strand breaks and about 70% of single-strand breaks. These effects are partially reversible. Inhibitors of poly(ADP-ribose) synthesis, such as 3-aminobenzamide, caffeine and nicotinamide have also been suggested as suppressors of PLD repair in plateau phase cells (Nakatsugawa and Sugahara, 1980; S. Nakatsugawa, unpublished data; O. Nikaido, personal communication; J. Brown, personal communication). Although these poly(ADP-ribose) synthesis inhibitors interfere with the ligation processes in DNA repair, they also alter the intracellular nucleotide pools (Ueda *et al.*, 1983; J. Cleaver, personal communication), an effect that may also result in inhibition of repair of PLD. Nucleoside pool size might also be altered by the above chain terminators or hydroxyurea. The action of hydroxyurea in fixing PLD after X-rays and in altering nucleotide pool size are known (Phillips and Tolmach, 1966), further supporting the hypothesis that these processes may be involved in PLD repair. These drugs and labeled compounds of these specific repair inhibitors will be useful tools to investigate further the molecular events in radiation- and chemically induced damage and the repair of these types of damage.

IV. Clinical Significance of PLD Repair

A. Clinical Significance of X-Ray PLD Repair in Cancer Cells

There have been numerous reports dealing with the role of PLD repair on radioresistance of cancer cells and the significance in radiotherapy for cancer (Little *et al.*, 1973; Hahn *et al.*, 1974b; Shipley *et al.*, 1975b; Weichselbaum *et al.*, 1977, 1980, 1982; Nakatsugawa and Sugahara, 1980). The existence of PLD repair after irradiation has been confirmed in various experimental tumors, and it was also observed that various types of anticancer drugs, mainly alkylating agents, induced PLD that can be repaired in murine tumors *in vivo*. From the point of view of cancer therapy, log phase PLD repair may be of less significance than plateau phase PLD repair. Therefore, plateau phase PLD repair is emphasized here.

In 1980, Nakatsugawa and Sugahara found that capacities in cells to perform X-PLD repair varies between the different cell growth phases, and they observed that the apparent increase of PLD repair was proportional to the increase of noncycling or quiescent (Q) cells, which was in agreement with the findings of others (Little *et al.*, 1973; Hahn *et al.*, 1974b). As shown in Fig. 3, the magnitude of PLD repair during 10 h in Hanks' BSS after 1000 rads increases from 2 to 3 in log phase to about 20

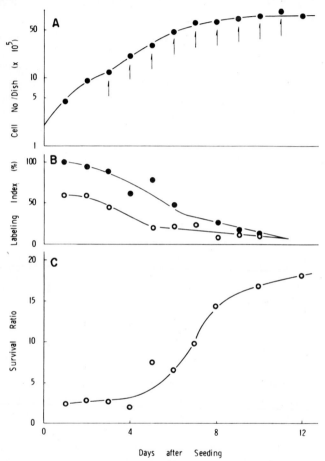

Fig. 3. The relationship between the growth phase and the magnitude of PLD repair after exposure to 1000 R of X rays in *hai* cells. (A) Growth curve of *hai* cells after seeding 2×10^5 cells per dish. (B) Labeling indices after 24 h of incubation in complete medium and Hanks' BSS containing 0.1 μCi/ml of [³H]TdR. (C) Variation in the capacity of the cells to perform PLD repair at different stages of growth, after 10 h of postirradiation incubation in Hanks' BSS. The magnitude of PLD repair is expressed as the survival ratio, in which the surviving fraction immediately after X irradiation is taken to be 1.0. Arrows indicate daily medium changes. (●) Changes in the cells incubated in complete medium. (○) Changes in the cells incubated in Hanks' BSS.

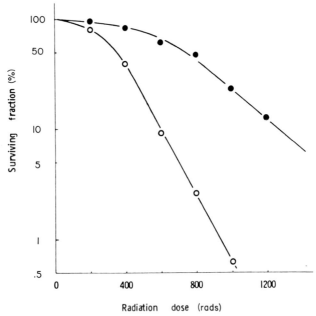

Fig. 4. Repair of PLD in X-ray dose–survival curves of the late stationary phases of Chinese hamster cells. Cells were either explanted immediately (○) or left in the Hanks' BSS for 10 h after X irradiation and then replated onto petri dishes for colony formation (●). Nakatsugawa *et al.* (1982b).

in the late stationary phase. The magnitude of PLD repair is expressed as the survival ratio (Fig. 3C), in which the cell survival of immediate explants is taken to be 1. In the late stationary phase, D_0 of the cells increased to more than twofold when held in the plateau phase for 10 h after irradiation (Fig. 4). Repair of PLD reportedly functions even under conditions of hypoxia (Hahn *et al.*, 1973b; Urano *et al.*, 1976). However, it is clinically well known that most rapidly growing cancers are often much more sensitive to radiotherapy and chemotherapy than are slow-growing tumors, which may have a large proportion of Q cells. Thus, one possible explanation for differences in responses to therapy may be the differences in cellular capacity to repair PLD, as proposed by Weichselbaum *et al.* (1977, 1980, 1982a,b). They found that tumor cells that are relatively nonradiocurable, as a group, may undergo much more X-PLD repair than normal diploid fibroblasts, whereas cancer cells from radiocurable tumors undergo almost the same PLD repair as normal fibroblasts. Tumor cells with the intermediate curability may have an intermediate capacity. According to their data, these differences may not be explained by cell kinetics or Q-cell population size, but may be due to the intrinsic cellular capacity to repair. These workers tested more than 10 different kinds of human cancers, and an additional number of specimens should reveal whether a generalization of this parallelism between the cancer cells' capacity to perform PLD repair and the curabilities of cancers is valid.

B. Clinical Significance of SLD Repair in Cancer Cells

Since the first discovery by Elkind and colleagues (Elkind and Sutton, 1959, 1960; Elkind *et al.*, 1967), SLD repair may be one of the most important factors influencing the curability of human cancers by radiation therapy. This is partly because the usual radiotherapy involves adoption of fractionated protocols of low-LET radiation. It would be reasonable to assume that during fractionation, SLD would be required (Elkind *et al.*, 1968). There are no data available showing the extraordinarily high or much higher capacity of human cancer cells to repair SLD than that of normal human diploid fibroblasts, which have rather a small extrapolation number, less than 2. Among the human cancer cells or their lines, only malignant melanoma cells have been reported to have a wide "shoulder," extrapolation number of 4 to 40.

Most reports on melanoma cells have suggested that the radioresistance of melanomas might be attributable to their large shoulder, that is, their higher capacity to repair SLD. However, Weichselbaum *et al.* (1982) reported that in melanoma and osteosarcoma cells, cell survival is increased only up to twofold, even during a sufficient interval between the fractionations. This suggests that the melanoma and osteosarcoma cells have a low capacity to repair SLD, although they are radioresistant. Chavaudra *et al.* (1981) suggested that the radioresistance might be due to the greater population of hypoxic cells, as determined using two human melanomas transplanted into *nude* mice. Their data and the data mentioned in the previous section suggest that the very low radiocurability of melanomas may not be attributable to SLD repair capacity but rather to PLD repair or to hypoxic-cell population. Thus, the role of SLD repair on cancer cells' radioresistance may be considerably less than is sometimes assumed.

C. Normal Tissue: X-PLD Repair and SLD Repair

There are few reports on repair of PLD or of SLD in normal tissues and its role in cancer radiotherapy. Some findings have suggested that in normal tissues, both PLD and SLD repairs probably are operative, but the magnitude may be small. Gould and Clifton (1979), reported that in mammary glands and the thyroid, *in situ* repair, probably similar to PLD repair, may function in radiation damage during the period of holding *in situ* and result in a great increase in the shoulder. Thomas and Gould (1982) suggested that even in bone marrow PLD repair may function, but in their case, after 9 h of holding *in situ,* the extrapolation number decreased to 1 and D_0 did not change.

Nakatsugawa *et al.* (1982b) found that radiation-induced bone marrow death may not be enhanced by a specific PLD repair inhibitor, cordycepin. In bone marrow, the magnitude of PLD repair may be small. Using a new technique, Lin *et al.* (1982) found that lung alveolar macrophage colony-forming cells may repair not PLD but rather SLD. Deschavanne *et al.* (1981) also used a new technique and studied the repairs of both PLD and SLD. Kidney cells showed less than a fourfold increase in survival during 8 h of holding *in situ* after 12 Gy of γ irradiation, and then survival decreased. Immediately explanted cells, those delayed for 8 h, and those delayed for 24 h had D_0 values of 1.56, 2.31, and 1.92 Gy, respectively. The authors suggested that the magnitude of SLD repair during 8 h of interval between two 6-Gy doses may be 2.7-fold of cell survival increase. Similar PLD and SLD repair was observed in mouse lungs. After 10.5 Gy of irradiation and *in vivo* holding, survival of lung cells increased for 6 h but then decreased to the level of 0 h, 24 h later, K. Ono (personal communication) observed that radiation-induced oral mucosal death (OMD) of mice was not enhanced by an inhibitor of PLD repair, N^6-butyrylcordycepin (N^6-BC). These specific inhibitors of PLD repair may be effective tools for measuring the capacity of normal tissues or cells as well as cancer cells to repair PLD.

D. Significance of Chemical-PLD Repair in Cancer Therapy

Bleomycin, 5-FU, CCNU, L-PAM, cyclophosphamide, mechlorethamine, methylmethane sulfonate, and actinomycin D reportedly induce PLD (Hahn *et al.*, 1973a; Barranco *et al.*, 1975; Takabe *et al.*, 1974; Hahn, 1975, 1976; Braun and Hahn, 1975; Barranco, 1976; Law *et al.*, 1981; Horsman *et al.*, 1982).

One exception among the DNA-damaging agents seems to be adriamycin. It is postulated that this drug may intercalate between bases of DNA chain, resulting in the inhibition of synthesis of DNA and RNA (Calendi *et al.*, 1965). Hahn *et al.* (1975), T. Miyamoto (personal communication), and Barranco (1976) suggested that adriamycin might not induce PLD. A large number of cancer chemotherapeutic agents do appear to be DNA-damaging chemicals. Thus, the repair of chemical-induced PLD may play an important role in the resistance of human cancer cells against antitumor drugs. It is well known that slow-growing cancers, particularly solid tumors, are much more resistant against any combination of anticancer chemical than are rapid-growing cancers such as leukemia. In consideration of cell kinetics, fixation of PLD may take place readily in rapidly growing cancers, because the relative lag period between the treatment and the first DNA synthesis is shorter. Involvement of hypoxia in the chemoresistance (resistance against chemotherapy) of cancer cells has been suggested (Martin *et al.*, 1981; Law *et al.*, 1981; Horsman *et al.*, 1982). However, the role of hypoxia in chemoresistance may be much smaller than its role in radioresistance.

V. Significance of PLD Repair Inhibition in Radiotherapy and Chemotherapy

A. Inhibition of X-PLD Repair

The magnitude of PLD repair *in situ* in human nonradiocurable cancer may be much larger than in cells in normal tissues. Therefore, complete inhibition of PLD repair would lead to a differential or selective radiosensitization of cancer cells. Using specific inhibitors, purine nucleoside analogs, the magnitude of PLD repair in tumors or normal tissues can be assessed. Moreover, with application of PLD repair inhibitors as radiosensitizers, there may be a selective sensitization of tumors. The significance of PLD repair inhibitor in cancer radiotherapy has been partly confirmed using experimental tumors. Hypoxic-cell sensitizers such as misonidazole have different molecular mechanisms of radiosensitization from those of PLD repair inhibitors. The combination of a hypoxic-cell sensitizer, radiation, and a PLD repair inhibitor is worthy of consideration.

Other than the specific chemical inhibitors mentioned already, there have been a few reports on the inhibition of plateau phase PLD repair (Evans *et al.*, 1974). One is the inhibition by hyperthermia as Li *et al.* first reported (1976), and another is that by actinomycin D, as reported by Dritschilo *et al.* (1979), the inhibition of which is reversible and therefore less applicable in cancer therapy. It is interesting that both may suppress SLD repair as well as PLD repair (Elkind *et al.*, 1964; Elkind and Kano, 1970; Ben-Hur *et al.*, 1974; Li *et al.*, 1976; Dritschilo *et al.*, 1979). The purine nucleoside analogs may not suppress SLD repair. Another radiosensitizing alkylating agent, ICRF-159 (Hellmann and Murkin, 1974; Ryall *et al.*, 1974), has been reported to suppress SLD but not PLD repair (Taylor and Bleehen, 1977a,b).

In bacterial LHR, Yonei (1980), suggested that membrane-binding drugs, which modify or change the membrane fluidity of cells, inhibit the LHR in *E. coli* after UV exposure. They used chlorpromazine, procaine, and quinidine as the membrane drugs. In cultured mammalian cells, (L5178Y cells), these drugs reportedly sensitize hypoxic cells to X ray in order to protect the oxic cells and to potentiate hyperthermic cell killing (Yau and Kim, 1980). Shenoy and Singh (1980) also indicated that chlorpromazine may have cytotoxic and radiosensitizing effects in sarcoma 180A tumors in male Swiss albino mice. However, C. Y. Mitsutani (personal communication) suggested that the effects of membrane drugs on radiosensitivity may depend on the cell strain, and such effects were not observed in HeLa cells or Chinese hamster cells but only in mouse L1210 or L5178Y cells. Raaphorst and Azzam (1981) suggested that polyamines such as spermine and spermidine may fix the X-ray-induced PLD in both log and plateau phase, of Chinese hamster V-79 cells.

High-LET radiation therapy has attracted attention of radiotherapists; the advantages include low oxygen enhancement ratio, high RBE (relative biological effectiveness), low cell cycle dependency of radiosensitivity, and small repair after exposure. Thus, low PLD or SLD repair can be achieved by high-LET radiation. Because the application of high-LET radiation therapy requires a considerable expense, large facilities, and experts for operation and maintenance, the number of facilities now available is limited. Hypoxic-cell radiosensitizers may complement the disadvantages of low-LET radiation. Fragyl and misonidazole at clinically applicable doses have not achieved the high enhancement ratio (ER). Desmethylmisonidazole (Ro-07-9963), Ro-03-8799, and SR-2508, which may be less toxic than misonidazole, are undergoing clinical trials (Brown, 1982). Inhibitors of PLD repair may complement the defect of low-LET radiations and may achieve higher ER, in combination with hypoxic-cell sensitizers.

Another significance of the inhibition of PLD repair may be related to the problems of secondary tumors induced by X ray. Clark *et al.* (1981) suggested that preirradiation hyperthermia increased the frequency of X-ray-induced malignant transformation by a factor of 4 to 5. Gilman and Thilly (1977) suggested that heat might increase the mutability of human diploid lymphoblasts. In contrast, Harisiadis *et al.* (1980) suggested that postirradiation heat treatment reduced oncogenic transformation. M. Watanabe (personal communication) suggested that if heat is given concomitantly with irradiation, the induction of X-ray carcinogenesis was reduced. Postirradiation hyperthermia reportedly inhibits the X-PLD repair in the plateau phase. Spiro *et al.* (1982) stated that heat may decrease the activity of DNA polymerase β, which has been regarded as one of the repair enzymes (Waser *et al.*, 1979; Wawra and Dolejs, 1979; Siedlecki *et al.*, 1980).

These data suggest that if PLD repair is inhibited, there may be a reduction in X-radiation carcinogenesis. Misonidazole has been reported to increase the X-ray-induced oncogenic transformation and to be mutagenic at bacterial levels (Miller and Hall, 1978). Therefore, misonidazole may be called a "nonclean sensitizer." One of the PLD repair inhibitors, cordycepin, reportedly reduces the 3-methylcholanthrene-induced carcinogenesis (Price *et al.*, 1975); thus it can be called a "clean sensitizer." Problems of secondary tumorigenesis after radiotherapy and chemotherapy are often related to complications of cancer treatment. In this sense, inhibition of X- and chemical-PLD repairs should be of great importance.

B. Chemical-PLD Repair Inhibition

Hyperthermia may influence the frequency of malignant transformation induced by X ray. Braun and Hahn (1975) reported that bleomycin-induced PLD repair is inhibited by postirradiation heat treatment, but not by preirradiation heat treatment. Most of the anticancer drugs, especially DNA-damaging agents, are mutagenic or oncogenic. The data on the effect of hyperthermia on PLD repair suggest that if the antitumor drug-induced PLD is inhibited by specific inhibitors, the chemical carcinogenesis may be reduced.

The lack of reports on the inhibition of chemically induced PLD repair is possibly due to the underestimation of PLD repair in chemotherapy. Other than the inhibition by heat (Braun and Hahn, 1975; Hahn *et al.*, 1975), Nakatsugawa and Sugahara (1982) suggested that the specific inhibitors of X-ray-induced PLD repair may inhibit the antitumor drug-induced PLD repair. M. R. Horsman (personal communication) indicated that inhibitors may suppress L-PAM PLD repair of RIF-1 tumor cells. Ishii and Bender (1978) reported the inhibitory effect of caffeine on prereplication repair of mitomycin C-induced DNA damage. Byfield *et al.* (1981) found that caffeine, theophylline, and theobromine may sensitize tumor cells to alkylating agents. Mizuno and Ishida (1982) reported that local anesthetics (membrane-related drugs) such as dibucaine, tetracaine, butacaine, lidocaine, and procaine enhance cell killing by bleomycin, but not by adriamycin, mitomycin C, and *cis*-chlorodiamineplatinum (II). These data suggested a possible clinical application as potentiators of chemotherapy. However, data on experimental tumor systems using these agents have not been reported.

VI. Possibility of Clinical Application of PLD Repair Inhibitors as Radio- and Chemosensitizers in Human Cancer Therapy

A. Studies in Experimental Cancer Therapy

More than 100 chemicals have been tested in the screening system of PLD repair inhibitors *in vitro* (N. Nakatsugawa and T. Sugahara, unpublished; Iliakis, 1980, 1981; Sugahara and Nakatsugawa, 1981; Nakatsugawa *et al.*, 1982a; U *et al.*, 1982; M. Watanabe, personal communication). (Fig. 5). Among these chemicals, three purine nucleoside analogs—that is, 3'-deoxyadenosine (3'-dA, cordycepin), 1-β-D-arabinofuranosyladenine (Ara-A), and 3'-deoxyguanosine (3'-dG) were selected, as shown in Fig. 6. Among these three nucleoside analogs, 3'-dG was the least toxic when tested in experimental cancer therapy ($LD_{50} = 1.0$ g/kg), whereas 3'-dA, although a potent inhibitor, was comparatively toxic ($LD_{50} = 0.3$ g/kg) (S. Kodama, personal communication) and was readily inactivated by adenosine deaminase. To prevent the deamination of 3'-dA, N^6-butyryl-3'-dA (7904) was tested in experimental treatment of tumors. In experimental radiotherapy using EMT-6 tumors, as shown in

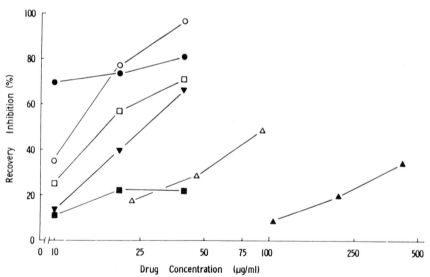

Fig. 5. Efficiencies of nucleoside analogs against PLD repair in Chinese hamster cells *in vitro,* with radiation dose of 1000 rads. (○) 3'-dA, (●) Ara-A, (□) 3'-dG, (▼) 7904; (△) 2',3'-ddT, (■) 3'-dC, (▲) 3'-dU.

Fig. 6, potent radiosensitization with ER = 2.2 was achieved by 7904 (U *et al.*, 1982; Nakatsugawa *et al.*, 1982b). However, in RIF-1 tumors in which PLD repair may be low (Rasey and Nelson, 1981), 7904 showed an ER of only 1.4. The applied dosage of PLD repair inhibitors was 80–100 mg/kg in experimental radiotherapy. Even in a dose of 300 mg/kg, Ara-A showed no radiosensitization in RIF-1 and SCCVII tumors, possibly because of the deamination (S. Nakatsugawa and T. Sugahara, unpublished).

In experimental chemotherapy using EMT-6 tumors, 50 mg/kg of 3'-dG potentiated the effects of some antitumor drugs such as ACNU, FT-207, and bleomycin (Nakatsugawa and Sugahara, 1982; U *et al.*, 1982; Nakatsugawa *et al.*, (1982b). In syngeneic SCCVII (SQ$_1$) tumors, Ara-A (16–32 mg/kg) and 3'-dG (32 mg/kg) enhanced the effects of alkylating agents such as ACNU (12 mg/kg) and cyclophosphamide (10–40 mg/kg), which were given ip daily (Nakatsugawa, 1982; S. Nakatsugawa and T. Sugahara, unpublished). In particular, with the combination of cyclophosphamide and 3'-dG, the ER value obtained from the dose–growth delay time curve was 3.0 in large syngeneic SCCVII tumors (initial mean diameter = 8–11 mm). In small SCCVII tumors (initial mean diameter = 3–5 mm), complete regression (CR) occurred in the groups given the combined treatment (cyclophosphamide dose = 20 or 40 mg/kg), whereas CR was nil in the groups treated with cyclophosphamide alone even at 40 mg/kg/day for 5 days. The dose of cyclophosphamide used is in the range of clinically prescribed dosage for human patients, 10–50 mg/kg.

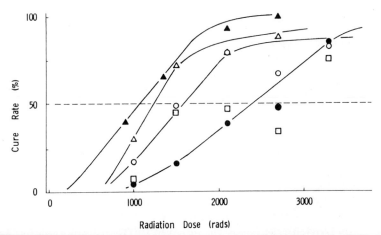

Fig. 6. Tumor cure dose assay of EMT-6 tumors in BALB/c mice using PLD repair inhibitors. (▲) 7904 (100 mg/kg), (△) 3'-dG (100 mg/kg), (○) 3'-dA (100 mg/kg), (□) 3'-dA (pre), (●) control. From U *et al.* (1982).

In the combination treatment groups, there appears to be a tumor size dependence of the chemosensitization (S. Nakatsugawa and T. Sugahara, unpublished). The potentiation by the inhibitor seems to be greater in large than in small tumors. Shipley *et al.* (1975b) reported the tumor size dependence of the response in a case of Lewis lung tumor. Similarly, Steel *et al.* (1976) and Steel and Adams (1975) noted a tumor size dependence in the case of cyclophosphamide and BCNU treatment. Hagemann *et al.* (1973) also suggested the dependence of efficacy of chemotherapy on the mode of growth of tumors. These data indicate that the level of cell killing by chemotherapy is much greater in small, rapidly growing tumors. The resistance of large tumors against chemotherapy might be at least partly due to the repair of chemotherapeutic agent-induced PLD (Barranco, 1976; Law *et al.*, 1981; Horsman *et al.*, 1982).

Thus, the tumor size dependence of chemosensitization by PLD repair inhibitors might be of great use in chemotherapy of human cancers and in the elucidation of the role of PLD repair on the resistance of large and slow-growing tumors to chemotherapy. There are no reported data suggesting the enhancement of normal tissue toxicity by 3'-dG. Toxicological studies on 3'-dG are under way in Japan, and 3'-dG may be more stable than adenosine analogs such as 3'-dA and Ara-A. Thus, even at lower doses of antitumor drugs, the potent chemosensitization may be achieved by PLD repair inhibitors, and even in large and slowly growing tumors, the potentiation might be available, if the repair inhibitors are sufficiently stable to penetrate the peripheral or hypoxic portions of tumors.

B. Prospects of PLD Repair Inhibitors as Clinically Applicable Sensitizers

In screening tests of PLD repair inhibitors, M. Watanabe, (personal communication) found several nontoxic but potent inhibitors of radiation-induced PLD repair. On the basis of these data, a research group was organized in Japan by Sugahara in 1978 to test the effects of PLD repair inhibitors at various levels. The phase II study of Ara-A as a radio- and chemosensitizer is under way in Japan (Nakatsugawa, 1982). Developed as an antiviral agent for diseases such as herpes encephalitis or H.B. hepatitis in both the United States and Japan Ara-A has been marketed in the United States. However, before the drug can be used routinely as a radio- and chemosensitizer, there are obstacles to be overcome, such as stability and toxicity. In Japan, the effect of PLD repair inhibitor has been tested clinically, and this may be the first clinical trial to determine the significance of PLD repair and its inhibition. If inhibitors are clinically available, human cancer chemotherapy and radiotherapy should be greatly improved.

VII. Summary

This chapter reviewed various aspects of investigations on PLD and SLD repair. The possibility of a redefinition or a remodeling of classic concepts on the two types of repair has to be considered. Much more time will be required to clarify the molecular events of PLD and SLD repair. Mutant cells and specific repair inhibitors are now available as tools for study of these molecular mechanisms. Clinical implications of PLD repair in cancer therapy are now feasible as data on cellular levels and experimental therapy have been obtained. In Japan, the phase II study of PLD repair inhibitors for radio- and chemosensitization is under way, and the significance of PLD repair and its inhibition has been clinically studied.

Acknowledgments

Gratitude is extended to Drs. T. Sugahara, H. Takebe, M. Abe, and M. Takahashi for pertinent suggestions and discussion. Misses N. Odani, K. Katsuyama, S. Machida, K. Munemasa, N. Aoki, and E. Torii provided excellent technical assistance. Part of the work reported in this paper was done during the tenure of the International Fellowship of Cancer Research Campaign sponsored by the International Union Against Cancer.

References

Alper, T., and Gillies, N. E. (1960). The relationship between growth and survival after irradiation of E. coli strain B and two resistant mutants. *J. Gen. Microbiol.* **22,** 113–128.
Arlett, C. F. (1970). The influence of post-irradiation conditions on the survival of Chinese hamster cells after gamma-irradiation. *Int. J. Radiat. Biol.* **17,** 515–526.
Balis, M. E. (1968). "Antagonists and Nucleic Acids." North-Holland, Amsterdam.
Barranco, S. C. (1976). *In vitro* responses of mammalian cells to drug-induced potentially lethal and sublethal damage. *Cancer Treat. Rep.* **60,** 1799–1810.
Barranco, S. C., Novak, J. K., and Humphrey, R. M. (1975). Studies on recovery from chemically-induced damage in mammalian cells. *Cancer Res.* **35,** 1194–1204.
Belli, J. A., and Shelton, M. (1969). Potentially lethal radiation damage: repair by mammalian cells in culture. *Science (Washington, D.C.)* **165,** 490–492.
Belli, J. A., Dicus, G. J., and Bonte, F. J. (1967). Radiation response of mammalian tumor cells. I. Repair of sublethal damage *in vivo*. *J. Natl. Cancer Inst. (U.S.)* **38,** 673–682.
Ben-Hur, E., Elkind, M. M., and Bronk, B. V. (1974). Thermally enhanced radioresponse of cultured Chinese hamster cells: inhibition of repair of sublethal damage and enhancement of lethal damage. *Radiat. Res.* **58,** 38–51.

Braun, J., and Hahn, G. M. (1975). Enhanced cell killing by bleomycin and 43 C hyperthermia and the inhibition of recovery from potentially lethal damage. *Cancer Res.* **35,** 2921–2927.

Brown, J. M. (1982). Current status of SR-2508. *Radiosensitization Newsl.* **1,** 1.

Bryant, P. E., and Blocher, D. (1982). The effects of 9-beta-D-arabinofuranosyladenine on the repair of DNA strand breaks in X-irradiated Ehrlich ascites tumour cells. *Int. J. Radiat. Biol.* **42,** 385–394.

Byfield, J. E., Murnane, J., Ward, J. F., Calabro-Jones, P., Lynch, M., and Kulhanian, F. (1981). Mice, men, mustards and methylated xanthines: the potential role of caffeine and related drugs in the sensitization of human tumours to alkylating agents. *Br. J. Cancer* **43,** 669–683.

Calendi, E., Di Marco, A., Reggiani, M., Scarpinato, B., and Valentini, L. (1965). On physico-chemical interactions between daunomycin and nucleic acids. *Biochim. Biophys. Acta* **103,** 25–49.

Chavaudra, N., Guichard, M., and Malaise, E. P. (1981). Hypoxic fraction and repair of potentially lethal radiation damage in 2 human melanomas transplanted into *nude* mice. *Radiat. Res.* **88,** 56–68.

Clark, E. P., Hahn, G. M., and Little, J. B. (1981). Hyperthermic modulation of X-ray-induced oncogenic transformation in C3H 10T1/2 cells. *Radiat. Res.* **88,** 619–622.

Cleaver, J. E. (1978). DNA repair and its coupling to DNA replication in eukaryotic cells. *Biochim. Biophys. Acta* **516,** 489–516.

Cleaver, J. E. (1983). Structure of repaired sites in DNA synthesized in the presence of inhibitors of DNA polymerases alpha and beta in human fibroblasts. *Biochim. Biophys. Acta* (in press).

Cox, R., Masson, W. K., Weichselbaum, R. R., Nove, J., and Little, J. B. (1981). Repair of potentially lethal damage in X-irradiated cultures of normal and ataxia telangiectasia human fibroblasts. *Int. J. Radiat. Biol.* **39,** 357–366.

Deschavanne, P. J., Guichard, M., and Malaise, E.-P. (1981). Repair of sublethal and potentially lethal damage in lung cells using an *in vitro* colony method. *Br. J. Radiol.* **54,** 973–977.

Dewey, W. D., and Kight, N. (1969). Kinetics of cyclophosphamide damage-sublethal damage repair and cell-cycle-related sensitivity. *J. Natl. Cancer Inst. (U.S.)* **42,** 155–163.

Djordjevic, B., and Kim, J. H. (1969). Modification of radiation response in synchronized HeLa cells by metabolic inhibitors: effects of inhibitors of DNA and protein synthesis. *Radiat. Res.* **37,** 435–450.

Dritschilo, A., Piro, A. J., and Belli, J. A. (1976). Repair of radiation damage in plateau-phase mammalian cells: relationship between sub-lethal and potentially lethal damage states. *Int. J. Radiat. Biol.* **30,** 565–569.

Dritschilo, A., Piro, A. J., and Belli, J. A. (1979). Interaction between radiation and drug damage in mammalian cells. III. The effect of adriamycin and actinomycin-D on the repair of potentially lethal radiation damage. *Int. J. Radiat. Biol.* **35,** 549–560.

Elkind, M. M., and Kano, E. (1970). Actinomycin D and radiation fractionation studies in asynchronous and synchronized Chinese hamster cells. *Radiat. Res.* **44,** 484–487.

Elkind, M. M., and Sutton, H. (1959). X-ray damage and recovery in mammalian cells in culture. *Nature (London)* **184,** 1293–1295.

Elkind, M. M., and Sutton, H. (1960). Radiation response of mammalian cells grown in culture. I. Repair of X-ray damage in surviving Chinese hamster cells. *Radiat. Res.* **13,** 556–593.

Elkind, M. M., Whitmore, G. F., and Alescio, T. (1964). Actinomycin D: suppression of recovery in X-irradiated mammalian cells. *Science (Washington, D.C.)* **143,** 1454–1457.

Elkind, M. M., Sutton-Gilbert, H., Moses, W. B., and Kamper, C. (1967). Sub-lethal and lethal radiation damage. *Nature (London)* **214**, 1088–1092.

Elkind, M. M., Withers, H. B., and Belli, J. A. (1968). Intracellular repair and oxygen effect in radiobiology and radiotherapy. *Front. Radiat. Ther. Oncol.* **3**, 55–87.

Evans, R. G., Bagshaw, M. A., Gorden, L. F., Kurkjian, S. D., and Hahn, G. M. (1974). Modification of recovery from potentially lethal X-ray damage in plateau phase Chinese hamster cells. *Radiat. Res.* **59**, 597–605.

Ford, M. D., and Lavin, M. F. (1981). Ataxia telangiectasia: an anomaly in DNA replication after irradiation. *Nucleic Acids Res.* **9**, 1395–1404.

Frankenberg, D., and Frankenberg-Schwager, M. (1981). Interpretation of the shoulder of dose-response curves with immediate plating in terms of repair of potentially lethal lesions during a restricted time period. *Int. J. Radiat. Biol.* **39**, 617–632.

Ganesan, A. K., and Smith, K. C. (1968). Dark recovery processes in Escherichia coli irradiated with ultraviolet light. I. Effect of rec⁻ mutations on liquid holding recovery. *J. Bacteriol.* **96**, 365–373.

Gilman, M. Z., and Thilly, W. G. (1977). Cytotoxicity and mutagenecity of hyperthermia for diploid human lymphoblasts. *J. Therm. Biol.* **2**, 95–99.

Gould, M. N., and Clifton, K. H. (1979). Evidence for a unique *in situ* component of the repair of radiation damage. *Radiat. Res.* **77**, 149–155.

Hagemann, R. F., Schenken, L. L., and Lesher, S. (1973). Tumor chemotherapy: efficacy dependent on mode of growth. *J. Natl. Cancer Inst. (U.S.)* **50**, 467–474.

Hahn, G. M. (1968). Failure of Chinese hamster cells to repair sublethal damage when X-irradiated in the plateau phase of growth. *Nature (London)* **217**, 741–742.

Hahn, G. M. (1975). Radiation and chemically induced potentially lethal lesions in noncycling mammalian cells: recovery analysis in terms of X-ray- and ultraviolet-systems. *Radiat. Res.* **64**, 533–545.

Hahn, G. M. (1976). Recovery of cells from induced, potentially lethal damage. *Cancer Treat. Rep.* **60**, 1791–1798.

Hahn, G. M., and Little, J. B. (1972). Plateau phase cultures of mammalian cells: an *in vitro* model for human cancer. *Curr. Top. Radiat. Res.* **8**, 39–83.

Hahn, G. M., Ray, G. R., Gordon, L. F., and Kallman, R. F. (1973a). Response of solid tumor cells exposed to chemotherapeutic agents *in vivo:* cell survival after 2- and 24-hour exposure. *J. Natl. Cancer Inst. (U.S.)* **50**, 529–533.

Hahn, G. M., Bagshaw, M. A., Evans, R. G., and Gordon, L. F. (1973b). Repair of potentially lethal lesions in X-irradiated, density-inhibited Chinese hamster cells: metabolic effects and hypoxia. *Radiat. Res.* **55**, 280–290.

Hahn, G. M., Gordon, L. F., and Kurkjian, S. D. (1974a). Responses of cycling and noncycling cells to 1.3-bis (2-chloroethyl)-1-nitrosourea and to bleomycin. *Cancer Res.* **34**, 2373–2377.

Hahn, G. M., Rockwell, S., Kallman, R. F., Gordon, L. F., and Frindel, E. (1974b). Repair of potentially lethal damage *in vivo* in solid tumor cells after X-irradiation. *Cancer Res.* **34**, 351–354.

Hahn, G. M., Braun, J. B., and Har-Kedar, I. (1975). Thermochemotherapy: synergism between hyperthermia (42–43 °C) and adriamycin (or bleomycin) in mammalian cell inactivation. *Proc. Natl. Acad. Sci. USA* **72**, 937–940.

Hanawalt, P. C., Cooper, P. K., Ganesan, A. K., and Smith, C. A. (1979). DNA repair in bacteria and mammalian cells. *Annu. Rev. Biochem.* **48**, 783–836.

Harisiadis, L., Miller, R. C., Harisiadis, S., and Hall, E. J. (1980). Oncogenic transformation and hyperthermia. *Br. J. Radiol.* **53**, 479–482.

Hellmann, K., and Murkin, G. E. (1974). Synergism of ICRF 159 and radiotherapy in treatment of experimental tumors. *Cancer (Amsterdam)* **34**, 1033–1039.

Horowitz, A., Norwint, H., and Hall, E. J. (1975). Conditioned medium from plateau phase cells, effect on growth of proliferative cells and on repair of potentially lethal radiation damage. *Radiology (Easton, Pa.)* **114**, 723–726.

Horsman, M. R., Brown, J. M., and Schelley, S. L. (1982). The effect of misonidazole on the cytotoxicity and repair of potentially lethal damage from alkylating agents *in vitro*. *Int. J. Radiat. Oncol. Biol. Phys.* **8**, 761–765.

Iliakis, G. (1980). Effects of β-arabinofuranosyladenine on the growth and repair of potentially lethal damage in Ehrlich ascites tumor cells. *Radiat. Res.* **83**, 537–552.

Iliakis, G. (1981). Characterization and properties of repair of potentially lethal damage as measured with the help of arabinofuranosyladenine in plateau phase Ehrlich ascites tumor cells. *Radiat. Res.* **86**, 77–80.

Iliakis, G., and Nusse, M. (1982). Amphidicolin promotes repair of potentially lethal damage in irradiated mammalian cells synchronized in S phase. *Biochem. Biophys. Res. Commun.* **104**, 1209–1214.

Inoue, T., Hirano, K., Yokoiyama, A., Kada, T., and Kato, H. (1977). DNA repair enzymes in ataxia telangiectasia and Bloom's syndrome fibroblasts. *Biochim. Biophys. Acta* **479**, 497–500.

Inoue, T., Yokoiyama, A., and Kada, T. (1981). DNA repair enzyme deficiency and *in vitro* complementation of the enzyme activity in cell-free extracts from ataxia telangiectasia fibroblasts. *Biochim. Biophys. Acta* **655**, 49–53.

Ishii, Y., and Bender, M. A. (1978). Caffeine inhibition of prereplication repair of mitomycin C-induced DNA damage in human peripheral lymphocytes. *Mutat. Res.* **51**, 419–425.

Jain, V. K., Höltz, G. W., Pohlit, W., and Purohit, S. C. (1977). Inhibition of unscheduled DNA synthesis and repair of potentially lethal X-ray damage by 2-deoxy-D-glucose in yeast. *Int. J. Radiat. Biol.* **32**, 175–180.

Jaspers, N. G. J., and Bootzma, D. (1982). Genetic heterogeneity in ataxia-telangiectasia studied by cell fusion. *Proc. Natl. Acad. Sci. USA* **79**, 2641–2644.

Kada, T., Inoue, T., Yokoiyama, A., Mochizuk, H., Nakatsugawa, S., and Sugahara, T. (in press). Improvement in radiotherapy of cancer using modifiers of radiosensitivity of cells. *In* "DNA repair and cancer radiotherapy", Proc. Conf. Res. Biol. Individualisation Cancer Radiother. Probl. Developing Countries, Jülich F.R.G. 26–30 April, 1982 (J. S. Michell, ed.).

Law, M. P., Hirst, D. G., and Brown, J. M. (1981). Enhancing effect of misonidazole on the response of the RIF-1 tumor to cyclophosphamide. *Br. J. Cancer* **44**, 208–218.

Li, G. C., Evans, R. G., and Hahn, G. M. (1976). Modification and inhibition of repair of potentially lethal X-ray damage by hyperthermia. *Radiat. Res.* **67**, 491–501.

Lin, H. S., Kuhn, C. III, and Chen, D.-M. (1982). Radiosensitivity of pulmonary alveolar macrophage colony-forming cells. *Radiat. Res.* **89**, 283–290.

Little, J. B. (1969). Repair of sub-lethal and potentially lethal radiation damage in plateau phase cultures of human cells. *Nature (London)* **224**, 804–806.

Little, J. B. (1971). Repair of potentially-lethal radiation damage in mammalian cells: enhancement of conditioned medium from stationary cultures. *Int. J. Radiat. Biol.* **20**, 87–92.

Little, J. B., and Hahn, G. M. (1973). Life-cycle dependence of repair of potentially-lethal radiation damage. *Int. J. Radiat. Biol.* **23**, 401–407.

Little, J. B., Hahn, G. M., Frindel, E., and Tubiana, M. (1973). Repair of potentially lethal radiation damage *in vitro* and *in vivo*. *Radiology (Easton, Pa.)* **106**, 689–694.

Madoc-Jones, H., and Bruce, W. R. (1967). Sensitivity of L cells in exponential and stationary phase to 5-fluorouracil. *Nature (London)* **215**, 302–303.

Martin, W. M., McNally, N. J., and DeRonde, J. (1981). Enhancement of the effect of cytotoxic drugs by radiosensitizers. *Br. J. Cancer* **43**, 756–766.

Mauro, F., and Elkind, M. M. (1968). Comparison of repair of sublethal damage in cultured Chinese hamster cells exposed to sulfur mustard and X-rays. *Cancer Res.* **28,** 1156–1161.

McCormick, J. J., and Maher, V. M. (1981). Measurement of colony-forming ability and mutagenesis in diploid human cells. *In* "DNA Repair: A Laboratory Manual of Research Procedures" (E. C. Friedberg; and P. C. Hanawalt, eds.), pp. 501–521. Dekker, New York.

McNally, N. J. (1972). Recovery from sublethal damage by hypoxic tumor cells *in vivo. Br. J. Radiol.* **45,** 116–120.

Miller, R. C., and Hall, E. J. (1978). Oncogenic transformation *in vitro* by the hypoxic cell sensitizer misonidazole. *Br. J. Cancer* **38,** 411–417.

Mizuno, S., and Ishida, A. (1982). Selective enhancement of bleomycin cytotoxicity by local anesthetics. *Biochem. Biophys. Res. Commun.* **105,** 425–431.

Murnane, J. P., and Painter, R. B. (1982). Complementation of the defects in DNA synthesis in irradiated and unirradiated ataxiatelangiectasia cells. *Proc. Natl. Acad. Sci. USA* **79,** 1960–1963.

Murnane, J. P., Byfield, J. E., Chen, C.-T., and Hsia, C. (1981). The structure of methylated xanthines in relation to their effects on DNA synthesis and cell lethality in nitrogen mustard-treated cells. *Biophys. J.* **35,** 665–676.

Nakatsugawa, S. (1982). Ara-A as a radio- and chemosensitizer. *Radiosensitization Newsl.* **1,** 5–7.

Nakatsugawa, S., and Sugahara, T. (1980). Inhibition of X-ray-induced potentially lethal damage (PLD) repair by cordycepin (3'-deoxyadenosine) and enhancement of its action by 2'-deoxycoformycin in Chinese hamster *hai* cells in the stationary phase *in vitro. Radiat. Res.* **84,** 265–275.

Nakatsugawa, S., and Sugahara, T. (1982). Effects of inhibitors of radiation-induced potentially lethal damage repair on chemotherapy in murine tumors. *Int. J. Radiat. Oncol. Biol. Phys.* **8,** 1555–1559.

Nakatsugawa, S., Ishizaki, K., and Sugahara, T. (1978). The reduction in frequency of X-ray-induced sister chromatid exchanges in cultured mammalian cells during post-irradiation incubation in Hanks' balanced salt solution. *Int. J. Radiat. Biol.* **34,** 489–492.

Nakatsugawa, S., Sugahara, T., and Kumar, A. (1982a). Purine nucleoside analogues inhibit the repair of radiation-induced potentially lethal damage in mammalian cells in culture. *Int. J. Radiat. Biol.* **41,** 343–346.

Nakatsugawa, S., Kumar, A., Ono, K., Nishidai, T., Yukawa, Y., Takahashi, M., Abe, M., and Sugahara, T. (1982b). Increased tumor curability by radiotherapy combined with PLDR inhibitors in murine cancers. IAEA-SR-62, prospective methods of radiation therapy in developing countries. *IAEA-TECDOC,* **266,** 77–86.

Nolan, W. T., Thompson, J. E., Lepock, J. R., and Kruuv, J. (1981). Effect of membrane lipid perturbers on the temperature dependence of repair of sublethal and potentially lethal radiation damage. *Int. J. Radiat. Biol.* **39,** 195–206.

Painter, R. B. (1980). Effect of caffeine on DNA synthesis in irradiated and unirradiated mammalian cells. *J. Mol. Biol.* **143,** 289–301.

Painter, R. B. (1981). Radioresistant DNA synthesis: an intrinsic feature of ataxia telangiectasia. *Mutant. Res.* **84,** 183–190.

Painter, R. B., and Young, B. R. (1982). Effect of hypertonicity and X radiation on DNA synthesis in normal and ataxia-telangiectasia cells. *Radiat. Res.* **92,** 552–559.

Parry, E. M., and Parry, J. M. (1976). The genetic control of liquidholding recovery and U.V.-induced repair resistance in the yeast, Saccharomyces cerevisiae. *Int. J. Radiat. Biol.* **30,** 13–24.

Paterson, M. C., Smith, B. P., Lohman, P. H. M., Anderson, A. K., and Fishman, L.

(1976). Defective excision repair of γ-ray-damaged DNA in human (ataxia telangiectasia) fibroblasts. *Nature (London)* **260**, 444–447.

Paterson, M. C., Anderson, A. K., Smith, B. P., and Smith, P. J. (1979). Enhanced radiosensitivity of cultured fibroblasts from ataxia telangiectasia heterozygotes manifested by defective colony-forming ability and reduced DNA repair replication after hypoxic γ-irradiation. *Cancer Res.* **39**, 3725–3734.

Patrick, M. H., and Hayness, R. H. (1964). Dark recovery phenomena in yeast. II. Conditions that modify the recovery process. *Radiat. Res.* **23**, 564–579.

Patrick, M. H., Hayness, R. H., and Uretz, R. B. (1964). Dark recovery phenomena in yeast. I. Comparative effects with various inactivating agents. *Radiat. Res.* **21**, 144–163.

Phillips, R. A., and Tolmach, L. J. (1966). Repair of potentially lethal damage in X-irradiated HeLa cells. *Radiat. Res.* **29**, 413–432.

Pohlit, W., and Heyder, I. R. (1981). The shape of dose-survival curves for mammalian cells and repair of potentially lethal damage analysed by hypertonic treatment. *Radiat. Res.* **87**, 613–634.

Price, P. J., Suk, W. A., Peters, R. L., Martin, C. E., Bellew, T. M., and Huebner, R. J. (1975). Cordycepin inhibition of 3′-methylcholanthrene-induced transformation *in vitro* (39098). *Proc. Soc. Exp. Biol. Med.* **150**, 650–653.

Raaphorst, G. P., and Azzam, E. I. (1981). Fixation of potentially lethal radiation damage in Chinese hamster cells by anisotonic solutions, polyamines and dimethylsulfoxide. *Radiat. Res.* **86**, 52–66.

Raaphorst, G. P., and Dewey, W. C. (1979). A study of the repair of potentially lethal and sublethal radiation damage in Chinese hamster cells exposed to extremely hypo- or hypertonic NaCl solutions. *Radiat. Res.* **77**, 325–340.

Rasey, J. S., and Nelson, N. J. (1981). Repair of potentially lethal damage following irradiation with X-rays or cyclotron neutrons: response of the EMT-6/UW tumor system treated under various growth conditions *in vitro* and *in vivo*. *Radiat. Res.* **85**, 69–84.

Roberts, R. B., and Aldous, E. (1949). Recovery from ultraviolet irradiation in Escherichia coli. *J. Bacteriol.* **57**, 363–375.

Robertson, J. B., Oleson, Jr., F. B., Williams, J. R., and Little, J. B. (1977a). Survival of synchronized V79 cells treated with X-rays and cordycepin. *Int. J. Radiat. Biol.* **31**, 11–16.

Robertson, J. B., Williams, J. R., and Little, J. B. (1977b). Relative responses of an X-ray-resistant hybrid cell-line and its parent line to X-irradiation, ultraviolet light, actinomycin D and cordycepin. *Int. J. Radiat. Biol.* **31**, 529–539.

Robertson, J. B., Williams, J. R., and Little, J. B. (1978). Enhancement of radiation killing of cultured mammalian cells by cordycepin. *Int. J. Radiat. Biol.* **34**, 417–429.

Ryall, R. D. H., Hanham, I. W. F., Newton, K. A., Hellmann, K., Brinkley, D. M., and Hjertaas, O. K. (1974). Combined treatment of soft tissue and osteosarcomas by radiation and ICRF 159. *Cancer (Amsterdam)* **34**, 1040–1045.

Sato, C., and Kojima, K. (1971). Irreversible loss of negative surface charge and loss of colony-forming ability in Burkitt lymphoma cells after X-irradiation. *Exp. Cell Res.* **69**, 435–439.

Sato, C., Kojima, K., Onozawa, M., and Matsuzawa, T. (1972). Relationship between recovery of cell surface charge and colony-forming ability following radiation damage in three cell-lines. *Int. J. Radiat. Biol.* **22**, 479–488.

Sato, C., Kojima, K., and Nishizawa, K. (1975). Recovery from radiation-induced decrease in cell membrane charge by added adenosine triphosphate and its modification by colchicine or cytochalasin B. *Biochem. Biophys. Res. Commun.* **67**, 22–27.

Shenoy, M. A., and Singh, B. B. (1980). Cytotoxic and radiosensitizing effects of chlorpromazine hydrochloride in sarcoma 180A. *Indian J. Exp. Biol.* **18**, 791–795.

Shipley, W. U., Stanley, J. A., Courtenay, V. D., and Field, S. B. (1975a). Repair of radiation damage in Lewis lung carcinoma cells following *in situ* treatment with fast neutrons and γ-rays. *Cancer Res*. **35**, 932–938.

Shipley, W. U., Stanley, J. A., and Steel, G. G. (1975b). Tumor size dependency in the radiation response of the Lewis lung carcinoma. *Cancer Res*. **35**, 2488–2493.

Siedlecki, J. A., Szyszko, J., Pietrzykowska, I., and Zmudzka, B. (1980). Evidence implying DNA polymerase-β function in excision repair. *Nucleic Acids Res*. **8**, 361–375.

Silvestrini, R., Di Marco, A., Di Marco, S., and Dasdia, T. (1963). Azione Della Daunomicina sul metabolismo degli acidi nuclei di Cellule normali e neoplastiche coltivate *in vitro*. *Tumori* **49**, 399–411.

Spiro, I. J., Denman, D. J., and Dewey, W. C. (1982). Effect of hyperthermia on CHO DNA polymerases α and β. *Radiat. Res*. **89**, 134–149.

Steel, G. G., and Adams, K. (1975). Stem-cell survival and tumor control in the Lewis lung carcinoma. *Cancer Res*. **35**, 1530–1535.

Steel, G. G., Adams, K., and Stanley, J. (1976). Size dependence of the response of Lewis tumors to BCNU. *Cancer Treat. Rep*. **60**, 1743–1748.

Sugahara, T., and Nakatsugawa, S. (1981). Radiation sensitization studies in Japan. *Cancer Treat. Rep*. **8**, 51–61.

Suit, H., and Urano, M. (1969). Repair of sublethal radiation injury in hypoxic cells of a C3H mouse mammary carcinoma. *Radiat. Res*. **37**, 423–434.

Suzuki, E., Hoshi, H., and Horikawa, M. (1979). Repair of radiation-induced lethal and mutational damage in Chinese hamster cells *in vitro*. *Jpn. J. Genet*. **54**, 109–119.

Takabe, Y., Watanabe, M., Miyamoto, T., and Terasima, T. (1974). Demonstration of repair of potentially lethal damage in plateau phase cells of Ehrlich ascites tumor after exposure to bleomycin. *Gann* **65**, 559–560.

Taylor, I. W., and Bleehen, N. M. (1977a). Changes in sensitivity to radiation and ICRF 159 during the life of monolayer cultures of EMT-6 tumor line. *Br. J. Cancer* **35**, 587–594.

Taylor, I. W., and Bleehen, N. M. (1977b). Interaction of ICRF 159 with radiation, and its effect on sub-lethal and potentially lethal radiation damage *in vitro*. *Br. J. Cancer* **36**, 493–500.

Terzaghi, M., and Little, J. B. (1975). Repair of potentially lethal damage in mammalian cells is associated with enhancement of malignant transformation. *Nature (London)* **253**, 548–549.

Thomas, F., and Gould, M. N. (1982). Evidence for the repair of potentially lethal damage in irradiated bone marrow. *Radiat. Environ. Biophys*. **20**, 89–94.

Twentyman, P. R. (1976a). Dose fractionation does not prevent repair of potentially lethal damage induced by bleomycin *in vivo*. *Cancer Treat. Rep*. **60**, 259–260.

Twentyman, P. R. (1976b). Comparative chemosensitivity of exponential versus plateau phase cells in both *in vitro* and *in vivo* model systems. *Cancer Treat. Rep*. **60**, 1719–1722.

Twentyman, P. R., and Bleehen, N. M. (1973). The sensitivity of cells in exponential and stationary phases of growth to bleomycin and to 1.3-bis(2-chloroethyl)-1-nitrosourea. *Br. J. Cancer* **28**, 500–507.

Twentyman, P. R., and Bleehen, N. M. (1974). The sensitivity to bleomycin of a solid mouse tumour at different stages of growth. *Br. J. Cancer* **30**, 469–472.

Twentyman, P. R., and Bleehen, N. M. (1975). Studies of "potentially lethal damage" in EMT 6 mouse tumour cells treated with bleomycin either *in vitro* or *in vivo*. *Br. J. Cancer* **32**, 491–501.

U, R., Nakatsugawa, S., Kumar, A., Takahashi, M., Ono, K., Abe, M., Nagata, H., and Sugahara, T. (1982). The chemical inhibition of PLD (potentially lethal damage) repair *in vitro* and *in vivo* in cancer therapy. *Int. J. Radiat. Oncol. Biol. Phys*. **8**, 457–460.

Ueda, K., Ohashi, Y., Hatakeyama, K., and Hayaishi, O. (1983). Inhibition of DNA ligase activity by histones and its reversal by poly (ADP-ribose). *In* "ADP-Ribosylation, DNA Repair and Cancer (O. Hayaishi, M. Miwa, S. Shall, M. Smulson, and T. Sugimura, eds.) Jap. Sci. Soc. Press, Tokyo.

Urano, M., Nesumi, N., Ando, K., Koike, S., and Ohnuma, N. (1976). Repair of potentially lethal radiation damage in acute and chronically hypoxic tumor cells *in vivo*. *Radiology (Amsterdam)* **118**, 447–451.

Utsumi, H., and Elkind, M. M. (1979). Potentially lethal damage. Qualitative differences between ionizing and non-ionizing radiation and implications for "single-hit" killing. *Int. J. Radiat. Biol.* **35**, 373–380.

Utsumi, H., Hill, C. K., Ben-Hur, E., and Elkind, M. M. (1981). "Single-hit" potentially lethal damage: evidence of hit repair of mammalian cells. *Radiat. Res.* **87**, 576–591.

Waldren, C. A., and Rasco, I. (1978). Caffeine enhancement of X-ray killing in cultured human and rodent cells. *Radiat. Res.* **73**, 95–110.

Waser, J., Hübscher, U., Kuenzle, C. C., and Spadari, S. (1979). DNA polymerase β from brain neuron is a repair enzyme. *Eur. J. Biochem.* **97**, 361–368.

Wawra, E., and Dolejs, I. (1979). Evidences for the function of DNA polymerase β in unscheduled DNA synthesis. *Nucleic Acids Res.* **7**, 1675–1685.

Weichselbaum, R. R., Little, J. B., and Nove, J. (1977). Response of human osteosarcoma *in vitro* to irradiation: evidence for unusual cellular repair activity. *Int. J. Radiat. Biol.* **31**, 295–299.

Weichselbaum, R. R., Nove, J., and Little, J. B. (1978). Deficient recovery from potentially lethal radiation damage in ataxia telangiectasia and xeroderma pigmentosum. *Nature (London)* **271**, 261–262.

Weichselbaum, R. R., Nove, J., and Little, J. B. (1980). Radiation response of human tumor cells *in vitro*. *In* "Radiation Biology in Cancer Research" (R. E. Meyn and H. R. Withers, eds.), pp. 345–351. Raven, New York.

Weichselbaum, R. R., Malcolm, A. W., and Little, J. B. (1982). Fraction size and repair of potentially lethal radiation damage in a human melanoma cell line: possible implications for radiotherapy. *Radiology (Easton, Pa.)* **42**, 225–228.

Weichselbaum, R. R., Schmit, A., and Little, J. B. (1982b). Cellular repair factors influencing radiocurability of human malignant tumours. *Br. J. Cancer* **45**, 10–16.

Weiss, B. G., and Tolmach, L. J. (1967). Modification of X-ray-induced killing of HeLa S cells by inhibitors of DNA synthesis. *Biophys. J.* **7**, 779–795.

Whitmore, G. F., and Gulyas, S. (1967). Studies on recovery processes in mouse L cells. *Natl. Cancer Inst. Monogr.* **24**, 141–156.

Winans, L. F., Dewey, W. C., and Dettor, C. M. (1972). Repair of sublethal and potentially lethal X-ray damage in synchronous Chinese hamster cells. *Radiat. Res.* **52**, 333–351.

Yau, T. M., and Kim, S. C. (1980). Local anaesthetics as hypoxic radiosensitizers, oxic radioprotectors and potentiators of hyperthermic killing in mammalian cells. *Br. J. Radiol.* **53**, 687–692.

Yonei, S. (1979). Modification of radiation effects of E. coli B/r and a radiosensitive mutant Bs-1 by membrane-binding drugs. *Int. J. Radiat. Biol.* **36**, 547–551.

Yonei, S. (1980). Inhibitory effect of membrane-specific drugs on liquid-holding recovery in U.V.-irradiated E. coli cells. *Int. J. Radiat. Biol.* **37**, 685–689.

14 Repair of DNA Damage Induced by Ionizing Radiation in Ataxia Telangiectasia Cells and Potentially Lethal Damage Repair Inhibitors

Tsuneo Kada
Tadashi Inoue
Akiko Yokoiyama
Hajime Mochizuki

Department of Induced Mutation
National Institute of Genetics
Mishima 411, Japan

Shigekazu Nakatsugawa

Department of Experimental Radiology
Faculty of Medicine, Kyoto University
Kyoto 606, Japan

Tsutomu Sugahara

Kyoto National Hospital
Kyoto 612, Japan

I. Introduction

Elucidation of the nature of DNA damage produced by ionizing irradiation and its repair mechanisms allows us not only to evaluate hazards due to radiation but also to open new approaches to their use in cancer radiotherapy. This chapter reports the results of *in vivo* and *in vitro* studies on the repair of radiation-induced DNA damage and its chemical inhibition.

II. *In Vitro* Rejoining of Strand Breaks and Repair of Biological Capacity of γ-Ray-Induced DNA Damage in Toluenized Cells of *Bacillus subtilis*

In an attempt to understand the biochemical mechanisms involved in the repair of DNA damage induced by ionizing radiation, experiments were initiated by means of γ-irradiated and toluene-treated cells of *B. subtilis*. Toluene treatment of *Escherichia coli* at 37°C causes a nonselective permeability of bacterial membrane for substances of low molecular

TABLE I

Requirements for Repair of γ-Ray-Induced Damage of Transforming DNA in Toluene-Treated Cells of *B. subtilis*[a]

γ-Ray dose (krads)	Incubation medium[b]	Incubation time (min)	No. of transformants/ml of conpetent culture
0	Complete	0	11,460
0	Complete	10	7,320
0	−4dXTP	0	9,870
0	−4dXTP	10	6,300
30	Complete	0	1,100
30	Complete	10	6,440
30	−4dXTP	0	1,270
30	−4dXTP	10	740
30	−NAD	0	1,170
30	−NAD	10	1,370
30	−Mg^{2+}	0	1,360
30	−Mg^{2+}	10	980

[a] From Noguti and Kada (1972).
[b] The complete mixture contained, in phosphate buffer, 33 μM each of dATP, dGTP, dCTP, and TTP (4-dXTP); 150 μM of NAD, and 5 mM of MgCl$_2$.

weight and allows for the analysis of DNA metabolism (Jackson and De Moss, 1965; Moses and Richardson, 1970). Toluene treatment at 0°C is also effective in making *B. subtilis* cells accessible to substrates and cofactors of enzymes involved in the repair of damage induced by ionizing radiation.

Cells of *B. subtilis,* which are wild as to arginine biosynthesis, were exposed to γ rays from a ^{137}Cs source, then treated with 1% (v/v) toluene at 0°C in potassium phosphate buffer (pH 7.5). The cell suspension was then diluted appropriately with the phosphate buffer containing substrates and cofactors for the DNA repair. This solution was maintained at 37°C. The complete mixture for repair treatment contained dATP, dGTP, dCTP, dTTP, NAD, and MgCl$_2$. The repair reaction was terminated by cooling and by addition of EDTA to the system. Cells were then collected and lysed with lysozyme and detergents. Then DNA was extracted and analyzed as to transforming activity on competent Arg⁻ cells of *B. subtilis,* and molecular size was estimated by ultracentrifugation in an alkali-sucrose gradient. Table I shows that the transforming capacity of the DNA extracted from irradiated cells increased considerably during incubation of cells in the complete mixture but not in the absence of any one of the substrates or cofactors. Results shown in Fig. 1 indicate that the

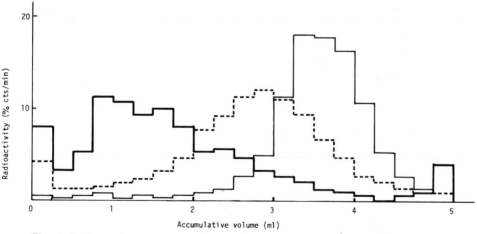

Fig. 1. Sedimentation analysis in alkali–sucrose gradient on repair of radiation-induced DNA single-strand breaks of toluenized cells in the presence of defined biochemical factors. Irradiated (30 krads) and toluene-treated cells of *B. subtilis* were incubated for 10 min at 37°C in a buffered (pH 8.0) mixture containing 33 μM each of 4dXTP (see Table I), 150 μM NAD, and 10 mM MgCl$_2$, then sedimented in alkali–sucrose gradient (10–30%) at 35,000 rpm for 140 min. (———) Neither irradiated nor incubated, (———) irradiated but not incubated, and (-------) irradiated and incubated. Similar shift of sedimentation profiles by incubation of toluenized cells was absent when the medium for incubation lacked one of the defined factors or when cells were not irradiated. For details see Noguti and Kada (1972).

molecular size of irradiated DNA increased in direct proportion to the recovery of biological activities.

III. Isolation and Characterization of Enzymes Involved Specifically in the Repair of γ-Ray-Induced DNA Damage of *B. subtilis* Cells

The results just outlined suggested that DNA polymerase I and DNA ligase are involved in DNA strand rejoining and the recovery of transforming capacity. Because γ irradiation will produce several kinds of breaks in the DNA strand (Fig. 2), involving those that do not serve as substrates for *in vitro* DNA synthesis with DNA polymerase I, we predicted the existence of enzymes that convert the broken termini to 3′-OH and that are essential as primers for *in vitro* DNA synthesis (Noguti and Kada, 1975a,b). Development of an assay system for the primer-activating (PA) enzyme, in which the capacity of cellular extracts enhances the priming activity of γ-irradiated colicin E1 DNA for purified DNA polymerase I can be measured, has enabled identification of two kinds of PA enzymes in extracts of *B. subtilis* (Fig. 3; Inoue and Kada, 1977). One was shown to be an apurinic site-specific endonuclease (Fig. 4), and the other was a "cleaning" exonuclease (Inoue *et al.*, 1981). Schemes of the repair processes of DNA damage induced by γ-irradiation are shown in Fig. 5.

IV. Characterization of the Repair Deficiency of Ataxia Telangiectasia Cells

Ataxia telangiectasia (AT) is an autosomal recessive disease characterized by telangiectasia, neurological degeneration, immunological deficiency, and predisposition to malignancy (for review see Paterson and Smith, 1979). A unique feature of this disease is that the patients and cells derived from these patients exhibit an extreme sensitivity to ionizing

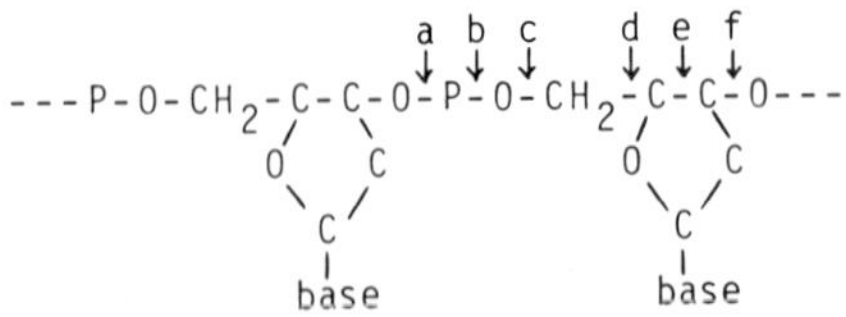

Fig. 2. Chemical structure of DNA strand. Arrows indicate possible breaks by radiation.

radiation. Therefore, this disease may be associated with defective repair mechanisms for ionizing radiation-induced DNA damage.

Ataxia telangiectasia and normal fibroblasts were compared with regard to the capacity of their cellular extracts to enhance the priming activity of γ-irradiated colicin E1 DNA for purified DNA polymerase I. It was observed that ataxia strains had a substantially lower capacity than normal strains, whereas the activities of apurinic site-specific endonuclease in these extracts were similar (Fig. 6; Inoue *et al.*, 1977). Then, three AT

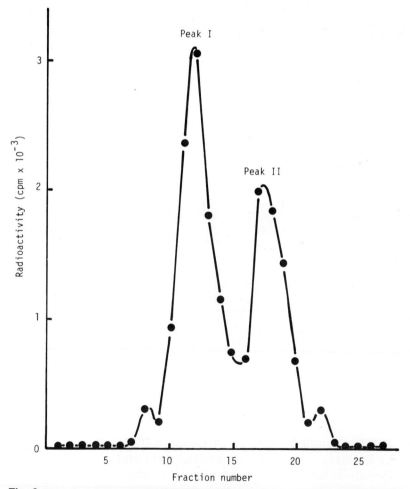

Fig. 3. Phosphocellulose chromatography profiles of primer-activating enzymes isolated from *B. subtilis*. Incorporated radioactivities into high molecular weight portions of DNA are measured. From Inoue and Kada (1977).

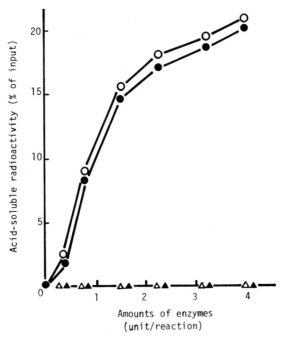

Fig. 4. Action of the apurinic endonuclease on native and heavily depurinated ³H-labeled DNA. The assays were done in the standard reaction mixtures or in mixtures containing 5 m*M* MgCl₂ instead of EDTA. (●, ○) Depurinated DNA, (▲, △) native DNA, (●, ▲) standard reaction mixture, and (○, △) same but with 5 m*M* MgCl₂ instead of EDTA. From Inoue and Kada (1978).

homozygotes, one heterozygote, and normal fibroblast strains were compared as to the capacity of their cellular extracts to enhance the priming activity of γ-irradiated colicin E1 DNA for purified DNA polymerase I of *E. coli*. The homozygotes had a substantially lower activity than normal strains, but differences between the heterozygote and normal strains were not apparent. *In vitro* complementation of the activity occurred between extracts of certain strains of homozygotes, allocating them to two complementation groups (Inoue *et al.*, 1981).

V. *In Vitro* Repair System of γ-Irradiated DNA by Extracts from DNA Repair-Proficient and Repair-Deficient Human Fibroblastic Cells

We reported that the transforming capacity of γ-ray-inactivated chromosomal or plasmid DNA of *B. subtilis* was recovered to a certain extent

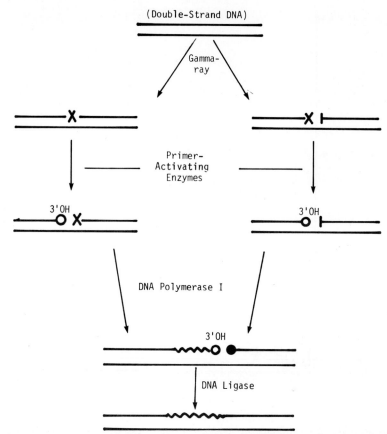

Fig. 5. Schemes of the repair processes of DNA damage induced by γ irradiation. (—X—) DNA damage, (—X ⊢—) DNA damage resulting in chain scission, (ⁿⁿⁿⁿ) newly synthesized region.

by *in vitro* treatment of irradiated DNA using a highly diluted extract obtained from human placental tissues or human fibroblast cells cultured *in vitro* (Fig. 7) (T. Kada and H. Mochizuki, unpublished). This activity was lost by heating the extract at 100°C or by treating it with EDTA; thus we assumed that certain enzymatic protein(s) were involved in the recovery. Here described are results of similar experiments where effects of extracts from DNA repair-proficient and repair-deficient human fibroblastic cells were studied.

Two normal fibroblast strains and three AT homozygotes were compared as to the capacity of their cellular extracts to enhance the activity of the γ-irradiated transforming DNA. We found that 50–60% of the DNA

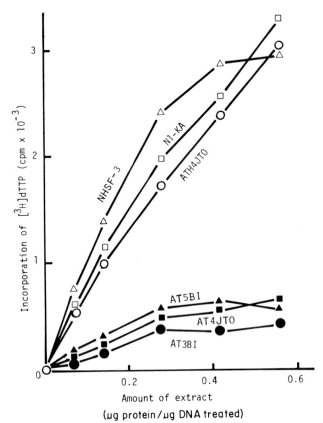

Fig. 6. Primer-activating enzyme activities in cellular extracts from AT (▲, ■, ●), AT heterozygote (○), and normal fibroblasts (△, □). Irradiated and unirradiated DNA were independently treated with the indicated amount of the extracts for 30 min at 37°C. After the incubation, a 3-μl sample was withdrawn from each reaction mixture and applied to the assay system for the priming activity of DNA. From Inoue *et al.* (1981).

damage induced by γ rays was repaired by *in vitro* reaction with the highly diluted extracts obtained from normal cells mentioned before, as estimated from gradual increases in the number of transformant colonies in the course of treatment of γ-irradiated DNA by the extracts. Extracts from cells of AT patients, however, showed no such activity (Table II). The repair activity in normal cells was lost by heating at 60°C for 30 min or by treating with EDTA, as in the case of human placenta tissues. When similar assays were carried out with DNA exposed to ultraviolet light, the recovery shown with normal fibroblast cells was not obtained (data not shown). These observations suggest that the recovery from radiation in-

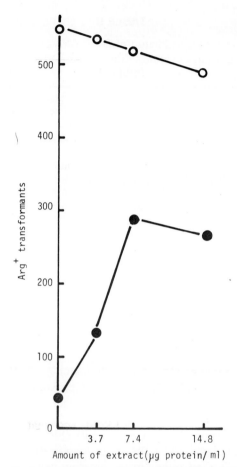

Fig. 7. *In vitro* repair of γ-irradiated transforming DNA of *B. subtilis* by treatment with diluted extract of human placental tissue. Unirradiated or irradiated DNA was incubated with extracts containing different amounts of protein at 37°C for 10 min and added to competent cultures of Arg⁻ recipient cells. After incubation at 37°C, the number of Arg⁺ transformant colonies was counted. (O———O) Unirradiated; (●———●) irradiated (10 krads).

jury in transforming DNA is specific to ionizing radiations and is closely related to the repair deficiency in AT cells.

VI.   Inhibition of the *in Vitro* Repair by Chemical PLD Inhibitors

Nakatsugawa *et al.* (1982) and Nakatsugawa and Sugahara (1980) studied the effect of growth phase and chemicals on potentially lethal damage

TABLE II

Recovery of γ-Irradiated pUB110 DNA by Treatment
with Extract of Human Fibroblastic Cells Cultured
in Vitro[a]

	Mean number of Km[r] colonies[b]	
Treatment of DNA	0 krads	10 krads
TKM-buffer	631	82
Extract (50 μg/ml protein) of:		
N1-KA[c]	610	376
NHSF-3[c]	613	394
AT3BI[d]	598	99
AT5BI[d]	609	84
AT4JTO[d]	613	110

[a] Treated DNA (37°C for 10 min) was used for transformation on competent cells of *B. subtilis* NIG17.

[b] Colonies formed by transformation with pUB110 DNA, with or without irradiation, then treated with one of the extracts.

[c] Normal.

[d] Ataxia telangiectasia.

(PLD) repair in X-irradiated Chinese hamster *hai* cells and found that cordycepin (3′-deoxyadenosine) is a strong inhibitor (Fig. 8). This chemical was later shown to be a good radiosensitizer in mice carrying EMT-6 tumor cells (Nakatsugawa and Sugahara, 1982). It has also been found that 3′-deoxyguanosine (3′-dG) is a good PLD inhibitor and radiosensitizer. Because a number of AT cells are lacking in PLD repair (Cox, 1982), the chemically inhibited repair in mammalian cells may possibly be related to a genetic deficiency in the DNA repair of human AT cells.

These chemical radiosensitizers act as DNA repair inhibitors, as evidenced in our *in vitro* repair study. Chromosomal DNA of *B. subtilis* cells was prepared, exposed to γ rays (10.8 krad, and treated, under appropriate conditions, with extracts of human placental tissues in the presence or absence of 3′-dA or 3′-dG. The recovery of biological activity of DNA by cellular extracts was totally lost in the presence of 3′-dA or 3′-dG (Fig. 9A and B).

VII. Discussion

Existence of DNA primer-activating (PA) enzymes working prior to partial DNA repair synthesis with DNA polymerase 1 and converting radiation-produced ends to 3′-OH termini that serve as priming substrates

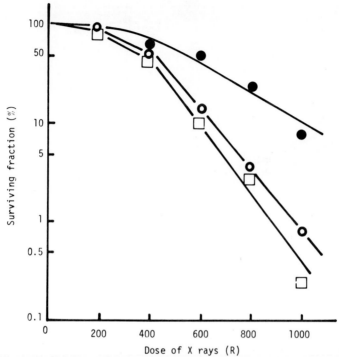

Fig. 8. The effect of cordycepin on PLD repair in X-irradiated Chinese hamster *hai* cells. Cells cultured for 10 days replated immediately or 10 h after various doses of X irradiation. From Nakatsugawa and Sugahara (1980). (○) Replated immediately after X rays; (●) replated after 10 h of postirradiation incubation in Hanks' BSS; (□) replated after 10 h postirradiation treatment with 250 μM cordycepin.

was first predicted from the study using toluene-treated bacteria. These enzymes were isolated, purified, and identified in *B. subtilis*. One was an apurinic site-specific endonuclease and the other was a "cleaning" exonuclease.

On the other hand, studies on repair-proficient (normal) and repair-deficient (ataxia telangiectasia) human fibroblastic cells revealed the following:

1. Ataxia telangectasia (AT) cells showed remarkably lower activities of PA enzymes than did normal cells.
2. Ataxia telangiectasia cells lack in the capacity to repair irradiated transforming DNA *in vitro*.
3. Ataxia telangiectasia cells of certain lines are lacking in PLD repair (Cox, 1982).
4. Mutations are noninducible by X ray in AT cells (Simons, 1982).

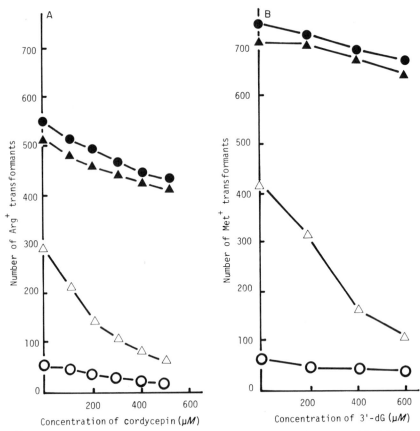

Fig. 9. *In vitro* repair of γ-irradiated DNA by human placental extract and its inhibition by cordycepin (A) or 3′-dG (B). Experiments similar to those shown in Fig. 7 were carried out. Cordycepin or 3′-dG was present at different concentrations in the course of incubation of irradiated DNA with the placental extract. ●, Unirradiated DNA; ▲, unirradiated DNA incubated with placental extract; ○, irradiated DNA incubated with placental extract; △, irradiated DNA.

Because 3′-dA and 3′-dG are potent inhibitors working in the *in vivo* PLD repair as well as in the *in vitro* recovery of irradiated transforming DNA, the following points must be considered:

1. Do 3′-dA or 3′-dG compounds inhibit the PA enzyme activities?
2. Are PA enzymes involved in the PLD repair?
3. Are 3′-dA and 3′-dG antimutagens involved in irradiated cells? (It has been found that 3′-dA and 3′-dG function as antimutagens in γ-irradiated Chinese hamster V-79 cells.)

References

Cox, R. (1982). A cellular description of the repair defect in ataxia-telangiectasia. *In* "Ataxia-Telangiectasia" (B. A. Bridges and D. G. Harnden, eds.), pp. 141–153. Wiley, New York.

Inoue, T., and Kada, T. (1977). Studies on DNA repair in *Bacillus subtilis*. III. Identification of an exonuclease which enhances the priming activity of γ-irradiated DNA by 'cleaning' damaged ends. *Biochim. Biophys. Acta* **478**, 234–243.

Inoue, T., and Kada, T. (1978). Purification and properties of a *Bacillus subtilis* endonuclease specific for apurinic sites in DNA. *J. Biol. Chem.* **253**, 8559–8563.

Inoue, T., Hirano, K., Yokoiyama, A., Kada, T., and Kato, H. (1977). DNA repair enzymes in ataxia telangiectasia and Bloom's syndrome fibroblasts. *Biochim. Biophys. Acta* **479**, 497–500.

Inoue, T., Yokoiyama, A., and Kada, T. (1981). DNA repair enzyme deficiency and *in vitro* complementation of the enzyme activity in cell-free extracts from ataxia telangiectasia fibroblasts. *Biochim. Biophys. Acta* **655**, 49–53.

Jackson, R. W., and De Moss, J. A. (1965). Effects of toluene on *Escherichia coli*. *J. Bacteriol.* **90**, 1420–1425.

Moses, R. E., and Richardson, C. C. (1970). Replication and repair of DNA in cells of *Escherichia coli* treated with toluene. *Proc. Natl. Acad. Sci. USA* **67**, 674–681.

Nakatsugawa, S., and Sugahara, T. (1980). Inhibition of X-ray-induced potentially lethal damage (PLD) repair by cordycepin (3'-deoxyadenosine) and enhancement of its action by 2'-deoxycoformycin in Chinese hamster hai cells in the stationary phase *in vitro*. *Radiat. Res.* **84**, 265–275.

Nakatsugawa, S., and Sugahara, T. (1982). Effects of inhibitors of radiation-induced potentially lethal damage repair on chemotherapy in murine tumors. *Int. J. Radiat. Oncol. Biol. Phys.* **8**, 1555–1559.

Nakatsugawa, S., Kumar, A., and Sugahara, T. (1982). Purine nucleoside analogues inhibit the repair of radiation-induced potentially lethal damage in mammalian cells in culture. *Int. J. Radiat. Biol.* **41**, 343–346.

Noguti, T., and Kada, T. (1972). Semi-*in vitro* repair of radiation-induced damage in transforming DNA of *Bacillus subtilis*. *J. Mol. Biol.* **67**, 507–512.

Noguti, T., and Kada, T. (1975a). Studies on DNA repair in *Bacillus subtilis*. I. A cellular factor acting on γ-irradiated DNA and promoting its priming activity for DNA polymerase I. *Biochim. Biophys. Acta* **395**, 284–293.

Noguti, T., and Kada, T. (1975b). Studies on DNA repair in *Bacillus subtilis*. II. Partial purification and mode of action of an enzyme enhancing the priming activity of γ-irradiated DNA. *Biochim. Biophys. Acta* **395**, 294–305.

Paterson, M. C., and Smith, P. J. (1979). Ataxia telangiectasia: an inherited human disorder involving hypersensitivity to ionizing radiation and related DNA-damaging chemicals. *Annu. Rev. Genet.* **13**, 291–318.

Simons, J. W. I. M. (1982). Studies on survival and mutation in ataxia-telangiectasia cells after X-irradiation under oxic and anoxic conditions. *In* "Ataxia-Telangiectasia" (B. A. Bridges and D. G. Harnden, eds.), pp. 155–167. Wiley, New York.

15 *Radiation Sensitivity and Intracellular cAMP*

Takashi Aoyama
Hiroshi Kimura
Toshiko Yamada
Department of Experimental Radiology
Shiga University of Medical Science
Otsu, 520-21, Japan

I. Introduction

Sutherland and Rall discovered cyclic adenosine 3′,5′-monophosphate (cAMP) in 1958, and this nucleotide was found to be a central regulator of various biological processes (Robison *et al.*, 1968; Pastan and Perlman, 1971). Mammalian cells were originally shown to have the intracellular "second messenger" for hormone-mediated cellular regulation (Robinson *et al.*, 1971). Many hormones act on their endocrine target issue through activation of adenylate cyclase in the cell membrane; intracellular cAMP levels are thus enhanced, and tissue-specific reactions to this high cAMP level are provoked (Willingham, 1976).

The morphology and growth of various cultured cell lines are influenced by cAMP or its derivatives. Treatment of several cell lines of transformed cells with cAMP, its butyryl derivatives, or agents that elevate intracellular cAMP levels changed the morphology of these cells significantly, making them look more like their normal parent cells (Hsie and Puck, 1971;

Modification of Radiosensitivity in Cancer Treatment

ISBN 0-12-676020-9

Hsie *et al.*, 1971; Johnson *et al.*, 1971a,b; Johnson and Pastan, 1971). Treatment with cAMP or the agents just mentioned decreased the growth rate of transformed cells in various lines and in several normal cell lines (Ryan and Heidrick, 1968; Bürk, 1968; Heidrick and Ryan, 1970; Hsie and Puck, 1971; Johnson and Pastan, 1971, 1972), but this treatment usually had no such effect in normal cell lines (Johnson *et al.*, 1971b). Intracellular cAMP levels are higher in density-inhibited culture of some cell lines (Heidreck and Ryan, 1971; Otten *et al.*, 1972; Anderson *et al.*, 1973), and in serum-restricted culture than in corresponding logarithmic phase cultures (Moens *et al.*, 1975). Concentrations of cAMP were higher in slowly growing cells than in rapidly growing cells, and the addition of dibutyryl cAMP to the culture medium decreased the growth rate (Otten *et al.*, 1971; Sheppard, 1972; Johnson and Pastan, 1972).

Factors modifying the survival of irradiated cells, including the rate of proliferation, the passage of the cell from exponential to stationary phase of growth, and the point in the cell cycle at which the cell is irradiated, are influenced by the level of intracellular cAMP. It therefore seems appropriate to study the relation of intracellular cAMP to the reproductive survival of irradiated cells.

In vitro and *in vivo* studies strongly suggested that cyclic nucleotides may be the important factors in determining the radiosensitivity of mammalian cells. This chapter is a general review of what is known of cAMP, as related to radiosensitivity of mammalian cells. Possible mechanisms underlying modifications of the effects of intracellular cAMP on cellular radiosensitivity are discussed.

II. Modification of Intracellular cAMP Levels

Cyclic AMP is produced intracellularly by the action of adenylate cyclase, which is bound with a cell membrane. This enzyme catalyzes the conversion of adenosine triphosphate (ATP) to cAMP. Cyclic AMP can then be degraded by a second enzyme (or enzymes), phosphodiesterase(s) (PDE), to yield the noncyclic derivative 5'-adenosine monophosphate (5'-AMP). Thus the level of cAMP in cells can be regulated through activities of these two enzymes; or its loss from the soluble cytoplasm by external excretion or binding by specific cAMP-binding proteins in the cell.

Intracellular cAMP levels can be altered artificially by several means (Willingham, 1976). One is to add cAMP itself to the culture medium. However, because cAMP itself does not readily pass through the cell membrane, analogs that do so more easily, such as N^2,O^2-dibutyryl-cAMP (Bt_2cAMP), N^6-monobutyryl-cAMP (BtcAMP), and the 8-bromo derivative of cAMP (8BrcAMP) are used. Although the actions of these agents are poorly understood, Bt_2cAMP seems to act through inhibition of the degradation enzyme PDE (Hsie *et al.*, 1975).

Another method of increasing intracellular cAMP levels in cells is to stimulate the activity of adenylate cyclase activity. Hormones such as epinephrine, ACTH, and glucagon function in such a manner in hormonally responsive cells *in vivo,* but cells in culture are often not hormonally responsive. Prostaglandins activate adenylate cyclase in cultured cells; one of the most effective of these is prostaglandin E_1 (PGE_1). Another method of elevating cAMP levels is through inhibition of its degradative enzyme PDE. Many drugs have this property, including xanthines—that is, aminophylline, theophylline, 1-methyl-3-isobutylxanthine (MIX), and papaverine—and other synthetic inhibitors (e.g., Roche compound 1724). Deprivation of serum factors also results in the elevation of cAMP levels in many cell types in culture.

Changes in cAMP levels in Chinese hamster ovary (CHO) cells in response to addition of Bt_2cAMP, caffeine, and PGE_1 to the medium are shown in Fig. 1. Addition of Bt_2cAMP to a final concentration of 1 mM produces a rapid increase in intracellular cAMP concentration, which peaks at 30 min, after which the concentration diminishes slowly over several hours. This result is consistent with the observation made by Lehnert (1979b) using MIX. However, we found that 1 mM caffeine and 10 mg/ml PGE_1 did not increase cAMP levels in CHO cells in our laboratory, as indicated in Fig. 1.

Lowering cAMP levels is more difficult. Fresh serum factors decrease cAMP levels in some lines of cells. Treating cells with proteases such as trypsin causes in a fall in cAMP levels. Insulin, with an activity in liver cells opposite to that of glucagon, causes lowered cAMP levels by inhibiting adenylate cyclase, activating cAMP PDE, or both. It can be seen that agents that decrease the intracellular levels of cAMP are often growth stimulators in culture systems.

III. Radioprotective Effects of cAMP

Historically, Langendorff and Langendorff (1971, 1972) reported initially that the effects of radioprotective agents might be mediated by increased formation of cAMP. They observed that the β-adrenergic blocking agent, LB 46 (Visken), decreased the radioprotective effects of S-(2-aminoethyl)isothiouronium bromide hydrobromide (AET), cystamine, or the bacterial lipopolysaccharide (LPS). The blocking agents decreased 30-day survival of mice after irradiation by factors of about 2 to

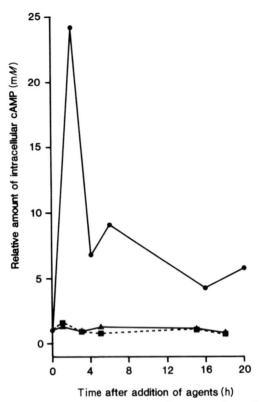

Fig. 1. Amount of intracellular cAMP in CHO cells expressed as a function of control values for various incubation times in medium containing (●) 1 mM Bt$_2$cAMP, (▲) 1 mM caffeine, and (■) 10 mg/ml PGE$_1$.

6, when the blocking agent was given before administration of the radio-protectors. They assumed that there was a certain relationship between the radioprotectors and the cAMP mechanism. They also examined the protective effects of 3'-AMP, 5'-AMP, ATP, and cAMP, or a combination of ATP and other nucleotides.

When the combination of ATP and cAMP was used, the mice irradiated to LD$_{98/30}$ were protected. Protection was also afforded by ATP, 3'-ATP, or 5'-AMP given alone. These investigators proposed that the protective substance is first transported to the effector cells where the drug interacts with regulatory subunits or receptors of the membrane-bound adenyl-cyclase system. This interaction between the receptors and the protective substance leads to an activation of the adenylcyclase system, resulting in an increase of the level of cAMP in the effector cell. They also assumed that this stimulation can be inhibited by blocking the receptors specific for the protector used.

Prasad (1972a,b) initially demonstrated *in vitro* that PGE_1 and Ro-20-1724 increased the survival of irradiated CHO cells and HeLa cells by about twofold when given before X irradiation. When given immediately after irradiation for a period of 1 or 4 h, these compounds affect the survival of irradiated cells. Prasad proposed the working hypothesis that the level of cAMP may be inversely related to the radiosensitivity of cells.

Pazdernik and Uyeki (1974) reported that agents that are known to alter cyclic nucleotide levels potentiated the radioprotective effects of 2-mercaptoethylamine (MEA, cysteamine). Development of granulocytic and monocytic colony-forming cells *in vitro* from BDF1 mouse bone marrow cells was markedly inhibited by exposing the cells to X ray before plating. Addition of 33 mM MEA before irradiation resulted in a 10–50% increase in survival of the irradiated cells. The radioprotective effects of MEA were greatly potentiated by incubating the cells for 1 h before adding MEA with agents known to alter cyclic nucleotide levels, such as 10^{-4} M isoproterenol, 10^{-4} M theophylline, 10^{-7} M imidazole, and 10^{-3}–10^{-5} M cAMP. No significant protection occurred if these agents were used in the absence of MEA.

Mitznegg (1973) reported that the administration of 150 mg/kg cysteamine leads to a transient inhibition of [^{3}H]thymidine incorporation into DNA of liver cells in white mice and that this functional suspension of DNA synthesis is probably responsible for cysteamine-induced radioprotective effects. Cysteamine induced the acceleration of DNA restoration and the prevention of loss in liver weight and in the total liver content of DNA, RNA, and protein, 4 and 8 days after a whole-body γ irradiation with 500 rads. In addition, Mitznegg found that administration of 200 mg/kg Bt_2 cAMP showed similar effects. Furthermore, cysteamine itself initiates an elevation of endogenous cAMP in the liver cells. Therefore, cysteamine-induced radioprotective effects seem to be mediated by cAMP. This means that cysteamine administration leads to the formation of cAMP, which might induce a transient functional suspension of DNA synthesis. Cells should be more resistant to ionizing radiation in this stage.

Kovář (1976) and Fremuth (1977) also studied the relationship between cyclic nucleotides and radiosensitivity. They found that the cAMP (100 mg/kg) decreases the radiosensitivity of Chinese hamster cells by a factor of 1.15 when given 10 min before the exposure and that Bt_2cAMP had a similar effect. It is interesting that cGMP inhibited the protective effect of cAMP when applied simultaneously and induced an increase in the radiosensitivity. They suggested that functional changes in the proliferation activity of the cells in critical radiosensitive tissue such as bone marrow after the application of cyclic nucleotides principally correlate with the change of the radiosensitivity of the organism.

Grant *et al.* (1976) followed up the results of Langendorff and Langendorff (1971, 1972) and confirmed the protective effect of adenine nucleotides. At the same time, they found that the administration of cAMP alone also induced radioresistance. This is consistent with the results of Kovář and Fremuth (1976). They found, however, that the protection by sulfur-containing compounds such as cysteamine and WR-2721 was not mediated by the increases in cAMP levels, as determined from the study of the small intestine and spleen.

IV. A Role of cAMP in Sublethal Damage Repair

Lehnert (1975) observed that reproductive survival of Chinese hamster V-79 lung cells and CHO cells after irradiation was influenced by the level of intracellular cAMP. Lehnert carried out the first experiments to determine the effect of exogenous cAMP or its derivatives on postirradiation survival. However, there was no effect on survival for a range of doses when cells were irradiated in medium containing 1 mM cAMP. Theophylline was used concomitantly with cAMP to eliminate the possibility that cAMP was being degraded by PDE, but the addition of theophylline did not increase the survival. Combining Bt_2cAMP and theophylline produced only a slight increase in D_0 value. Several inhibitors of cAMP PDE and PGE_1 were also tested. The agents Ro-20-1724, DL-152, and PGE_1 were all effective in elevating the level of intracellular cAMP. These three drugs and MIX, a very potent inhibitor of PDE, caused notable changes in postirradiation survival in treated cells, as shown in Fig. 2.

The effects of elevated cAMP levels on survival of irradiated cells are complex, because the amount of sublethal damage (SLD) accumulated and the slope of the exponential region of the survival curve increase simultaneously. Lehnert (1979a) found that the time of addition to the culture medium of the drugs that elevate intracellular cAMP, in relation to the time of irradiation, was an important factor in modification of radiation response of mammalian cells by these drugs.

When CHO cells were transferred to the medium containing 0.2 mM MIX immediately after irradiation (Fig. 3A), MIX-treated CHO cells showed a decrease in D_0 and some increase in the extrapolation number. If the cells were transferred to a MIX medium 60 min prior to irradiation,

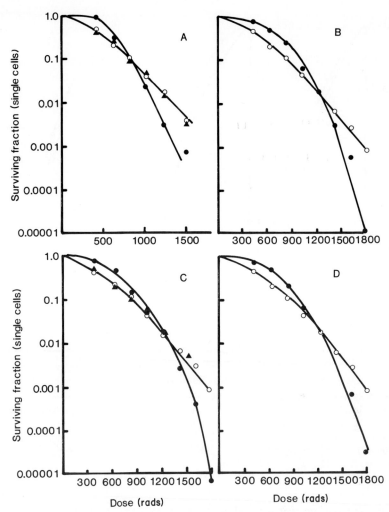

Fig. 2. Survival curves for V-79 cells treated with various drugs before X irradiation. (A) Control (○); 0.5 mM theophylline (▲); 0.5 mM MIX (●). (B) Control (○); 200 mg/ml Ro-20-1724 (●). (C) Control (○); 10^{-5} M reserpine (▲); 10^{-5} M DL-152 (●). (D) Control (○); 10 mg/ml PGE$_1$ (●). From Lehnert (1975).

there was also a decrease in D_0, a marked enhancement of the shoulder of the survival curve, and an increase in the extrapolation number (Fig. 3B). The cells grown in medium containing 0.2 mM MIX for 18 h prior to irradiation increased in extrapolation number, but the D_0 changed little (Fig. 3C). Exposure of CHO cells to 1 mM Bt$_2$cAMP or to 10 μg/ml PGE$_1$ for 3 h after irradiation also caused a decrease in D_0 and an increase in

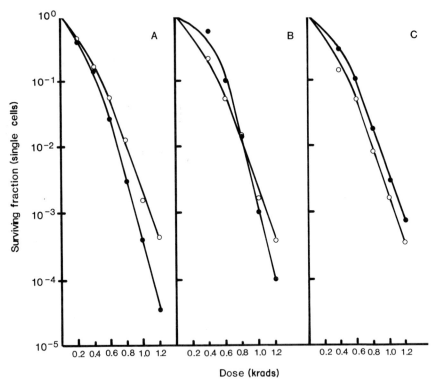

Fig. 3. Survival curves for CHO cells in various treatments with MIX in relation to the time of irradiation. (A) ($\bigcirc$) Control: $D_0 = 125$, $n = 6.5$. ($\bullet$) Cells transferred to medium containing 0.2 mM MIX immediately after irradiation: $D_0 = 96$, $n = 14$. (B) ($\bigcirc$) Control: $D_0 = 127$, $n = 7.0$. ($\bullet$) Cells transferred to MIX medium 60 min before irradiation: $D_0 = 87$, $n = 200$. (C) ($\bigcirc$) Control: $D_0 = 122$, $n = 6.5$. ($\bullet$) Cells grown in MIX medium for 18 h prior to irradiation: $D_0 = 128$, $n = 12$. From Lehnert (1979a).

extrapolation number. Reduction of cell survival by MIX after 1100 rads was most effective if it was added just before or just after irradiation. It was not necessary that MIX be present during irradiation for maximum effectiveness, because MIX added just after irradiation reduced survival to a slightly greater extent than did MIX added just before irradiation, as shown in Fig. 4.

Radiosensitization effect, as a reduction of D_0, by elevation of intracellular cAMP was examined as a function of the position of cell in the cell cycle. This effect was not seen for the cells irradiated up to the latter part of G_1 but occurred in late G_1 and S-phase cells treated with MIX by a factor of approximately 2.5, as shown in Fig. 5.

The survival curve for CHO cells grown in medium containing 0.2 mM

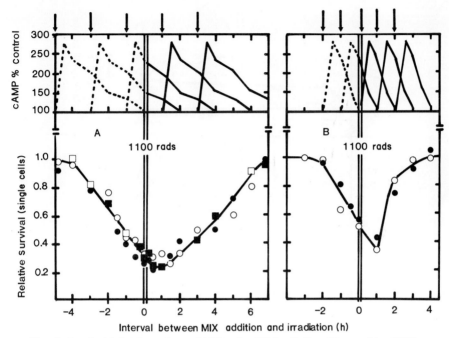

Fig. 4. Survival following a dose of 1100 rads of X irradiation. The xanthine MIX was added to the medium at various times before irradiation (values to the left of zero time) or after irradiation (values to the right of zero time). At each time, survival of MIX-treated cells is expressed as a proportion of the number of cells surviving radiation in replicate, non-MIX-treated flasks (relative survival). (A) MIX was added at the times indicated and remained in the medium for the duration of the experiment. Upper panel: Intracellular cAMP concentration (percentage of control) following addition of MIX at various times (indicated by arrows). Lower panel: Relative postirradiation survival of MIX-treated cells given 1100 rads of X irradiation. Different symbols represent data from different experiments. (B) Cells were incubated in medium containing 0.2 mM MIX for 60 min only, commencing at the time indicated by the position of the experimental point. Upper panel: Intracellular cAMP concentration during and after a 60-min exposure of cells to 0.2 mM MIX (times at which MIX was added to the medium indicated by arrows. Lower panel: Relative survival of cells exposed to MIX for 60 min at various times before or after irradiation. From Lehnert (1979a).

MIX for 18 h prior to irradiation is shown in Fig. 3C. The survival curve shows an enhanced shoulder and increased extrapolation number when compared with the survival curve for control cells, whereas the exponential slopes of both curves are similar. The survival of MIX-treated cells is increased by a factor of 2.1 to 2.3, over the whole dose range. The development of maximum radioresistance with MIX treatment required about 8 h in CHO cells irradiated with a dose of 600 rads at various points in time after addition of MIX to the medium (Lehnert, 1979b).

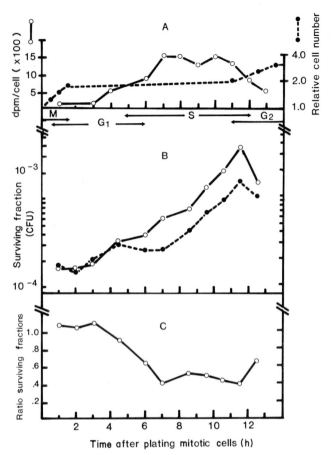

Fig. 5. Radiosensitization effect by elevation of intracellular cAMP examined as a function of the position of cells in cell cycle. (A) Duration of phases of the cell cycle in CHO cells, data derived from measurements of timing of cell division and DNA synthesis. (B) Surviving fraction of CHO cells after 1100 rads delivered at various times after plating mitotic cells. (○) Control. (●) Cells transferred to medium containing 0.2 mM MIX 30 min before irradiation. (C) Ratio of survival of MIX-treated cells to control cells calculated using data from (B). From Lehnert (1979a).

Enhancement of the shoulder on the survival curve of cells grown in medium containing MIX indicates an increased capacity of the cells to accumulate SLD. Lehnert (1979b) attempted to determine whether high intracellular levels of cAMP enhance the capacity to repair such damage by measuring the extent of recovery between the two doses of irradiation. Cells grown in control medium or those grown for 18 h in medium containing MIX were irradiated with a total dose of 1100 rads, either in a single

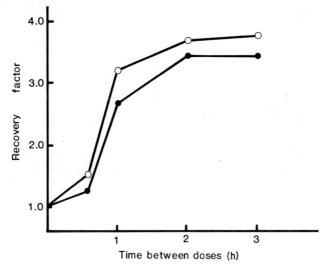

Fig. 6. Increase in survival obtained when CHO cells were irradiated with a total dose of 1100 rads as two 550-rad fractions. (○) Cells growing in control medium. (●) Cells grown in medium containing 0.2 mM MIX for 18 h prior to irradiation. From Lehnert (1979b).

dose or in two 550-rad fractions. The results of this experiment are shown in Fig. 6 and are expressed as a recovery factor (i.e., the ratio of the surviving fraction for a split dose to the surviving fraction for a single dose). Unexpectedly, the extent of repair of SLD seems to be similar in control and MIX-treated cells, as shown in Fig. 6. Lehnert analyzed the results using the method of Durand and Sutherland (1973) to assess the percentage of the accumulated SLD repaired during the period between the doses and clarified that the total amount of SLD accumulated was greater than in the control but that a much smaller portion was repaired.

Effects of MIX on postirradiation survival of synchronized cells were also observed (Fig. 7). A short exposure (e.g., 60 min) to MIX before irradiation at different times throughout the division cycle revealed that G_1- and early S-phase cells responded to the exposure most effectively and showed the highest surviving fraction. There was also another experiment in which MIX was added at 0, 3, or 6 h after plating mitotic cells. The result of the experiment indicated that culture of the cells in the MIX-containing medium for more than 6 h before irradiation was necessary to increase postirradiation survival. When the comparison was made between the mitotic cells collected from monolayers exposed to control and to medium containing MIX for the preceding 18 h, the survival of control and of MIX-treated cells was the same at the beginning and at the end of the experimental period. At all other times throughout the division cycle,

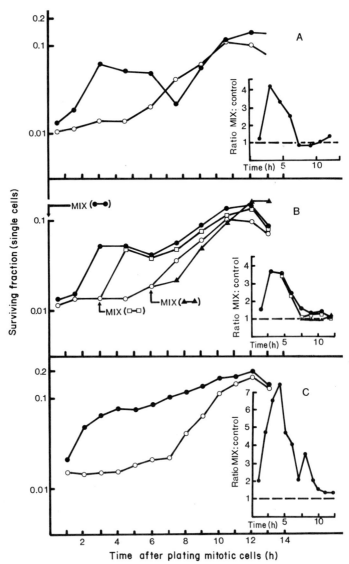

Fig. 7. Survival of CHO cells synchronized by mitotic selection and irradiated with a dose of 600 rads at various times after plating mitotic cells. The small graph inserted on the right-hand side of each panel shows the same data plotted as a ratio of surviving fractions, MIX: control. (A) (○) Control; (●) MIX added 60 min prior to irradiation. (B) (○) Control; (●) MIX added at 0 h, (□) at 3 h, and (▲) at 6 h after plating mitotic cells. (C) (○) Control; (●) mitotic cells selected from monolayers growing in 0.2 mM MIX for the 18 h preceding irradiation and mitotic cells plated in medium containing MIX. From Lehnert (1979b).

MIX-treated cells had a higher fraction of survivors than did the control cells, and the ratio of surviving fractions was again greatest during G_1 phase and declined during the S phase.

Lehnert (1979b) claimed that the increase in radioresistance was independent of cell cycle perturbation produced by MIX but was concomitant with MIX-induced morphological conversion of cells from an epithelial form to an elongated, fibroblast-like form. It has been known that numerous intracellular processes are involved in the morphological conversion of the cells just mentioned. There are difficulties, therefore, in finding the significant relationship between the altered radiosensitivity and the morphological change in MIX-treated cells.

V.   A Role of cAMP in Potentially Lethal
Damage Repair

Investigators have ascertained that there is another type of repair from radiation damage, that is, repair of potentially lethal damage (PLD) (Phillips and Tolmach, 1966; Hahn, 1975). Intracellular cAMP levels are high in density-inhibited cultures of some cell lines and serum-restricted cultures (Otten *et al.*, 1971; Heidrick and Ryan, 1971; Anderson *et al.*, 1973; Moens *et al.*, 1975). Thus attention should be given to a possible relationship between intracellular cAMP and the repair of PLD.

The survival curve of exponential phase JTC-11 cells, originally isolated from Ehrlich ascites tumor cells by Hamasaki (1964), had a D_0 of 71 rads and a D_q of 522 rads, as shown in Fig. 8. When cells were cultured in medium containing 1 mM Bt_2cAMP for 14 h before and 6 h after irradiation, the survival of X-irradiated JTC-11 cells increased considerably at higher doses. The D_q (528 rads) did not change, but the D_0 increased to 101 rads. When JTC-11 cells were incubated with Bt_2cAMP for 14 h and plated in the normal medium immediately after irradiation, there was no effect on survival. The D_0 of the survival curve was 78 rads, with the D_q equal to 506 rads. It was interesting that neither pre- nor postirradiation incubation of mouse L cells with Bt_2cAMP for 22 h increased the number of survivors. The kinetics of recovery from PLD in cells treated with Bt_2cAMP before and after X irradiation is shown in Fig. 9A and B. Recovery in JTC-11 cells reached a maximum 6 h after X irradiation, followed by a decrease in survival, although survival of nontreated JTC-11 cells was slightly increased 6 h after X irradiation. There was no apparent recovery from PLD in mouse L cells. Preincubation with 1 mM Bt_2cAMP for 6 h was sufficient for induction of maximum recovery from PLD. Recovery was not observed in either JTC-11 or mouse L cells, at any

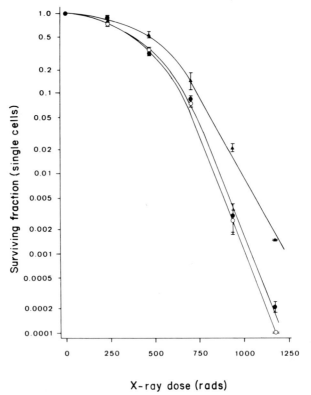

Fig. 8. Effect of dibutyryl cAMP on survival of JTC-11 cells exposed to X rays. The exponentially growing cells were exposed to various doses of X rays immediately followed by incubation in plastic dishes for assay of colony-forming ability (○). They were either incubated with 1 m*M* Bt$_2$cAMP for 14 h before irradiation and exposed to X rays immediately followed by incubation in plastic dishes (●), or incubated with Bt$_2$cAMP for 14 h before and 6 h after irradiation (▲). Each point is the mean of triplicate samples. Vertical bars indicate ±SEM. From Kimura *et al.* (1981).

postirradiation incubation time when X-irradiated (658 rads) exponentially growing cells were treated with the drug only after irradiation.

VI. Effect of cAMP on Radiosensitivity of Tumors and Normal Tissues

In vivo studies on radioprotective effects of cAMP have centered around the investigation of the indicators such as survival of animals or biochemical changes in normal tissue, but the effects on radiosensitivity

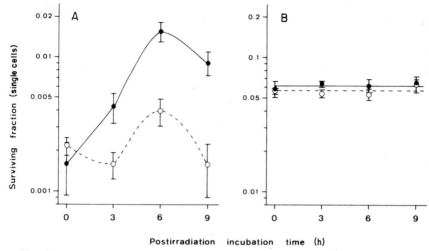

Fig. 9. Time course of repair of potentially lethal damage of (A) JTC-11 cells and (B) mouse L cells. The exponentially growing cells were either X irradiated (940 rads) and inoculated into plastic dishes for assay of colony-forming ability at each interval from irradiation (○), or incubated with 1 mM Bt$_2$cAMP for 14 h before and for each time after irradiation, and inoculated into plastic dishes (●). Vertical bars are standard errors. From Kimura *et al.* (1981).

of tumors and normal tissues have been given little attention. Dubravsky *et al.* (1978) compared the effect of Bt$_2$cAMP injected ip before irradiation on the radiation sensitivity of normal tissues (the proliferating hair follicle and small gut) and of tumors, micrometastases of fibrosarcoma cells in the lung and the 50% cure dose (TCD$_{50}$) of two different mammary carcinomas.

Survival curves for hair follicle cells were determined using the unique assay system shown in Fig. 10. The control survival curve for hair follicle cells is defined by a D_0 of 185 rads. The survival curve for hair follicle cells for mice injected ip with Bt$_2$cAMP (30 mg/kg) was biphasic and appeared to contain two different populations, A and B. Population A possessed the same sensitivity as the control, with a D_0 of 202 rads, but with a displacement to the right; population B was resistant, with a D_0 of 450 rads. The effect of Bt$_2$cAMP on the survival of cryptogenic cells of the jejunum after X irradiation was tested. As shown in Fig. 11, Bt$_2$cAMP given ip 4 h before irradiation led to a high survival of cryptogenic cells, by a factor of about 1.2 to 2.5. There was no significant change in the sensitivity, as determined by the D_0, in the untreated and treated cryptogenic cells.

In contrast to normal tissue, the response of malignant tissues to radiation did not change with a preinjection of Bt$_2$cAMP. When Bt$_2$cAMP was

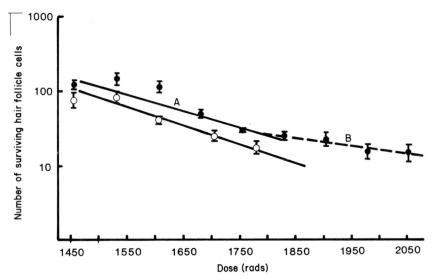

Fig. 10. Survival curves of hair follicle cells for mice exposed to γ irradiation on the third day after plucking with and without preinjection of Bt_2cAMP, 30 mg/kg. (○) Control, D_0 = 185 (range 141–267) rads. (●) Bt_2cAMP: Population A had the same sensitivity as the control with D_0 = 202 (range 140–359) rads, but with a displacement to the right; B was a resistant population with D_0 = 450 (range 347–641) rads. Vertical bars are standard errors. From Dubravsky *et al.* (1978).

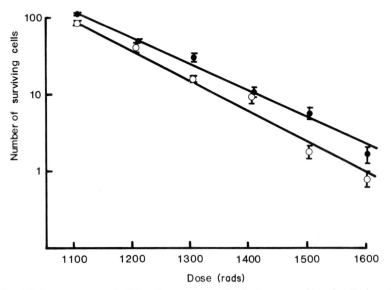

Fig. 11. Survival curves for jejunal crypt stem cells of mice exposed to γ irradiation with and without preinjection of Bt_2cAMP, 30 mg/kg. (○) Control, D_0 = 111 (range 99–126) rads; (●) Bt_2cAMP, D_0 = 129 (range 117–143) rads. Vertical bars are standard errors. From Dubravsky *et al.* (1978).

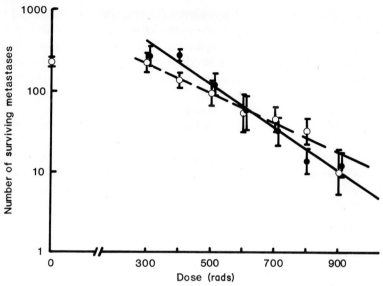

Fig. 12. Survival curves for artificial FSa metastases on the fourth day after transplantation, irradiated with and without preinjection of Bt_2cAMP, 30 mg/kg. ($\bigcirc$) Control, $D_0 = 238$ (range 205–284) rads; ($\bullet$) Bt_2cAMP, $D_0 = 162$ (range 136–201) rads. From Dubravsky *et al.* (1978).

injected before irradiation, the sensitivity of the fibrosarcoma (FSa) micrometastases in the lung irradiation seemed to be the same as in the control and when Bt_2cAMP was injected before irradiation (Fig. 12). Even though the D_0 was 162 rads in Bt_2cAMP-treated animals and the D_0 of the control was 238 rads, the sensitivity was mainly affected by the change in the shoulder width. The two tumors, mammary carcinoma MDA-MCa-4 and MCa-K, were also examined. There was no apparent effect of preinjection of Bt_2cAMP on the TCD_{50} at 120 days after irradiation. The MCa-4 control TCD_{50} is 6711 rads, that is, not much different from the value for the tumor treated with Bt_2cAMP (6720 rads). The TCD_{50} for MCa-K was lower than the other mammary carcinoma, but again there was no difference between the Bt_2cAMP-treated group and the nontreated group.

VII. Mechanisms Underlying the Modifications of Intracellular cAMP Effects on Radiosensitivity

Prasad (1972a,b) demonstrated the protective effect of cAMP in irradiated CHO cells and proposed that the level of this nucleotide may be inversely related to the radiosensitivity of cells. Prasad also stated that this hypothesis was consistent with the law of Bergonié and Tribondeau in the sense that it may provide a molecular basis for this law, as there is a striking correlation between the level of cAMP and the doubling time of cells; that is, fast-growing cells have a low cAMP level and slow-growing cells have high levels.

This hypothesis is quite interesting and acceptable in principle to us, but it is difficult to clarify the details of the mechanism underlying the cAMP action to the cellular radiosensitivity. To exaplain the radioprotective effects of cysteamine, Mitznegg (1973) speculated that cAMP might induce a transient functional suspension of DNA synthesis, which should make DNA more resistant to ionizing radiation. Kovář and Fremuth (1976) proposed the similar interpretation that functional changes in the proliferation activity of the cells caused by cAMP decrease the radiosensitivity. Dubravsky *et al.* (1978) noted that correlation of intracellular cAMP levels through the division cycle to radiation sensitivity revealed that the extrapolation number was highest during the period when intracellular cAMP level was at a maximum, namely S phase in V-79 cells. Conversely, mitotic cells in which cAMP was at a minimum have the smallest extrapolation number, 1.0. There was another correlation in HeLa cells in that S- and G_1-phase cells, having high cAMP contents, are less sensitive to radiation, whereas G_1–S boundary, G_2, and M cells are low in cAMP content and sensitive to radiation (Sinclair, 1968; Friedman, 1976). Dubravsky *et al.* (1978) therefore thought that because transformed cells contain less cAMP than normal controls in general, this might explain why a short exposure to Bt_2cAMP protected the normal tissue and did not affect the tumors.

Lehnert (1979a) attempted to clarify a mechanism underlying the correlation between increased concentrations of cAMP and the effect of reduction in D_0 and enhancement of postirradiation survival. Lehnert noted the findings of reduced survival following postirradiation treatment of HeLa cells with caffeine (Busse *et al.*, 1977), because caffeine, a methylxanthine, is structurally similar to MIX, the most potent drug having the D_0-reduction effect, and both are inhibitors of cAMP phosphodiesterase. However, caffeine apparently does not induce elevation of cAMP in cultured cells (Zeilig *et al.*, 1976), as we confirmed (cf. Fig. 1). The radiosensitization by caffeine differs from that produced by MIX in that caffeine requires 8 h postirradiation exposure to produce a maximal effect (Busse *et al.*, 1977), whereas MIX does so in less than 1 h.

The involvement of cAMP in the regulation of the cell cycle may explain the D_0-reduction effect (Lehnert, 1979a). The transient cessation in cell division observed when MIX was added to exponentially growing

CHO cells may be attributed to the arrest of cells in G_2 for period roughly equivalent in duration to the period for which intracellular cAMP is elevated. However, the D_0 reduction of MIX-treated CHO cells is not directly attributable to this type of cell cycle effect, in that the effect does not depend on cAMP being elevated with preirradiation treatment. However, cAMP-induced changes in cell cycle after irradiation could result in altered radiation response.

The enhancement effect of postirradiation survival with MIX is independent of the level of intracellular cAMP at the time of irradiation, because in cells exposed to MIX for a prolonged period, cAMP concentration is similar to that of controls. Therefore, MIX enhances survival of CHO cells by factors other than changes in cAMP level. The arrest of cells in G_2 would hardly explain the enhancement effect. However, it is interesting that MIX reacts on G_1- and early S-phase cells to increase postirradiation survival (Lehnert, 1979b).

The enhanced repair capacity for sublethal damage seen with high intracellular levels of cAMP was examined by measuring the extent of recovery between the two doses of radiation, as the survival curve for CHO cells treated with MIX before irradiation showed enhanced shoulder and increased extrapolation number. However, the extent of repair of SLD seems to be quite similar in control and MIX-treated cells (Lehnert, 1979b).

It is also difficult to explain the mechanism in potentially lethal damage repair induced by pre- and postirradiation incubation of cells with BT_2cAMP. We observed the repair in JTC-11 cells. Analysis of the difference between JTC-11 and mouse L cells may lead to clarification of the mechanism. The effects of Bt_2cAMP on growth of exponentially growing JTC-11 and mouse L cells were also compared. Growth curves of untreated exponentially growing JTC-11 and mouse L cells and those treated with BT_2cAMP are showin in Fig. 13A and B. Growth of JTC-11 cells was inhibited by Bt_2cAMP, and the decrease was constant throughout the drug treatment. In contrast, the growth rate of mouse L cells was reduced almost to zero for the first 16 h, after which the rate was much the same as that seen in the control. The mitotic index of JTC-11 cells did not change except for a slight decline 5 h after the treatment, but that of mouse L cells increased 1.5 h after the cells had been returned to the control medium and there was a decrease to the level of exponentially growing cells.

The peak of the mitotic index 1.5 h after treatment was possibly caused by release of the cells from a Bt_2-cAMP-induced G_2 arrest, as shown in Fig. 14A and B. According to the hypothesis proposed by Little (1973), G_2 arrest was irrelevant to PLD repair induction. Overall growth of JTC-11 cells was decreased with the treatment shown in Fig. 13A. It seems likely

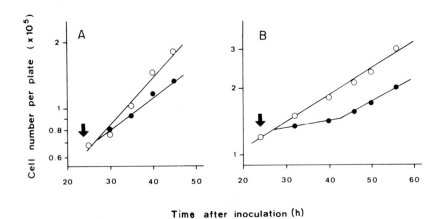

Fig. 13. Growth inhibition by 1 mM Bt$_2$cAMP of (A) JTC-11 and (B) mouse L cells. Cells were grown with (●) or without (○) 1 mM Bt$_2$cAMP. Arrow indicates the addition of Bt$_2$cAMP. Similar results were obtained in duplicate experiments. From Kimura *et al.* (1981).

that the rate at which the cells proceed from G_1 to S phase may be reduced considerably and that the duration of G_1 is longer in the treated cells, although we had no evidence that the ratio of cell population arrested in G_1 was increased.

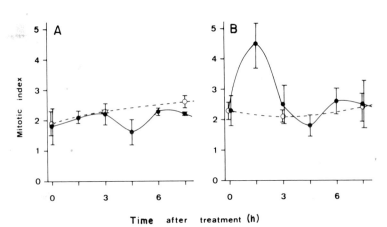

Fig. 14. Changes in mitotic index of (A) JTC-11 or (B) mouse L cells after treatment with 1 mM Bt$_2$cAMP. The cells were grown with (●) or without (○) 1 mM Bt$_2$cAMP for 14 h after 1-day culture in control medium and were returned to control medium at time 0 indicated in the figure. The mitotic index is defined as the percentage of the total cells counted that were at metaphase. The experiments were (A) duplicated or (B) tripled. Vertical bars, ±SD. From Kimura *et al.* (1981).

We found that the survival of CHO cells exposed to mitomycin C decreased three times as much as that of the cells treated with 1 mM Bt$_2$cAMP before mitomycin C treatment as compared to the absence of treatment with the cyclic nucleotide (Shinohara *et al.*, 1983). This sensitization effect of Bt$_2$cAMP began at 3 to 4 h after the start of pretreatment with this agent, reached a maximum at around 10 h, then continued. The increase of intracellular cAMP level by Bt$_2$cAMP treatment began immediately after the treatment and reached a peak after 2 h, the increase being 25 times that of the controls. The level then decreased quickly, reached several times that of the control level 4 h after the treatment, and thereafter decreased gradually as shown in Fig. 1. The maximum sensitization to the effect of mitomycin C by the pretreatment with Bt$_2$cAMP may be attained 8 h after the intracellular cAMP level has reached the maximum. Therefore, intracellular events that occur in 1 to 6 h after the maximum cAMP level may possibly be responsible for this sensitization. Because the action mechanism of mitomycin C is claimed to be on the cross-link (Iyer and Szybalski, 1963), the effect of mitomycin C may be exerted more strongly when the chromatin structure of the cell is relaxed rather than tight. Langan (1971) proposed that the chromatin structure may be altered by phosphorylation of histone when the intracellular cAMP level was increased. If such is the case, then the structure of chromatin may relax with this intracellular mechanism.

This assumption about the molecular mechanism may partially explain the effects of cAMP on the modification of radiosensitivity. From this aspect, it should be noticed that G$_1$- and early S-phase cells are responsible for the increase effect of postirradiation survival, and late G$_1$- and S-phase cells are responsible for the radiosensitization effect of this cyclic nucleotide.

When the structure of chromatin in G$_1$ phase is relaxed by increased intracellular cAMP, access of ligase to damaged places on DNA strands may be facilitated in this extended structure as opposed to the tight structure in original G$_1$ phase. It has been proposed that poly(ADP-ribose) participates in such actions as DNA repair (Durkacz *et al.*, 1980; Edwards and Taylor, 1980; Berger and Sikorski, 1981) through activation of ligase and its localization on damaged points of DNA strands (Creissen and Shall, 1982). Szumiel proposed that poly(ADP-ribosylation) of chromatin would be enhanced by the inhibitory action of cAMP on (ADP-ribose) glycohydrolase, although this has not been analyzed (Szumiel, 1983).

Poirier *et al.* (1982) observed that poly(ADP-ribosylation) of rat pancreatic polynucleosomes causes relaxation of chromatin structure by electron microscopy. Jump *et al.* (1979) found that ADP-ribosylation mainly occurred in regions of chromatin undergoing DNA synthesis. Therefore, the structure of chromatin in S phase, which is already relaxed for replication, may become more relaxed by increased intracellular cAMP. This may disturb access of the enzymes onto the break points of DNA strand and rejoining of DNA strands.

This may result in sensitization by increased cAMP. This simple hypothesis is not sufficient to explain the entire mechanism, but it may throw some light on the puzzle of the very complex effects of cAMP on cellular radiosensitivity.

Acknowledgment

We extend our thanks to M. Ohara for reading the manuscript.

References

Anderson, W. B., Russell, T. R., Carchman, R. A., and Pastan, I. (1973). Interrelationship between adenylate cyclase activity, adenosine 3′:5′ cyclic monophosphate levels, and growth of cells in culture. *Proc. Natl. Acad. USA* **70**, 3802–3805.

Berger, N. A., and Sikorski, G. W. (1981). Poly(adenosine diphosphoriose) synthesis in ultraviolet irradiated xeroderma pigmentosum cells reconstituted with micrococcus luteus UV endonuclase. *Biochemistry* **20**, 3610–3614.

Bürk, R. R. (1968). Reduced adenyl cyclase activity in a polyoma virus transformed cell line. *Nature (London)* **219**, 1272–1275.

Busse, P. M., Bose, S. K., Jones, R. W., and Tolmach, L. J. (1977). The action of caffeine on X-irradiated HeLa cells. II. Synergistic lethality. *Radiat. Res.* **71**, 666–677.

Creissen, D., and Shall, S. (1982). Regulation of DNA ligase activity by poly(ADP-ribose). *Nature (London)* **296**, 271–272.

Dubravsky, N. B., Hunter, N., Mason, K., and Withers, H. R. (1978). Dibutyryl cyclic adenosine monophosphate: effect on radiosensitivity of tumors. *Radiology (Easton, Pa.)* **126**, 799–802.

Durand, R. E., and Sutherland, R. M. (1973). Growth and radiation survival characteristics of V79-171b Chinese hamster cells: a possible influence of intercellular contact. *Radiat. Res.* **56**, 513–527.

Durkacz, B. W., Omidiji, O., Gray, D. A., and Shall, S. (1980). (ADP-ribose)n participates in DNA excision repair. *Nature (London)* **283**, 593–596.

Edwards, M. J., and Taylor, A. M. R. (1980). Unusual levels of (ADP-ribose)n and DNA synthesis in ataxia telangiectasia cells following γ-ray irradiation. *Nature (London)* **287**, 745–747.

Fremuth, F. (1977). Changes in radiosensitivity induced by cyclic nucleotides and chemical radioprotection. *Folia Biol. (Prague)* **23**, 212–217.

Friedman, D. L. (1976). Role of cyclic nucleotides in cell growth and differentiation. *Physiol. Rev.* **56**, 652–708.

Grant, G. A., Barlow, J. A., and Leach, K. E. (1976). Modification of survival of gamma irradiated by adenosine nucleotides. *Strahlentherapie* **152**, 285–291.

Hahn, G. M. (1975). Radiation and chemically induced potentially lethal lesion in noncycling mammalian cells: recovery analysis in terms of X-ray and ultraviolet-like-systems. *Radiat. Res.* **64,** 533–545.

Hamasaki, M. (1964). On the properties of an established cell strain, JTC-11, from ascites tumor in tissue culture. I. The characteristics of the standard strain K-strain. *Okayama Igakkai Zasshi* **76,** 1–11.

Heidrick, M. L., and Ryan, W. L. (1970). Cyclic nucleotides on cell growth in vitro. *Cancer Res.* **30,** 376–378.

Heidrick, M. L., and Ryan, W. L. (1971). Adenosine 3',5'-cyclic monophosphate and contact inhibition. *Cancer Res.* **31,** 1313–1315.

Hsie, A. W., and Puck, T. T. (1971). Morphological transformation of Chinese hamster cells by dibutyryl adenosine cyclic 3':5'-monophosphate and teststerone. *Proc. Natl. Acad. Sci. USA* **68,** 358–361.

Hsie, A. W., Jones, C., and Puck, T. T. (1971). Further changes in differentiation state accompanying the conversion of Chinese hamster cells to fibroblastic form by dibutyryl adenosine cyclic 3':5'-monophosphate and hormones. *Proc. Natl. Acad. Sci. USA* **68,** 1648–1652.

Hsie, A. W., Kawashima, K., O'Neill, J. P., and Schroder, C. H. (1975). Possible role of adenosine cyclic 3':5'-monophosphate phosphodiesterase in the morphological transformation of Chinese hamster ovary cells mediated by $N^6,O^{2'}$-dibutyryl adenosine cyclic 3':5'-monophosphate. *J. Biol. Chem.* **250,** 984–989.

Iyer, V. N., and Szybalski, W. (1963). A molecular mechanism of mitomycin action: linking of complementary DNA strands. *Proc. Natl. Acad. Sci. USA* **50,** 355–362.

Johnson, G. S., and Pastan, I. (1971). Change in growth and morphology of fibroblasts by prostaglandins. *J. Natl. Cancer Inst. (US)* **47,** 1357–1364.

Johnson, G. S., and Pastan, I. (1972). Role of 3'5' adenosine monophosphate in regulation of morphology and growth of transformed and normal fibroblasts. *J. Natl. Cancer Inst. (US)* **48,** 1377–1383.

Johnson, G. S., Friedman, R. M., and Pastan, I. (1971a). Cyclic AMP-treated sarcoma cells acquire several morphological characteristics of normal fibroblasts. *Ann. N.Y. Acad. Sci.* **185,** 413–416.

Johnson, G. S., Friedman, R. M., and Pastan, I. (1971b). Restoration of several morphological characteristics of normal fibroblasts in sarcoma cells treated with adenosine 3'5'-cyclic monophosphate and its derivatives. *Proc. Natl. Acad. Sci. USA* **68,** 425–429.

Jump, D. B., Butt, T. R., and Smulson, M. E. (1979). Nuclear protein modification and chromatin structure. 3. Relationship between poly(adenosine diphosphate) ribosylation and different function forms of chromatin. *Biochemistry* **18,** 983–990.

Kimura, H., Yasui, T., and Aoyama, T. (1981). Modification of radiation sensitivity of cultured cells by pre- and post-irradiation incubation with dibutyryl cyclic AMP. *Radiat. Res.* **85,** 207–214.

Kovář, J., and Fremuth, F. (1976). Control effects of cyclic nucleotides on the proliferation activity of the bone marrow cells of the Chinese hamster in vivo and their relation to the radiosensitivity. *Acta Univ. Carol. Med.* **22,** 329–366.

Langan, T. A. (1971). Cyclic AMP and histone phosphorylation. *Ann. N.Y. Acad. Sci.* **185,** 166–185.

Langendorff, H., and Langendorff, M. (1971). Chemical radiation protection and the cAMP mechanism. *Int. J. Radiat. Biol.* **19,** 493–495.

Langendorff, H., and Langendorff, M. (1972). Adenosin-nukleotide und Strahlenempfindlichkeit. *Strahlentherapie* **144,** 451–456.

Lehnert, S. (1975). Modification of postirradiation survival of mammalian cells by intracellular cyclic AMP. *Radiat. Res.* **62**, 107–116.

Lehnert, S. (1979a). Modification of radiation response of CHO cells by methylisobutyl xanthine. I. Reduction of D_0. *Radiat. Res.* **78**, 1–12.

Lehnert, S. (1979b). Modification of radiation response of CHO cells by extrapolation number. *Radiat. Res.* **78**, 13–24.

Little, J. B. (1973). Factors influencing the repair of potentially lethal radiation damage in growth-inhibited human cells. *Radiat. Res.* **56**, 320–333.

Mitznegg, P. (1973). On the mechanism of radioprotection by cysteamine. II. The significance of cyclic 3',5'-AMP for the cysteamine-induced radioprotective effects in white mice. *Int. J. Radiat. Biol.* **24**, 339–344.

Moens, W., Vokaer, A., and Kram, R. (1975). Cyclic AMP and cyclic GMP concentration in serum- and density-restricted fibroblast cultures. *Proc. Natl. Acad. Sci. USA* **72**, 1063–1067.

Otten, J., Johnson, G. S., and Pastan, I. (1971). Cyclic AMP levels in fibroblasts: relationship to growth rate and contact inhibition of growth. *Biochem. Biophys. Res. Commun.* **44**, 1192–1198.

Otten, J., Bader, J., Johnson, G. S., and Pastan, I. (1972). A mutation in a Rous sarcoma virus gene that controls adenosine 3',5'-monophosphate levels and transformation. *J. Biol. Chem.* **247**, 1632–1633.

Pastan, I., and Perlman, R. L. (1971). Cyclic AMP in metabolism. *Nature New Biol.* **229**, 5–7.

Pazdernik, T. L., and Uyeki, E. M. (1974). Enhancement of the radioprotective effects of 2-mercaptoethylamine on colony forming cells by agents which alter cyclic nucleotide levels. *Int. J. Radiat. Biol.* **26**, 331–340.

Phillips, R. A., and Tolmach, L. J. (1966). Repair of potentially lethal damage in X-irradiated HeLa cells. *Radiat. Res.* **29**, 413–432.

Poirier, G. G., de Murica, G., Jongstra-Bilen, J., Niedergang, C., and Mandel, P. (1982). Poly(ADP-ribosyl)ation of polynucleosomes causes relaxation of chromatin structure. *Proc. Natl. Acad. Sci. U.S.A.* **79**, 3423–3427.

Prasad, K. N. (1972a). Radioprotective effect of prostaglandin and an inhibitor of cyclic nucleotide phosphodiesterase on mammalian cells in culture. *Int. J. Radiat. Biol.* **22**, 187–189.

Prasad, K. N. (1972b). Cyclic AMP and the radiosensitivity of HeLa cells in culture. *Radiat. Res.* **51**, 520–521.

Robinson, G. A., Nahas, G. G., and Triner, L. eds. (1971). Cyclic AMP and Cell Function. *Ann., N.Y. Acad Sci.* **185**, 1–556.

Robison, G. A., Butcher, R. W., and Sutherland, E. W. (1968). Cyclic AMP. *Annu. Rev. Biochem.* **37**, 149–174.

Ryan, W. L., and Heidrick, M. L. (1968). Inhibition of cell growth in vitro by adenosine 3',5'-monophosphate. *Science (Washington, D.C.)* **162**, 1484–1485.

Sheppard, J. R. (1972). Difference in cyclic adenosine 3',5' monophosphate levels in normal and transformed cells. *Nature New Biol.* **236**, 14–16.

Shinohara, S., Otsu, Y., Yamada, T., Kimura, H., and Aoyama, T. (1983). Modification of the sensitivity of CHO cells to mitomycin C by dibutyryl cyclic AMP. *Biochem. Biophys. Res. Commun.* **111**, 247–252.

Sinclair, W. K. (1968). Cyclic X-ray response in mammalian cells in vitro. *Radiat. Res.* **33**, 620–643.

Sutherland, E. W., and Rall, T. W. (1958). Fractionation and characterization of a cyclic adenosine ribonucleotide formed by tissue particles. *J. Biol. Chem.* **232**, 1077–1091.

Szumiel, I. (1983). Ca^{2+},Mg^{2+} and (Adenosine diphosphate ribose)$_n$ in cellular response to irradiation. *J. Theor. Biol.* **101,** 441–451.

Willingham, M. C. (1976). Cyclic AMP and cell behavior in cultured cells. *Int. Rev. Cytol.* **44,** 319–363.

Zeilig, C. E., Johnson, R. A., Sutherland, E. W., and Friedman, D. L. (1976). Modulation of intracellular adenosine 3' : 5'-monophosphate levels in HeLa cells. *J. Cell Biol.* **71,** 515–534.

16 Modification of Radiosensitivity of Bacterial and Mammalian Cells by Membrane-Specific Drugs

Shuji Yonei
Clara Yukie Mitsutani
Takeshi Todo

Laboratory of Radiation Biology
Department of Zoology
Faculty of Science, Kyoto University
Kyoto 606, Japan

Ohtsura Niwa

Department of Experimental Radiology
Faculty of Medicine, Kyoto University
Kyoto 606, Japan

I. Introduction

Ionizing radiation induces many forms of cellular damage including interphase death, mitotic death, division delay, giant cell formation, inhibition of DNA synthesis, chromosome aberrations, mutation, and transformation. It is commonly accepted that the molecular basis for some of these cellular responses involves damage to the DNA genome (Okada, 1970; Ahnström and Ehrenberg, 1980; Chadwick and Leenhouts, 1981).

Modification of Radiosensitivity in Cancer Treatment
Copyright © 1984 by Academic Press Japan, Inc.
All rights of reproduction in any form reserved.
ISBN 0-12-676020-9

Numerous studies have stressed that the DNA probably represents the critical target in radiation-induced cell death (Okada, 1970; Burki, 1976; Cremer *et al.*, 1976; Chadwick and Leenhouts, 1981). However, there is substantial evidence indicating that membrane may be an important site for radiation damage (Bacq and Alexander, 1961; Patrick, 1977; Alper, 1979; Köteles, 1979).

The cell membrane is also considered to be a critical site for the modification of radiation response of cells (Alper, 1979; Köteles, 1979; Yau, 1979; Yonei, 1982). For example, Alper (1971, 1979) concluded that oxygen enhances the expression of radiation damage to DNA to a relatively small extent compared to its effect on cell survival, and that other sites may be more affected by the presence of oxygen at the time of irradiation. Alper suggested that the latter may be located in cell membranes. Support of this view has come from Watkins (1970) and Yonei (1982) with regard to the development and oxygen enhancement ratio of radiation damage to lysosomal and plasma membranes. Studies on the time scale of oxygen effects in bacterial and mammalian cells with the fast-flow rapid-mix technique (Shenoy *et al.*, 1975a) further emphasized the role of cell membranes in cellular radiosensitization by oxygen. A possible means of gaining further insight into the role of membranes may be by studying the combined effects of radiation and an agent that interacts specifically with membrane components.

The rationale often cited for the importance of the oxygen effect is that hypoxic cells are contained in many types of tumors, both animal and human (Withers, 1975; Koch, 1979; Fowler, 1980), and these hypoxic cells would be resistant to radiation therapy (Withers, 1975; Adams, 1979; Fowler, 1980; Sugahara and Nakatsugawa, 1981). Theoretically, in order to minimize the effect of an unfavorable oxygen distribution, one might apply either agents that preferentially radiosensitize the hypoxic fractions of tumors or agents that selectively radioprotect normal tissues (Adams, 1979; Fowler, 1980; Yau and Kim, 1980; Sugahara and Nakatsugawa, 1981).

The drugs in the former list, hypoxic-cell radiosensitizers, can be broadly classified into two subgroups (Shenoy and Gopalakrishna, 1977). The first subgroup consists of electron-affinic compounds including nitroimidazoles such as misonidazole (Brown and Yu, 1979; Whillans and Whitmore, 1981; Korbelik *et al.*, 1981). The second subgroup subsumes what are commonly known as "membrane-specific drugs," such as local anesthetics, analgesics, and tranquilizers (Shenoy *et al.*, 1975b; Singh *et al.*, 1980; Yonei, 1982). These drugs specifically interact with cell membranes, causing alterations in their structural and functional organization (Seeman, 1972; Sheetz and Singer, 1974; Papahadjopoulos *et al.*, 1975; Silva *et al.*, 1979; Yonei and Todo, 1982), and therefore may mimic the modifying effects of oxygen on cellular radiosensitivity. These drugs are used widely in clinical practice, and information on related toxicology and pharmacology is available. Therefore, if these drugs are effective radiosensitizers, they may prove effective for radiation therapy.

The present chapter summarizes our own observations plus studies of the published reports of other authors, emphasizing that membrane-specific drugs such as chlorpromazine, procaine, and lidocaine can modify the lethal effect of ionizing radiation on bacterial and mammalian cells, both *in vitro* and *in vivo*. The modifying effects of the drugs are discussed in terms of possible mechanisms. In addition, it should be noted that the membrane-specific drugs exhibit toxicity preferentially toward cells under conditions of hypoxia and that they can potentiate hyperthermic killing in bacterial and mammalian cells *in vitro* and *in vivo*.

II. Radiosensitizing Effect of Membrane-Specific Drugs on Bacterial Cells

Bacteria have been used to investigate various phenomena in radiobiology, and they remain the most suitable test systems for investigating many of the biological effects of radiation.

Carbonyl compounds, by virtue of their electron affinity to $C=O$ groups, are good radiosensitizers in bacterial and mammalian cells (Adams and Cooke, 1969; Barnes *et al.*, 1969). The electron charge distribution at the carbonyl bond of some local anesthetics also plays an important role in their anesthetic activity (Shenoy *et al.*, 1974). These same authors tested procaine hydrochloride, a common local anesthetic, and found that *E. coli* B/r irradiated while in contact with the drug were sensitized only when irradiation was carried out under hypoxic conditions. There was considerable sensitization also of hypoxically irradiated *E. coli* B/r treated with procaine immediately after irradiation. It is well established that the action of anesthetic drugs is associated with their binding to cell membranes (Seeman, 1972, 1975; Sheetz and Singer, 1974; Papahadjopoulos *et al.*, 1975). Therefore, the discovery of Shenoy *et al.* (1974) gave rise to a new class of hypoxic radiosensitizers derived from membrane-specific drugs. This class of compounds also includes other local anesthetics, analgesics, and tranquilizers. Shenoy *et al.* (1975b) found that other membrane-specific drugs enhanced radiation lethality of *E. coli* B/r, only under hypoxic conditions.

We also investigated the radiosensitizing action of such membrane-specific drugs on *E. coli* cells, especially with regard to the molecular mechanisms involved in this process (Yonei, 1979, 1982; Yonei *et al.*, 1981). We used local anesthetics such as procaine and lidocaine, and also a common tranquilizer, chlorpromazine (CPZ), as a potent radiosensitiz-ing drug. Exponentially growing cells of *E. coli* were irradiated with vari-ous doses of X rays at room temperature, under both oxic and hypoxic conditions. Solutions of the drugs were added to the cell suspensions just before irradiation. Immediately after irradiation, the cell suspensions were serially diluted and plated on nutrient agar to estimate cell survival. Chlorpromazine at a concentration of up to 0.1 mM affected neither the colony-forming ability of unirradiated *E. coli* B$_{s-1}$ (a DNA repair-defec-tive mutant, UvrB$^-$ExrA$^-$Lon$^-$) nor that of *E. coli* B/r (wild type for DNA repair). Loss of colony-forming ability in both strains was observed when the drug was added at higher concentrations such as 10 mM, but there was no significant difference between the sensitivity of *E. coli* B$_{s-1}$ to the drug and that of B/r. Furthermore, CPZ alone induced no mutation in the *E. coli* cells. These results demonstrate that CPZ induces no direct damage on the DNA genome in the cell. This conclusion was confirmed by the experimental results. In the absence of EDTA there appeared to be no significant induction of mutation on near-UV irradiation in the pres-ence of CPZ; however, when EDTA-treated cells were subjected to near-UV plus CPZ, the induced mutation frequency increased with the time of irradiation (Yonei and Todo, 1982). Therefore, CPZ specifically binds to the cell membrane.

Figure 1 shows that CPZ at 0.1 mM markedly sensitized *E. coli* B/r under hypoxic conditions of irradiation, and no sensitization by the drug was evident when X irradiation was carried out under oxic conditions (Yonei, 1979). Similar results were obtained when other drugs were used as "membrane-specific radiosensitizers" (Shenoy *et al.*, 1975b; Yonei, 1979, 1982). Among the compounds tested, CPZ was the most effective. Irradiated CPZ or irradiated procaine proved nontoxic to unirradiated cells of *E. coli* B/r, but addition of the drugs to hypoxically irradiated cells immediately after irradiation had a considerable sensitizing effect (She-noy *et al.*, 1974, 1975b; George *et al.*, 1975; Yonei, 1982). This would rule out the involvement of stable toxic products and/or short-lived transients of the drugs in this process. Therefore, we postulated that radiosensitiza-tion induced by the drugs may be the consequence of alterations in the cell membrane organization.

As can be seen in Fig. 2, there was no significant sensitization by CPZ at 0.1 mM under either oxic or hypoxic conditions of irradiation in *E. coli* B$_{s-1}$, cells genetically unable to repair radiation damage to DNA (Yonei, 1979). Similar observations were obtained with *E. coli* polA mutant (Yonei, 1982). These findings strongly suggest that the ultimate enhance-ment of lethality of X-irradiated *E. coli* B/r cells by CPZ and other mem-brane-specific drugs may be ascribed to inhibition of postirradiation DNA

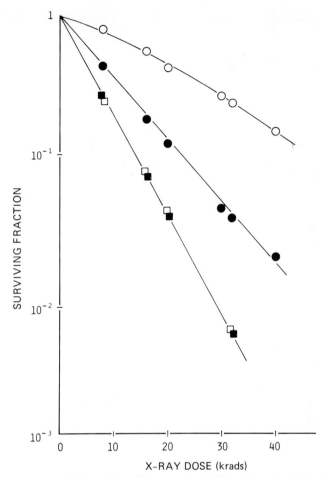

Fig. 1. The effects of CPZ on the radiation response of hypoxic and oxic *E. coli* B/r cells. The concentration of CPZ used was 0.1 m*M*. Open symbols, irradiation without drug; closed symbols, irradiation with drug. (○, ●) Hypoxic conditions. (□, ■) Oxic conditions. Reproduced from Yonei (1979), with permission of Taylor & Francis Ltd.

repair in the cells. This argument is supported by the following experimental results (Yonei *et al.*, 1981):

1. The frequencies of X-ray-induced mutation significantly increased in CPZ-treated *E. coli* cells under hypoxic conditions of irradiation.
2. Patterns of sedimentation of DNA in alkaline–sucrose density gradient centrifugation revealed that rejoining repair of DNA strand breaks was inhibited almost completely by the presence of CPZ at the time of irradiation and postirradiation incubation.

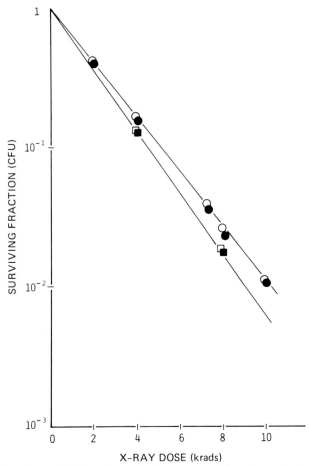

Fig. 2. The effects of CPZ on the radiation response of hypoxic and oxic *E. coli* B_{s-1}. Symbols are the same as those for Fig. 2. Reproduced from Yonei (1979), with permission of Taylor & Francis Ltd.

In earlier articles, damage to cell membranes by iodine compounds (Myers, 1971; Myers and Chetty, 1973) or phenethyl alcohol (Nair *et al.*, 1975) has also been shown to inhibit post-irradiation repair of single-strand breaks in bacterial DNA. These data indicate that the structural integrity of the cell membrane is essential for DNA repair in the cells. Furthermore, this view is comparable to studies of Yatvin (1976) and Yatvin *et al.* (1979a) in which the DNA repair and ultimate survival of *E. coli* cells following exposure to γ rays was influenced by the physical state (fluidity) of the cell membrane. However, it is also claimed that drugs such as procaine may modify only the "repair" of membrane, which in turn results in inhibition of DNA repair (Singh *et al.*, 1980). However, the nature of critical membrane damage and the mechanism of its repair remain speculative. The modification of repair by membrane-specific drugs requires further study.

George *et al.* (1975) reported that membrane-specific drugs did not modify the post-UV survival of *E. coli* B/r cells when added during irradiation. However, we found that CPZ, procaine, and lidocaine markedly inhibited the repair of UV-induced DNA damage and recovery of cell survival when UV-irradiated cells of *E. coli* were treated with the drugs through postirradiation incubation (Yonei, 1980; Todo and Yonei, 1982). It is therefore possible that the repair of DNA in *E. coli* is partly associated with the cell membrane. The mechanism of the relationship between cell membrane and DNA repair is currently under investigation in our laboratory. Furthermore, membrane-specific drugs can also sensitize the lethal effect of antitumor drugs such as mitomycin C and diethylmaleate on *E. coli* (S. Yonei, C. Y. Mitsutani, T. Todo, and O. Niwa, unpublished).

In addition to the drugs mentioned previously, Anderson and Patel (1977) and Anderson *et al.* (1978) suggested that some bipyridinium compounds sensitized the anoxic bacteria by action at a site associated with the outer membrane.

III. Modifying Effects of Membrane-Specific Drugs on Radiation Response of Mammalian Cells *in Vitro* and *in Vivo*

Local anesthetics belong to a class of clinically useful compounds that exert pharmacological effects by blocking nerve impulse propagation (Seeman, 1972, 1975, Ritchie, 1975; Strichartz, 1976). Although the molecular mechanisms of these drug actions are not fully understood, the involvement of cell membranes, as the critical site for the drug actions, has been commonly accepted (Seeman, 1972, 1975; Sheetz and Singer, 1974; Papahadjopoulos *et al.*, 1975). This type of drug–membrane interaction is not limited to the neural membrane. Local anesthetics have been used in studies to modify membrane-mediated cellular processes and regulatory mechanisms (Poste *et al.*, 1975; Papahadjopoulos *et al.*, 1975; Yau *et al.*, 1979; Schwarz *et al.*, 1982). The finding that local anesthetics radiosensitize hypoxic bacterial cells (Shenoy *et al.*, 1974, 1975b; Yonei, 1979) led to investigations of drugs that also modify the radiosensitivity of mammalian cells *in vitro*. Shenoy *et al.* (1975b) and George *et al.* (1975)

found that procaine at 25 m*M* was nontoxic to either Yoshida ascites tumor cells or rat thymocytes and that, under hypoxic conditions of irradiation, procaine sensitized both cell systems to much the same extent. No sensitization was observed under oxic conditions (George *et al.*, 1975). In contrast, Yau and Kim (1978) reported the radioprotective effect of procaine on oxic mammalian cells *in vitro*, using techniques of dye exclusion, growth extrapolation, and colony formation. Accordingly, Yau and Kim (1980) looked to see if this drug would also simultaneously radiosensitize mammalian cells *in vitro* and under hypoxia. It became evident that lidocaine, a commonly used local anesthetic, exhibited a dramatic radiosensitization to hypoxic mouse L5178Y lymphoma cells, whereas under oxic conditions of irradiation, this drug protected the cells against radiation-induced lethality (Yau and Kim, 1980). Thus the anesthetic drugs possess a "differential radiation-modifying capacity" between oxic and hypoxic mammalian cells.

Similar results were obtained using cultured mammalian cells. We compared the radiation-modifying effects of membrane-specific drugs in several types of mammalian cells, in particular in mouse L5178Y and L1210 lymphoma cells, and also in human HeLa cells. Two types of mouse lymphoma cell lines were maintained in Eagle's minimum essential medium supplemented with 10% calf serum as a suspension culture, and HeLa cells were cultured in the same medium, in monolayers. The cells were irradiated with various doses of X rays, diluted serially, and then incubated in soft agar for L5178Y and L1210 cells or in tissue culture flasks, in order for the HeLa cells to form viable colonies. The solutions of drugs were added to oxic or hypoxic cells immediately before irradiation. Figure 3 shows our experimental results with lidocaine. It is apparent that the local anesthetic drug can simultaneously radiosensitize L1210 cells as well as L5178Y cells under hypoxic conditions, and radioprotect them under oxic conditions. Under the specified experimental conditions, radioprotection of oxic cells or radiosensitization of hypoxic cells depends on concentration of the drugs. This differential effect of lidocaine between oxic and hypoxic cells was also observed with procaine (Fig. 4) and CPZ (Fig. 5) on mouse L5178Y cells. In contrast, there was no significant modification of the radiation response of HeLa cells in the presence of lidocaine during irradiation, under both conditions (Fig. 3A). The reason for this discrepancy was not determined. However, it is unlikely that the radiation-modifying effect can be specifically detected in mouse lymphoma cell lines, because radioprotective effects of procaine were observed in Chinese hamster ovary cells, under aerobic conditions (Yau, 1979). The modifying effect of local anesthetic drugs and tranquilizers on cellular radiation response is thus cell type specific and most likely involves the cell membranes.

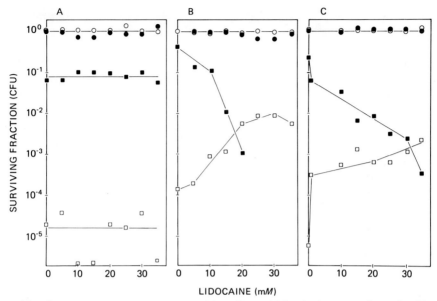

Fig. 3. Dose-dependent radiation-modifying effects of lidocaine in mammalian cells. (A) HeLa cells, (B) L1210 cells, (C) L5178Y cells. (○) Unirradiated in air; (□) 10 Gy-irradiated in air; (●) unirradiated in N_2 (hypoxia); (■) 10 Gy-irradiated in N_2.

Djordjevic (1979) reported that when present during irradiation only, procaine minimally protected HeLa cells from radiation damage, but postirradiation treatment of the cells with the procaine increased lethality in the cells, an effect that was dose dependent. With a 4.5-h treatment with 1 mM procaine, a dose-modifying effect of 1.3 was obtained. The results indicate that the structural integrity of cellular membrane is essential for repair processes, including DNA repair, in mammalian cells as well as in bacterial cells (Yonei, 1979, 1982a). It is therefore possible that membrane-specific drugs may inhibit repair of potentially lethal radiation damage (PLDR), and such is considered to be an important factor for resistance of tumors to radiation therapy (Withers, 1975; Weichselbaum et al., 1977; Koch, 1979; Nakatsugawa and Sugahara, 1980). Related studies are in progress in our laboratory.

The mechanisms whereby membrane-specific drugs play a dual role in modifying the radiation response of mammalian cells are not clear. There may be an inhibition of postirradiation repair processes in the cells. Yau and Kim (1980) pointed out that such drugs sensitize mammalian cells by the same mechanism seen with many carbonyl compounds. The finding that CPZ and procaine radioprotect oxic mammalian cells, but not oxic bacteria, indicates that they may be modulating a cell component(s) or process(es) unique to oxic mammalian cells (Yau and Kim, 1980).

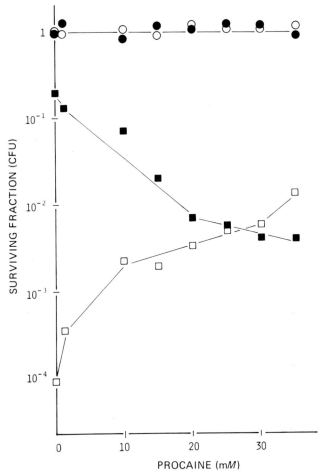

Fig. 4. Dose-dependent radioprotection of oxic and radiosensitization of hypoxic L5178Y cells by procaine. Symbols are the same as those for Fig. 3.

Chlorpromazine reduces the cellular ATP level and inhibits the generation of ATP, under conditions of anoxia (Lahrichi *et al.*, 1977; Shenoy and Singh, 1980). The reduction of ATP level in cells may result in inhibition of cellular repair processes and enhanced radiation lethality to cells (Shenoy and Gopalakrishna, 1977; Shenoy and Singh, 1980).

Hypoxic cells in tumors are believed to be the cause of tumor recurrences after radiation therapy (Withers, 1975; Adams, 1979; Koch, 1979; Sugahara and Nakatsugawa, 1981). Because such cells retain their proliferating ability and remain viable, deriving energy through anaerobic gly-

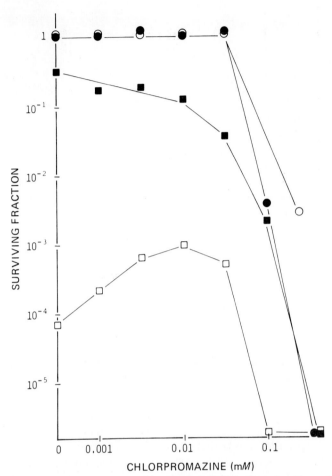

Fig. 5. Dose-dependent radioprotection of oxic L5178Y cells and radiosensitization of hypoxic ones by CPZ. Symbols are the same as those for Fig. 3.

colysis, drugs such as CPZ might prove useful in cancer radiotherapy. Shenoy and Singh (1980) investigated the radiosensitizing effect of CPZ in solid sarcoma 180A transplantable in Swiss mice. When CPZ was administered before irradiation at a single intratumor dose of 10 mg/kg, there was a definite tumor regrowth delay. With a dose of 20 mg/kg, the injection of CPZ resulted in a much slower tumor growth followed by a remarkable regression of the tumor, in all the animals (Shenoy and Singh, 1980). On Day 36 following radiotherapy, there was no palpable tumor, in any animal. These results clearly indicate the radiosensitizing effect of the drug in sarcoma 180A in mice. In addition, George *et al.* (1980) observed

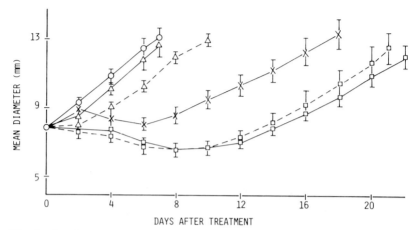

DAYS AFTER TREATMENT

Fig. 6. The effect of CPZ and radiation on the unclamped mouse fibrosarcoma. The drug was given 5 min before irradiation. The starting diameter is given as 8 mm, although there were minor variations (7–9 mm) from this. (O——O) Control; (△——△) CPZ 20 mg/kg; (△---△) CPZ 40 mg/kg; (×——×) 20 Gy X rays; (□——□) CPZ (20 mg/kg, before irradiation) plus 20 Gy; (□– –□) CPZ (40 mg/kg; before irradiation) plus 20 Gy. Vertical bars are standard deviations. Reproduced from George *et al.* (1980), with permission of Taylor & Francis Ltd.

that CPZ radiosensitized both chronically hypoxic (unclamped; see the results in Fig. 6) and acutely hypoxic (clamped) fibrosarcoma in mice when the drug was given 5 min before irradiation. Radiosensitization by CPZ *in vivo* was noted in mouse melanomas (see references in Shenoy and Singh, 1980). In these tissues CPZ causes radiosensitization by way of decreased transplantability and a lower incidence of metastasis (Shenoy and Singh, 1980). Whether there is a similar occurrence in the two transplantable tumors, sarcoma 180A and fibrosarcoma in mice (Shenoy and Singh, 1980; George *et al.*, 1980), is uncertain.

IV. Cytotoxicity of CPZ in Bacterial and Mammalian Cells *in Vitro* and *in Vivo*

The selective cytotoxicity of a drug toward hypoxic cells is of interest to radiotherapists. If such drugs prove to be effective radiosensitizers as well, their use in combination with radiation is expected to increase the cure rate in cancer treatment. Shenoy and colleagues investigated the cytotoxic effect of CPZ on *E. coli* and mammalian cells *in vivo*. In *E. coli* cells, CPZ is preferentially toxic toward hypoxic cells, depending on the drug concentration, and the hypoxic cytotoxicity is dependent on the temperature during treatment (i.e., the toxicity increases with temperatures above 30°C) (Shenoy and Singh, 1978). The finding that CPZ cytotoxicity was reduced when the cells were pretreated with N-ethylmaleimide only under hypoxic conditions indicates the inactivation of certain SH enzymes (Shenoy and Singh, 1978). Such enzymes are probably intimately associated with the cell membrane as are ATPase or glyceraldehyde phosphate dehydrogenase, the latter a rate-limiting enzyme in anaerobic glycolysis (Lahrichi et al., 1977). Thus the cytotoxicity of CPZ toward hypoxic cells may be the result of an inhibition of glycolysis (Lahrichi et al., 1977; Shenoy and Singh, 1978).

Shenoy and Singh (1980) found that CPZ administered ip to mice bearing a solid form of sarcoma 180A and in a dose of 40 mg/kg reduced the growth rate of tumors in treated animals. Shenoy et al. (1982) also found that the drug exhibits a carcinostatic effect on spontaneous mammary adenocarcinoma in breeding female CBA mice when the longevity of the tumor-bearing mice is taken as the criterion. Although there were no regressions in the tumor size, as compared to untreated controls, the incidence of secondaries in the treated groups was lower compared to the untreated controls. Whether this observation indicates a lower incidence and/or slower spreading of metastasis has yet to be determined (Shenoy et al., 1982). In contrast, CPZ was not effective for the ascites form of sarcoma 180A (Shenoy and Singh, 1980) and lymphosarcoma (Shenoy et al., 1982). The authors concluded that the ineffectiveness of CPZ might be the result of the absence of hypoxic cells in these tumors. Shenoy et al. (1982) investigated the distribution of CPZ in plasma and tumor tissue in sarcoma 180A and found that the peak level of the drug in tumor tissue was 2.5 times greater than the peak level in the plasma and was observed at 90 min following a single ip injection. The high tumor:plasma ratio suggests that the drug reaches the hypoxic tumor cells at concentrations greater than those in the plasma. Shenoy et al. (1982) also reported that CPZ has an inhibitory effect on oxygen utilization by different mammalian cells in vitro. They also found that in Chinese hamster V-79-171B spheroids (an in vitro tumor model), CPZ sensitizes by affecting the slope of the survival curve, thus indicating reoxygenation of the spheroids.

V. Potentiation of Hyperthermic Killing of Bacterial and Mammalian Cells in Vitro and in Vivo by Membrane-Specific Drugs

Hyperthermia and ionizing radiation in combination synergistically kill mammalian cells (Ben-Hur et al., 1974; Dewey et al., 1980; Miyakoshi et *al.*, 1982). These data plus advances in the localized heating of tumors (Marmor *et al.*, 1978; Sandhu *et al.*, 1978) provide rationale for the treatment of cancer in humans with combined hyperthermia and radiation therapy. Hyperthermia alone is also being applied as an additional or adjunctive mode of cancer therapy. The effects of hyperthermia on normal and malignant cells are under investigation (Bronk, 1976; Dewey *et al.*, 1980; Miyakoshi *et al.*, 1982). The nature of the hyperthermic target is of particular interest. A considerable body of evidence suggests that cellular membranes are involved in hyperthermic killing (Wallach, 1978, Yau, 1979, Dewey *et al.*, 1980; Stevenson *et al.*, 1981; Yatvin *et al.*, 1982). Yatvin (1977) and Dennis and Yatvin (1981) have presented evidence that supports the view that membrane lipid fluidity critically determines survival after thermal insult. Small elevations in temperature tend to increase the fluidity of cell membranes, and procaine and lidocaine are shown to be membrane-fluidizing agents (Yatvin, 1977; Yatvin and Dennis, 1978; Yau, 1979; Yonei, 1982a). Therefore, it is particularly interesting to find out if membrane-specific drugs will potentiate the hyperthermic killing of cells. In bacterial cells, procaine was found to enhance the hyperthermic killing (Yatvin, 1977; Yatvin and Dennis, 1978). These authors suggested that the drug- and nutrition-related decreases in the extent of membrane organization appear to increase susceptibility to hyperthermic killing of *E. coli* auxotrophs, whose membrane fatty acid composition can be partially controlled. They are unable to synthesize or degrade unsaturated fatty acids (Yatvin, 1977; Yatvin and Dennis, 1978; Dennis and Yatvin, 1981).

In mammalian cells *in vitro,* Yau (1979) found that procaine greatly potentiates the process of hyperthermic killing at 43°C in mouse L5178Y cells, as shown in Fig. 7. Potentiation was evident with a 1.0 m*M* concentration. Other local anesthetics such as lidocaine and dibucaine (Yau and Kim, 1980), as well as CPZ (Shenoy *et al.*, 1982), were found to have similar potentiating effects on the hyperthermic killing in L5178Y cells. Among the local anesthetics tested, dibucaine was the most and procaine the least effective (Yau and Kim, 1980). The potentiating capacity was dependent on the temperature of treatment and concentration of the drugs (Shenoy *et al.*, 1982). Compared to other drugs that enhance the hyperthermia-induced lethality, a lower concentration of CPZ in the micromolar range is required (Shenoy *et al.*, 1982). Using scanning electron microscopy, Yau (1979) and Mulcahy *et al.* (1981) presented evidence to indicate that procaine may induce a modification of heat-induced effects through unknown membrane-mediated mechanisms. The similarities in cellular response to hyperthermia and to membrane-specific drugs could be explained by the existence of a common site of action.

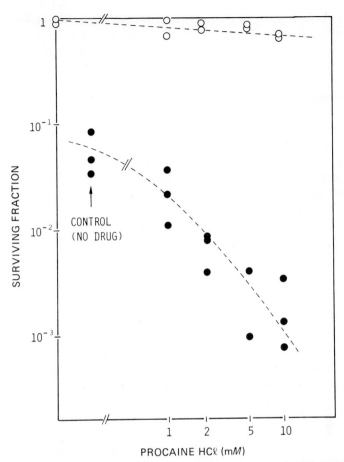

Fig. 7. Dose dependency of procaine in potentiating hyperthermic killing (43°C for 60 min) of mouse L5178Y-R₁ cells. (○) Incubation at 37°C; (●) incubation at 43°C. Reproduced from Yau (1979), with permission of Academic Press.

On the basis of these observations, it has been postulated that local anesthetics and CPZ might potentiate the therapeutic effect of hyperthermia in treatment of malignant disease. Yatvin *et al.* (1979b) reported potentiation by an anesthetic drug, lidocaine, of the tumor-inhibiting effect of local hyperthermia. They used young adult BDF₁ mice grafted with mammary adenocarcinoma strain CA755. Tumors were transplanted from donor mice and grown in the hind leg. The tumor-bearing legs were exposed to bath temperatures of 42 or 43.5°C for 1 h. Lidocaine was infused into three areas of the tumor within 5 min before heat treatment. Mean survival of the mice with lidocaine-infused tumors heated at 43.5°C was significantly greater than that of all other groups (Yatvin *et al.*, 1979b). Of 31 mice treated, 4 survived with complete control of the tumors.

VI. Summary and Conclusions

It is generally believed that cellular membranes as well as the DNA genome may be important sites for radiation-induced cellular response. A drug that induces various disorganizations of membrane structure and its functions may be capable of modifying the radiation response of cells. This class of compounds, called membrane-specific drugs, includes local anesthetics, analgesics, and tranquilizers. These compounds have been used in various studies to modify membrane-mediated cellular processes and regulatory mechanisms in bacterial and mammalian cells. Our observations and radiobiological studies of others can be summarized as follows:

1. Membrane-specific drugs such as procaine, lidocaine, and CPZ are found to sensitize radiation-induced lethality of *E. coli* cells, only under hypoxic conditions of irradiation. Sensitization is not observed when irradiation is carried out under oxic conditions.
2. These drugs simultaneously radiosensitize hypoxic mammalian cells and radioprotect oxic ones *in vitro*. The characteristic "differential radiation-modifying effect" is cell type specific.
3. In both bacterial and mammalian cells, the addition of the drugs to hypoxically irradiated cells within 1 min after irradiation has a considerable sensitizing effect. It appears that membrane-specific drugs inhibit postirradiation repair processes in the cells.
4. Chlorpromazine exerts a radiosensitizing effect on sarcoma 180A and fibrosarcoma *in vivo* when the drug is given 5 min before irradiation of the tumor-bearing mice. Therefore, the drug active *in vitro* is also potent *in vivo*.
5. Chlorpromazine has a cytotoxic effect, preferentially toward bacterial and mammalian cells under hypoxic conditions. Furthermore, the drug exhibits a carcinostatic effect on mammary adenocarcinoma in mice.
6. The membrane-specific drugs can potentiate the hyperthermic killing in bacterial and mammalian cells *in vitro*. The potentiation of hyperthermic damage is also observed *in vivo,* in terms of prolonged survival of tumor-bearing mice, when the local anesthetic lidocaine is injected into the tumor prior to heating. Such drugs may play an important role for clinical application of hyperthermia.

7. In addition, the membrane-specific drugs can sensitize the lethal effect of anticancer drugs on *E. coli* cells. Mizuno and Ishida (1982) found that cell killing by bleomycins, a group of antibiotics currently applied in the treatment of human cancer, is markedly potentiated by exposing mammalian cells to local anesthetics either before or after treatment with bleomycins.

Thus membrane-specific drugs can fulfill all or most of the stringent requirements needed for a compound to be of any practical use in radiation and hyperthermic therapy. Because the same compound is capable of exerting its radiation-modifying effects in opposite directions with hypoxic and oxic mammalian cells, the dose necessary to produce a given therapeutic result may be smaller when the drug is used in radiation therapy of partially hypoxic tumors *in vivo*. Furthermore, because such drugs are pharmacologically acceptable, the lapse of time between toxicological evaluation and clinical trials can be minimized. This new type of radiosensitizing compounds, with CPZ and procaine as their prototype, may be clinically applicable as an adjuvant to radiation treatment of human cancer. The present experimental results provide information of radiobiological importance. In particular, the structural integrity may be essential for cellular repair processes, including DNA repair.

Acknowledgments

We express our gratitude to Drs. T. Sugahara and M. Kato, Kyoto University for pertinent discussions and advice during the course of this research. Thanks are also owed to Dr. M. A. Shenoy, Bhabha Atomic Research Center of India, for helpful discussions. These studies were supported in part by grants from the Ministry of Education, Science and Culture, Japan.

References

Adams, G. E. (1979). The role of radiosensitizing drugs in the management of cancer. *Invest. Cell Pathol.* **2,** 303–308.

Adams, G. E., and Cooke, M. S. (1969). Electron-affinic sensitization. I. A structural basis for chemical radiosensitizers in bacteria. *Int. J. Radiat. Biol.* **15,** 457–471.

Ahnström, G., and Ehrenberg, L. (1980). The nature of the target in the biological action of ionizing radiations. *Adv. Biol. Med. Phys.* **17,** 129–172.

Alper, T. (1971). Cell death and its modification: the roles of primary lesions in membranes and DNA. *In* Proceedings of a Symposium (Biophysical Aspects of Radiation Quality) held by the IAEA in Lucas Heights, Australia, pp. 171–184.

Alper, T. (1979). Targets and mechanisms for cell killing. *In* "Cellular Radiobiology" (T. Alper, ed.), pp. 205–226. Cambridge Univ. Press, Cambridge.

Anderson, R. F., and Patel, K. B. (1977). Radiosensitization of *Serratia marcescens* by bipyridinium compounds. *Int. J. Radiat. Biol.* **32,** 471–479.

Anderson, R. F., Patel, K. B., and Smithen, C. E. (1978). Radiosensitization of *Serratia marcescens* by nitropyridinium compounds. *Br. J. Cancer* **37** (Suppl. 3), 103–106.

Bacq, Z. M., and Alexander, P. (1961). "Fundamentals of Radiobiology." Pergamon, London.

Barnes, J. H., Ashwood-Smith, M. J., and Bridges, B. A. (1969). Radiosensitization of bacterial cells by carbonyl compounds. *Int. J. Radiat. Biol.* **15,** 285–288.

Ben-Hur, E., Elkind, M. M., and Bronk, B. V. (1974). Thermally enhanced radio-response of cultured Chinese hamster cells: inhibition of repair of sublethal damage and enhancement of lethal damage. *Radiat. Res.* **58,** 38–51.

Bronk, B. V. (1976). Thermal potentiation of mammalian cell killing; clues for understanding and potential for tumor therapy. *Adv. Radiat. Biol.* **6,** 267–318.

Brown, J. M., and Yu, N. Y. (1979). Cytotoxicity of misonidazole *in vivo* under conditions of prolonged contact of the drug with the tumour cells. *Br. J. Radiol.* **52,** 893–896.

Burki, H. J. (1976). Critical DNA damage and mammalian cell reproduction. *J. Mol. Biol.* **103,** 559–610.

Chadwick, K. H., and Leenhouts, H. P. (1981). The molecular model for cell survival following radiation. *In* "The Molecular Theory of Radiation Biology" (K. H. Chadwick and H. P. Leenhouts, eds.), pp. 25–50. Springer-Verlag, Berlin.

Cremer, C., Cremer, T., Zorn, C., and Schoeller, L. (1976). Effects of laser UV-microirradiation ($\lambda = 2573$ Å) on proliferation of Chinese hamster cells. *Radiat. Res.* **66,** 106–121.

Dennis, W. H., and Yatvin, M. B. (1981). Correlation of hyperthermic sensitivity and membrane microviscosity in *E. coli* K1060. *Int. J. Radiat. Biol.* **39,** 265–271.

Dewey, W. C., Freeman, M. L., Raaphorst, P., Clark, E. P., Wong, R. S. L., Highfield, D. P., Spiro, I. J., Tomasovic, S. P., Denman, D. L., and Cross, R. A. (1980). Cell biology of hyperthermia and radiation. *In* "Radiation Biology in Cancer Research" (R. E. Meyn and H. R. Withers, eds.), pp. 589–621. Raven, New York.

Djordjevic, B. (1979). Differential effect of procaine on irradiated mammalian cells in culture. *Radiology (Easton, Pa.)* **13,** 515–519.

Fowler, J. F. (1980). Hypoxic cell radiosensitizers, present status and future promise. *In* "Radiation Biology in Cancer Research" (R. E. Meyn and H. R. Withers, eds.), pp. 533–546. Raven, New York.

George, K. C., Shenoy, M. A., Joshi, D. S., Bhatt, B. Y., Singh, B. B., and Gopal-Ayengar, A. R. (1975). Modification of radiation effects on cells by membrane-binding agents-procaine HCl. *Br. J. Radiol.* **48,** 611–614.

George, K. C., Srinivasan, V. T., and Singh, B. B. (1980). Cytotoxic effect of chlorpromazine and radiation on a mouse fibrosarcoma. *Int. J. Radiat. Biol.* **38,** 661–665.

Koch, C. J. (1979). The effect of oxygen on the repair of radiation damage by cells and tissues. *Adv. Radiat. Biol.* **8,** 273–315.

Korbelik, M., Palcic, B., and Skarsgard, L. D. (1981). Radiation-enhanced cytotoxicity of misonidazole. *Radiat. Res.* **88,** 343–353.

Köteles, G. J. (1979). New aspects of cell membrane radiobiology and their impact on radiation protection. *At. Energy Rev.* **17,** 3–30.

Lahrichi, M., Houpert, Y., Tarallo, P., Loppinet, V., and Siest, G. (1977). Protein and enzyme release from human leucocytes: influence of phenothiazine derivatives. *Chem. Biol. Interact.* **19,** 173–183.

Marmor, J. B., Pounds, D., Hahn, N., and Hahn, G. M. (1978). Treating spontaneous tumors in dogs and cats by ultrasound-induced hyperthermia. *Int. J. Radiat. Oncol. Biol. Phys.* **44,** 967–973.

Miyakoshi, J., Heki, S., Furukawa, M., and Kano, E. (1982). Recovery kinetics from the damage by step-up and step-down heatings in combination with radiation in Chinese hamster cells. *J. Radiat. Res.* **23**, 187–197.

Mizuno, S., and Ishida, A. (1982). Selective enhancement of bleomycin cytotoxicity by local anesthetics. *Biochem. Biophys. Res. Commun.* **105**, 425–431.

Mulcahy, R. T., Gould, M. N., Hidvegi, E., Elson, C. E., and Yatvin, M. B. (1981). Hyperthermia and surface morphology of P388 ascites tumour cells: effects of membrane modifications. *Int. J. Radiat. Biol.* **39**, 95–106.

Myers, D. K. (1971). DNA repair in *E. coli* B/r after X-irradiation in the presence of iodine of iodoacetamide. *Int. J. Radiat. Biol.* **19**, 293–295.

Myers, D. K., and Chetty, K. G. (1973). Effect of radiosensitizing agents on DNA strand breaks and their rapid repair during irradiation. *Radiat. Res.* **53**, 307–314.

Nair, C. K. K., Pradhan, D. S., and Sreenivasan, A. (1975). Rejoining of radiation-induced single-strand breaks in deoxyribonucleic acid of *Escherichia coli:* effect of phenetyl alcohol. *J. Bacteriol.* **121**, 392–395.

Nakatsugawa, S., and Sugahara, T. (1980). Inhibition of X-ray-induced potentially lethal damage (PLD) repair by cordycepin (3′-deoxyadenosine) and enhancement of its action by 2′-deoxycoformycin in Chinese hamster *hai* cells in the stationary phase *in vitro. Radiat. Res.* **84**, 265–275.

Okada, S. (1970). "Cells." Academic Press, New York.

Papahadjopoulos, D., Jacobson, K., Poste, G., and Sheperd, G. (1975). Effects of local anesthetics on membrane properties. I. Changes in fluidity of phospholipid bilayers. *Biochim. Biophys. Acta* **394**, 504–519.

Patrick, G. (1977). The effects of radiation on cell membranes. *In* "Mammalian Cell Membranes" (G. A. Jamieson and D. M. Robinson, eds.), Vol. 5, pp. 72–104. Butterworth, London.

Poste, G., Papahadjopoulos, D., Jacobson, K., and Vail, W. J. (1975). Local anaesthetics increase susceptibility of untransformed cells to agglutination by concanavalin A. *Nature (London)* **253**, 552–554.

Ritchie, J. M. (1975). Mechanism of action of local anesthetic agents and biotoxins. *Br. J. Anaesth.* **47**, 191–198.

Sandhu, T. S., Kowal, H. S., and Johnson, R. J. R. (1978). The development of microwave hyperthermia applicators. *Int. J. Radiat. Oncol. Biol. Phys.* **4**, 515–519.

Schwarz, M. A., Harper, P. A., and Juliano, R. L. (1982). Interactions of lectins with CHO cell surface membranes. II. Differential effects of local anesthetics on endocytosis of ConA and WGA binding sites. *J. Cell. Physiol.* **111**, 264–274.

Seeman, P. (1972). The membrane actions of anesthetics and tranquillizers. *Pharmacol. Rev.* **24**, 583–655.

Seeman, P. (1975). The actions of nervous system drugs on cell membranes. *In* "Cell Membranes Biochemistry, Cell Biology and Pathology" (G. Weissman and R. Claiborne, eds.), pp. 239–247. HP Publ., New York.

Sheetz, M. P., and Singer, S. J. (1974). Biological membranes as bilayer couples. A molecular mechanism of drug-erythrocyte interactions. *Proc. Natl. Acad. Sci. USA* **71**, 4457–4461.

Shenoy, M. A., and Gopalakrishna, K. (1977). Biochemical aspects of radiation sensitization of *E. coli* B/r by chlorpromazine. *Int. J. Radiat. Biol.* **33**, 587–593.

Shenoy, M. A., and Singh, B. B. (1978). Hypoxic cytotoxicity of chlorpromazine and the modification of radiation response in *E. coli* B/r. *Int. J. Radiat. Biol.* **34**, 595–600.

Shenoy, M. A., and Singh, B. B. (1980). Cytotoxic and radiosensitizing effects of chlorpromazine hydrochloride in Sarcoma 180A. *Indian J. Exp. Biol.* **18**, 791–795.

Shenoy, M. A., Singh, B. B., and Gopal-Ayengar, A. R. (1974). Enhancement of radiation lethality of *E. coli* B/r by procaine hydrochloride. *Nature (London)* **248**, 415–416.

Shenoy, M. A., Asquith, J. C., Adams, G. E., Michael, B. D., and Watts, M. E. (1975a). Time-resolved oxygen effects in irradiated bacteria and mammalian cells: a rapid-mix study. *Radiat. Res.* **62**, 498–512.

Shenoy, M. A., George, K. C., Singh, B. B., and Gopal-Ayengar, A. R. (1975b). Modification of radiation effects in single-cell systems by membrane-binding agents. *Int. J. Radiat. Biol.* **28**, 519–526.

Shenoy, M. A., Biaglow, J. E., Varnes, M. E., and Daniel, J. W. (1982). A biochemical basis for the radiosensitizing and cytotoxic effects of chlorpromazine hydrochloride *in vitro* and *in vivo*. *Int. J. Radiat. Oncol. Biol. Phys.* **8**, 725–728.

Silva, M. T., Sousa, J. C. F., Polónia, J. J., and Macedo, P. M. (1979). Effects of local anesthetics on bacterial cells. *J. Bacteriol.* **137**, 461–468.

Singh, B. B., Shenoy, M. A., and George, K. C. (1980). Nature of radiation and chemically induced lesions and role of cellular mechanisms in cell survival and mutagenesis. I. Membrane and cellular repair. *Adv. Biol. Med. Phys.* **17**, 109–113.

Stevenson, M. A., Minton, K. W., and Hahn, G. M. (1981). Survival and concanavalin A-induced capping in CHO fibroblasts after exposure to hyperthermia, ethanol, and X irradiation. *Radiat. Res.* **86**, 467–478.

Strichartz, G. (1976). Molecular mechanisms of nerve block of local anesthetics. *Anesthesiology* **45**, 421–441.

Sugahara, T., and Nakatsugawa, S. (1981). Radiation sensitization studies in Japan. *Cancer Treat. Rev.* **8**, 51–61.

Todo, T., and Yonei, S. (1983). The inhibitory effect of membrane-binding drugs on excision repair of DNA damage in UV-irradiated *Escherichia coli*. *Mutat. Res.* **112**, 97–107.

Wallach, D. F. H. (1978). Action of hyperthermia and ionizing radiation on plasma membranes. *In* "Cancer Therapy by Hyperthermia and Radiation" (C. Streffer, ed.), pp. 19–28. Urban & Schwarzenberg, Baltimore and Munich.

Watkins, D. K. (1970). High o.e.r. for the release of enzymes from isolated mammalian lysosomes after ionizing radiation. *Adv. Biol. Med. Phys.* **13**, 289–306.

Weichselbaum, R. R., Little, J. B., and Nove, J. (1977). Response of human osteosarcoma *in vitro* to irradiation: evidence for unusual cellular repair activity. *Int. J. Radiat. Biol.* **31**, 295–299.

Whillans, D. W., and Whitmore, G. F. (1981). The radiation reduction of misonidazole. *Radiat. Res.* **86**, 311–324.

Withers, H. R. (1975). The four R's of radiotherapy. *Adv. Radiat. Biol.* **5**, 241–271.

Yatvin, M. B. (1976). Evidence that survival of gamma-irradiated *Escherichia coli* is influenced by membrane fluidity. *Int. J. Radiat. Biol.* **30**, 571–574.

Yatvin, M. B. (1977). The influence of membrane lipid composition and procaine on hyperthermic death of cells. *Int. J. Radiat. Biol.* **32**, 513–521.

Yatvin, M. B., and Dennis, W. H. (1978). Membrane lipid composition and sensitivity to killing by hyperthermia, procaine and radiation. *In* "Cancer Therapy by Hyperthermia and Radiation" (C. Streffer, ed.), pp. 157–159. Urban & Schwarzenberg, Baltimore and Munich.

Yatvin, M. B., Gipp, J. J., and Dennis, W. H. (1979a). Influence of unsaturated fatty acids, membrane fluidity and oxygenation on the survival of an *E. coli* fatty acid auxotroph following -irradiation. *Int. J. Radiat. Biol.* **35**, 539–548.

Yatvin, M. B., Clifton, K. H., and Dennis, W. H. (1979b). Hyperthermia and local anesthetics: potentiation of survival of tumor-bearing mice. *Science (Washington, D.C.)* **205**, 195–196.

Yatvin, M. B., Cree, T. C., Elson, C. E., Gipp, J. J., Tegmo, I.-M., and Vorpahl, J. W. (1982). Probing the relationship of membrane "fluidity" to heat killing of cells. *Radiat. Res.* **89,** 644–646.

Yau, T. M. (1979). Procaine-mediated modification of membranes and of the response to X irradiation and hyperthermia in mammalian cells. *Radiat. Res.* **80,** 523–541.

Yau, T. M., and Kim, S. C. (1978). Radioprotection of mammalian cells by procaine. *Br. J. Radiol.* **51,** 551–552.

Yau, T. M., and Kim, S. C. (1980). Local anaesthetics as hypoxic radiosensitizers, oxic radioprotectors and potentiators of hyperthermic killing in mammalian cells. *Br. J. Radiol.* **53,** 687–692.

Yau, T. M., Kim, S. C., and Grissman, H. A. (1979). Selection and characterization of a variant of murine L5178Y lymphoma resistant to local anesthetics. *J. Cell. Physiol.* **99,** 239–246.

Yonei, S. (1979). Modification of radiation effects on *E. coli* B/r and a radiosensitive mutant B_{s-1} by membrane-binding drugs. *Int. J. Radiat. Biol.* **36,** 547–551.

Yonei, S. (1980). Inhibitory effect of membrane-specific drugs on liquid-holding recovery in UV-irradiated *E. coli* cells. *Int. J. Radiat. Biol.* **37,** 685–689.

Yonei, S. (1982). Membranes. *In* "Mechanisms of Radiation Injury -Physically Initial Step to Cell-Molecular Damages" (O. Yamamoto, ed.), pp. 273–303. Japan Sci. Soc. Press, Tokyo (in Japanese).

Yonei, S., and Todo, T. (1982). Enhanced sensitivity to the lethal and mutagenic effects of photosensitizing action of chlorpromazine in ethylenediaminetetraacetate-treated *Escherichia coli*. *Photochem. Photobiol.* **35,** 591–592.

Yonei, S., Todo, T., Furui, H., and Wada, T. (1981). Mechanisms for radiosensitizing action of membrane-specific drugs on *E. coli*. *J. Radiat. Res.* **22,** 32 (Abstr.).

PART FIVE

Hyperthermia

17 Instruments and Measurements

Hirokazu Kato

Department of Radiology
Shimane Medical University
Izumo 693, Japan

I. Heating Method

A. Measurement of Absorbed Power

The measurement of absorbed power distribution in the phantom is of the utmost importance when considering characteristics of applicators. The distribution of absorbed power can be derived from the distribution of rise in temperature if the heat diffusion in the phantom is minimal to the point of neglect. When the temperature gradient in the heating material is steep and/or a long period of time is required from heating to start of the temperature measurement, the heat diffusion may distort the distribution of rise in temperature from the distribution of absorbed power.

Conditions in which heat diffusion can be safely neglected are discussed in this chapter, on the basis of data obtained in experiments on capacitive heating (Ishida *et al.*, 1980). Agar, the heating material used, was composed of 2.0% w/w agar powder, 0.87% w/w NaCl, and 97.15% w/w water. The agar was trimmed into a cubic shape of $10 \times 10 \times 10$ cm. Two aluminum electrodes of 5.0 cm diameter were attached to the centers of the opposite faces of the agar. A cotton thread following a fine C–C thermocouple was run through from the center of one of the electrodes to

Modification of Radiosensitivity in Cancer Treatment
Copyright © 1984 by Academic Press Japan, Inc.
All rights of reproduction in any form reserved.
ISBN 0-12-676020-9

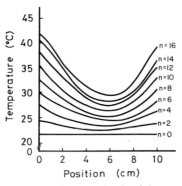

Fig. 1. Temperature profiles along the central axis of the agar. Radiofrequency heating for 10 sec in 120-mA plate current was repeated at about 10-sec intervals. The n values represent the repeated heating cycle. The 0-cm position is at one of the electrodes; the 10-cm position is at the other electrode.

the center of the other electrode, via a central axis of the agar. The agar was contained in a Styrofoam container. The RF current at 40.46 MHz was applied for 10 sec. Immediately after the heating, the thread was drawn at a speed of 2 cm/sec to record the temperature profile along the central axis of the agar. The RF heating for 10 sec followed by immediate measurement of the temperature profile was carried out once every 20 sec, and this procedure was repeated 25 times. Figure 1 shows the sequential temperature profiles along the central axis of the agar. Position "0 cm" represents the position at one of the electrodes, and "10 cm" that at the other electrode. The n values represent the repeated heating cycle. Sequential changes of temperature at three positions are shown in Fig. 2. Open circles, closed circles, and open triangles represent the temperatures at the positions 0, 5.9, and 10.0 cm, respectively. The increment of temperature at position 0 cm is linear within 4 min of heating time, followed by a downward swerving from the linearity. However, the linear increase in temperature at the position 5.9 cm is maintained over the experiment, where the temperature gradient is nearly zero, as shown in Fig. 1.

Causes of deviation from the linear relationship between the absorbed power profile and the distribution of rise in temperature can be enumerated as follows:

1. Finite spatial resolution in thermometry occurs as a result of finite response time due to heat capacity and heat conduction of the temperature probe and the time constant of the thermometer system.
2. The temperature profile is altered as a result of heat transfers within or out of the agar.

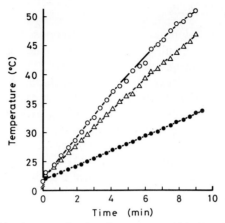

Fig. 2. Relationships between heating time course and temperatures in a variety of positions within the agar. The abscissa is the time during which cycles of 10-sec heating followed by about 10-sec intervals are repeated. (○) Temperatures at one of the electrodes. (●) Temperatures at 5.9 cm from one of the electrodes, where temperature was the lowest. (△) Temperatures at the other electrode.

3. Electric constants of the agar are altered concomitantly with the temperature increment. When the temperature is increased 1°C, the electroconductivity of an electrolyte increases about 2.5% while the dielectric constant decreases about 0.5% (Johnson and Guy, 1972).

The causes just enumerated appear negligible when the linear temperature increment is maintained, therefore the absorbed power profile would be the same as the profile of the increment of temperature. This linearity of temperature increment holds when the difference of the temperature over the agar is less than 3°C and less than 4 min of heating time, and when the temperature gradient in the agar is less than 3.2°C/cm.

B.   Capacitive Heating

Although the capacity heating occasionally induces overheating in the subcutaneous fatty layer, this heating is used for hyperthermia, as deep heating is feasible. Because the deep heating with this method varies with the size of the electrodes and the thickness of the heating material, it is essential to discuss the relationships between the size of the electrodes and the distribution of absorbed power, and between the thickness of heating material and the distribution of absorbed power (Tanaka *et al.*, 1981a).

1. Materials and Methods

The agar used, in columnar form, was composed of 2.0% w/w agar powder, 0.5% w/w NaCl, and 97.5% w/w water. The conductivity and the dielectric constant of the agar, at 13.56 MHz and 22°C, were 0.94 S/m and 76, respectively. The agar was 37.7 cm in diameter and 5, 10, 15, or 20 cm thick (L). Two electrodes, 5, 10, or 15 cm in diameter (D) were attached on the centers of both the bases of the agar. A thread bound to the C–C thermocouple of 0.1 mm in diameter was run through from the center of one of the electrodes to the center of the other electrode, via the central axis of the agar. The RF current at 13.56 MHz was supplied to the electrodes. Absorbed powers along the central axis were measured by the method described previously.

2. Results and Discussion

The distribution of absorbed power is shown in Fig. 3A, B, and C. The solid, dotted, and dashed lines represent different electrode diameters (D = 5, 10, and 15 cm). The absorbed power at the center of the agar increased according to both increase in the size of the electrode and decrease in the thickness of the agar. Figure 4 shows the relationship between the absorbed power at the midpoint on the central axis of the agar, which is normalized by the absorbed power at 1 cm from the base, and the thickness of the agar relative to the diameter of the electrodes (L/D). The open and solid circles and open triangles correspond to D = 5, 10, and 15 cm, respectively. The absorbed power exponentially decreased in accordance with the increase in the relative thickness of the agar. The three nearly concurrent curves suggest that the electric field distribution in the agar corresponds to the parallel relationship between the interelectrode interval and the electrode size, as discussed by Moon and Spencer (1961). The apparent linearities shown in Fig. 4 suggest that the deep heating is more feasible in a single radiofrequency (RF) heating by one pair of large electrodes than in multiportal RF heating using a few small electrodes (Suggar and LeVeen, 1979).

C. Inductive Heating

Considerable attention has been given to RF inductive heating as a noninvasive method of deep heating. The energy absorption in the fat layer is slight, penetration to the deeper regions is fairly good, noncontact heating is feasible, and the equipment can be easily adjusted. In some instances of inductive heating, the heating material is either inserted into a

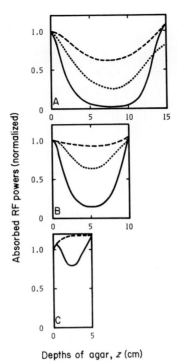

Fig. 3. Normalized distributions of absorbed RF power along Z axis in the agar of $L = 15$ (A), 10 (B), and 5 cm (C), respectively, with electrodes of various diameters. Curves are normalized at $z = 0$ cm. Diameters: (——) 5 cm; (·····) 10 cm; (-----) 15 cm.

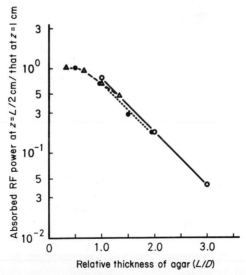

Fig. 4. Relationship between absorbed RF power at $z = L/2$ cm, normalized by that at $z = 1$ cm, and thickness of the agar, normalized by the diameter (D) of electrodes. Diameters: (○) 5 cm; (●) 10 cm; (△) 15 cm.

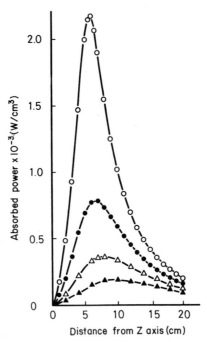

Fig. 5. Distributions of absorbed power in calculation by a cylindrical coil, 6 cm in radius and 24 cm in height. z Values: (○) 1 cm; (●) 3 cm; (△) 5 cm; (▲) 7 cm.

one-turned cylindrical coil or placed in front of the coil, as in the case of a pancake-type coil or a cylindrical coil (Hahn *et al.*, 1980).

Figure 5 shows the distributions of absorbed power in a cylindrical coil. The calculation was performed under conditions that the coil (6 cm in radius and 24 cm in height), in which flowed the surface current (10 A/cm, at 1 MHz), was placed 1 cm from the surface of a semi-infinitive plane absorber, the conductivity of which is 0.6 S/m, and that the potential around the coil is neglected. In Fig. 5, the abscissa indicates the distance from the coil (Z) axis, and the ordinate absorbed power in W/cm³. Parameters (z values) represent the distance from the base of the coil. There is no absorbed power in the region of the coil axis, and the maximum absorbed powers appear in annular regions at a radius corresponding to the coil. Although a more uniform absorbed power pattern can be achieved using a pancake-type coil, the amount of absorbed power at the depth is smaller than that by a cylindrical coil, which has the same radius as that of the outer coil in the pancake-type coil. The absorbed power at the depth can be improved by increasing the radius and/or the height of the coil. A deeper and more uniform heating can be achieved by moving the coil.

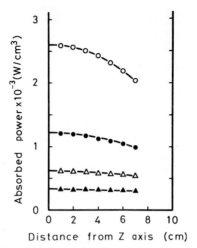

Fig. 6. Distribution of absorbed power in calculation by the cylindrical coil, 6 cm in radius and 24 cm in height. The coil axis is uniformly moved in the region within the radius of 12 cm. Symbols for z values are as in Fig. 5.

Figure 6 shows the distribution of the absorbed power obtained by uniformly moving the axis of the cylindrical coil, which is the same as the coil mentioned previously, in the region within a radius of 12 cm. Parameters (z values) represent the distance from the base of the coil. The maximum absorbed powers appear in the region of the central (Z) axis of the moving area. Figure 7 shows distributions of the absorbed power obtained by rotating the axis of the cylindrical coil, which is the same as the coil mentioned previously, at constant speed around an axis (Z axis), parallel to the coil axis, which is 12 cm away from the Z axis. Parameters (z values) represent the distance from the base of the coil. At $z = 1$ cm, the maximum absorbed power appears in an annular region at a radius of 6.5 cm. Taking these considerations into account, the latter method appears more suitable for deep heating.

D. Rectangular Coil

1. Theoretical Treatment

In inductive heating, the absorbed power in the region of the coil axis becomes zero, because the elementary vector potentials that originate from the elementary RF currents of the coil cancel out each other on the coil axis. Figure 8 shows the rectangular coil (Kato and Ishida, 1982), in which there is no cancellation of the elementary vector potentials in the

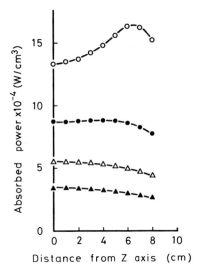

Fig. 7. Distributions of absorbed power in calculation by the cylindrical coil, 6 cm in radius and 24 cm in height. The coil axis is rotated around the Z axis in parallel to the coil axis, which is 12 cm apart from the Z axis. Symbols for z values are as in Fig. 5.

region of the heating material. This rectangular coil is composed of a one-turned square column-like coil, and the heating material is placed outside of and separate from the coil. Absorbed powers are calculated under conditions that the surface current, $\mathbf{J}[A/m]$, flows in a unit width of the one-turned square column-like coil, $h[m]$ in height, $W[m]$ in width, and $l[m]$ in length, as shown in Eq. (1).

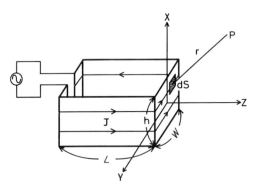

Fig. 8. Schematic illustration of the applicator devised in our department, which includes a one-turned square column-like coil.

$$J = \sqrt{2}\, J_e \cos 2\pi f t \tag{1}$$

where $J_e[A/m]$ indicates the effective current, $f[sec^{-1}]$ the frequency of the current, and $t[sec]$ the time. Vector potential **A** at the point P can be expressed as the sum of the vector potential attributable to the small area, dS, of the coil at a distance of r from P as shown in Eq. (2) (Feynman *et al.*, 1971).

$$\mathbf{A} = \frac{\mu}{4\pi} \int \frac{\mathbf{J}}{r}\, dS \tag{2}$$

where μ is permeability. When **A** changes with time, the electric field **E** occurs, shown in Eq. (3) (Smythe, 1950).

$$\mathbf{E} = -\frac{d\mathbf{A}}{dt} \tag{3}$$

Therefore, the electric field at the point P is shown as in Eq. (4).

$$\mathbf{E} = -\frac{\mu}{4\pi}\frac{d}{dt} \int \frac{\mathbf{J}}{r}\, dS \tag{4}$$

The absorbed power, $Q[W/m^3]$, per unit volume of heating material that has a conductivity $\sigma[S/m]$, is approximated to be

$$Q = \sigma \int_0^1 \mathbf{E} \cdot \mathbf{E}\, dt \tag{5}$$

$$= 4\pi^2 \sigma f^2 J_e^2 \left[\int \frac{dS}{r}\right]^2 \times 10^{-14} \tag{6}$$

provided that the electric field in the heating material is not influenced by the secondary effect of the induced eddy current and μ of the material is μ_0. Figure 9 shows the distributions of absorbed power in the semi-infinitive plane absorber on Y–Z plane in Fig. 8. The calculations were performed under conditions that h, w, l, J_e, f, and σ were substituted into 20 cm, 20 cm, 60 cm, 1 A/cm, 1 MHz, and 0.6 S/m, respectively. The abscissa represents the position y in cm shown in Fig. 8, and the ordinate represents the absorbed power in W/cm³.

2. Experiments

Radiofrequency current at 13.56 MHz was supplied to the one-turned square column-like coil, 20 cm in height, 20 cm in width, and 60 cm in length. The highly conductive material, which is muscle-equivalent phantom, was composed of 2.0% w/w agar powder, 0.43% w/w NaCl, and 97.57% w/w water. The electric conductivity and the dielectric constant of this phantom were 0.83 S/m and 75 at 13.56 MHz and 22°C, respec-

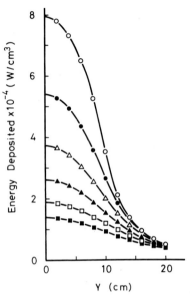

Fig. 9. Distributions of energy deposition. The abscissa represents the y axis shown in Fig. 8, and the ordinate represents the energy deposited per unit volume. Dimensions of the one-turned square column-like coil are 20 cm in height, 20 cm in width, and 60 cm in length. Parameters (z values) represent the distance shown in Fig. 8. Symbols for z values are as in Fig. 5, plus ($\square$) $z = 9$ cm, and ($\blacksquare$) 11 cm.

tively. The poorly conductive material was composed of 2.0% w/w agar powder and 98.0% w/w water. The conductivity and the dielectric constant were 0.019 S/m and 78 at 13.56 MHz and 22°C.

The configuration of the muscle-equivalent phantom is a column, 38.0 cm in diameter and 20.0 cm in height. The phantom was placed at a point $z = 2$ cm, shown in Fig. 8, and the central axis of the phantom coincided with Z axis in Fig. 8. Figures 10 and 11 show the distributions of increases in temperatures when the phantom was heated for 2 min. Figure 10 shows the distribution of increase in temperature on the Z axis and Fig. 11 the distribution of increases in temperature in the Y direction at $z = 3$ cm (corresponding to the depth of 1 cm), $x = 0$ cm. Figure 12 shows the distribution of increase in temperature in the X direction at $z = 3$ cm, $y = 0$ cm, when the phantom was heated for 3 min. The distribution of increase in temperature in the Y direction shown in Fig. 11 coincides with the theoretical distribution of absorbed power shown in Fig. 9. However, the distribution of increase in temperature in the X direction shown in Fig. 12 differs from the theoretical distribution of absorbed power shown in Fig. 9. The main peak is a double-peak type, which is attributable to the

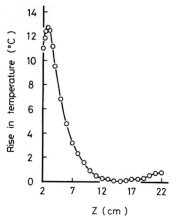

Fig. 10. Distribution of energy deposition on Z axis when the muscle-equivalent phantom is heated for 2 min. The abscissa represents Z axis (the phantom is placed at $z = 2$ cm), and the ordinate is the rise in temperature.

skin effect in the coil. The two side roves at $x = \pm18$ cm are due to the reverse portion of the eddy current, which is generated at the main peak. In Fig. 10, the small rise in temperature appears at a deep region near $z = 22$ cm, which is probably a result of the reverse portion of the eddy current that is generated in the shallow region. In Fig. 10, the penetration depth, which is defined as the range in which energy deposited decreases to a factor of e^{-2} (≈ 0.14), is 5.8 cm. However, the penetration depth is calculated to be 11.7 cm. This discrepancy is attributable to the finding that the electric field generated by the reverse portion of eddy current

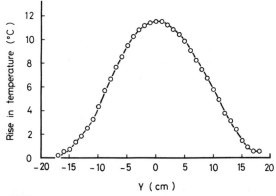

Fig. 11. Distribution of energy deposition in Y direction at $z = 3$ cm, $x = 0$ cm, obtained during the same experiment as in Fig. 10. The abscissa represents Y axis and the ordinate the rise in temperature.

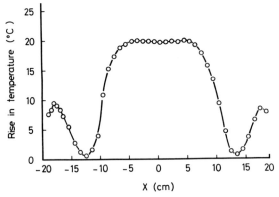

Fig. 12. Distribution of energy deposition in X direction at $z = 3$ cm, $y = 0$ cm, when the muscle-equivalent phantom is heated for 3 min. The abscissa represents X axis and the ordinate the rise in temperature.

offsets the electric field in the deeper region that is generated by the time variation of the vector potential.

Figure 13 shows the distribution of rise in temperature in the double-layered material. The double-layered material, 38.0 cm in diameter, consisted of the poorly conductive material 1.5 cm in thickness and the highly conductive material 20.0 cm in thickness. The double-layered material was placed at a point $z = 2$ cm, shown in Fig. 8, and heated for 3 min. The abscissa represents the Z axis. Absorbed power in the poorly conductive layer is smaller than that in the highly conductive layer. Thus, in the case

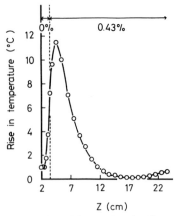

Fig. 13. Distribution of energy deposition on Z axis when the double-layered material (0% NaCl layer 1.5 cm thick + 0.43% NaCl layer 20.0 cm thick) is heated for 3 min. The abscissa indicates z values and the ordinates the rise in temperature.

of the human body, the rise in temperature in the fat layer would be smaller than that in muscles in the deeper regions.

Inductive heating essentially produces less heat in fat and bone, which have lower conductivities (Lehmann, 1965). Moreover, this type of heating is not influenced by an aerial layer as is ultrasound heating. Furthermore, the matching circuit of the instrument can be readily adjusted. The aperture size (h cm $\times$ W cm) can be chosen arbitrarily, depending on the requirement, as the resonance frequency of the coil is determined by inductance and capacitance of the coil circuit. The inductance of the one-turned square column-like coil is so small that the electric potential, which causes an overheating near the surface of the heating material, is little induced around the coil. It is considered that the one-turned square column-like coil is suitable for deep heating.

II. Thermometry

A. Invasive Thermometry

The metallic probe is not generally suitable for electromagnetic heating (Cetas, 1975; Cetas *et al.*, 1978), because it gives rise not only to erroneous indications on the thermometer but also to a hot spot in the heating material or heating of the probe itself. Therefore, investigations were carried out on the nonperturbing probes, either using high-impedance leads (Bowman, 1976) or utilizing changes in the transmission of either temperature-dependent liquid crystals (Johnson *et al.*, 1975) or the light through a thin-layer GaAs semiconductor (Christensen, 1977). Further investigation was made on a phosphor probe (Wickersheim and Alves, 1979), which utilizes the change in the color of the emitted light with phosphor temperature under ultraviolet irradiation.

Below a few decades of megahertz, however, the metallic probe can be used for temperature measurement without erroneous reading and production of a hot spot. The causes of noises and hot spot in this frequency region are considered to be as follows:

1. Radiofrequency flows into the thermometer.
2. When the resistances of the two kinds of metals in the thermocouple differ (Chakrabarty and Brezovich, 1980), RF current is sent to the junction and the exothermic reaction is produced.
3. When the rectifying function appears in the junction (Eno *et al.*, 1981), the inflow of RF current gives rise to the development of the voltage in addition to the thermal electromotive force.

4. When the metallic probe is placed in the heating material, electric current converges on this probe.
5. When the metallic probe is inserted into the material to be heated, an electric current flows from the probe to the ground by way of the thermometer or is sent to the ground by a stray effect. Thus electric current converges on the probe, and a hot spot is produced around the probe.

Figure 14 is a diagram of the developed thermometer system (Eno *et al.*, 1981), in which the phenomena just listed are taken into account. The system consists of (1) a digital thermometer, (2) two 380-μH choke coils made of chromel and alumel wires, respectively, (3) three 25-μH choke coils made by winding the cable of the probe around three toroidal cores, and (4) the aluminum foil used as a shield. The structure of the probe is shown at the lower part of Fig. 14. An enameled C–A thermocouple (5), 0.1 mm in diameter, connects to the choke coils (2); the junction of the thermocouple (6) is shown; a copper tube (7), 0.3 mm in inner diameter and 0.4 mm in outer diameter, connects to the aluminum foil (4) and a Teflon tube (8), 0.5 mm in inner diameter and 1.0 mm in outer diameter. Figure 15 shows the distribution of increase in temperature when the improved probe is held between the two severed column-like agars. Radiofrequency current at 13.56 MHz and a power rate of 365 W was supplied for 1 min to the two electrodes that were attached on the agars. Temperature profiles were measured along the probe before and after the heating. The abscissa indicates the distance from the central axis of the agars (Z axis). The solid line indicates the distribution of increase in temperature at the time when the probe was held, and the dotted line indicates the distribution of increase in temperature at the time of control (i.e., without the probe). The arrow indicates the range in which the probe

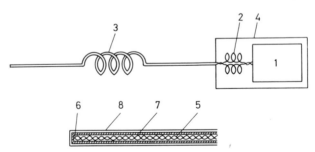

Fig. 14. Developed thermometer system. (1) Digital thermometer; (2) choke coils made of chromel and alumel wires; (3) choke coil made of probe cable; (4) aluminum foil; (5) C–A thermocouple; (6) junction of thermocouple; (7) copper tube that connects to the aluminum foil (4); (8) Teflon tube.

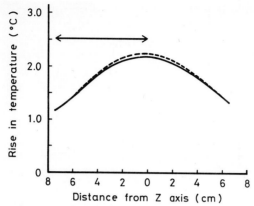

Fig. 15. Distribution of temperature increase. Solid line and dotted line represent temperature increases with and without probe, respectively. Arrow indicates the range for probe insertion.

was held. Because there is little difference between the two curves, it is assumed that the probe does not produce any modification of RF field or hot spot. Figure 16 shows the values indicated on the digital thermometer. The solid circles indicate the values obtained during RF heating and the open circles the values obtained at the time when RF is blocked. No change in the values indicated on the thermometer was seen at the time when RF was blocked at 60 sec, thus indicating that there will be no noise. Furthermore, because no change in the indicated temperature after RF blocking was seen, the production of a hot spot was not expected.

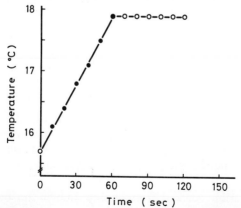

Fig. 16. Indicated values on the digital thermometer. (●) Values obtained during RF heating; (○) values obtained at the time when RF is blocked.

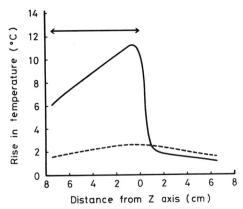

Fig. 17. Distributions of temperature rises. Solid line represents insertion of grounded copper wire in the agar. Dotted line represents control without insertion of grounded wire.

The solid line in Fig. 17 indicates the distribution of increase in temperature at the time when the grounded copper wire (1 mm diameter) was held in the agars. The agar in the region around the copper wire became extremely hot at this stage. The dashed line in the figure indicates the control without the copper wire.

Another probe was manufactured by modifying this improved probe (shown in Fig. 14). The copper tube and the choke coils were removed, and ferromagnetic powder was added to the space between the thermocouple and the inside of the Teflon tube. In this probe also, no detectable hot spot or erroneous reading could be seen at the time when the RF current at 8 MHz was supplied at a rate of 350 W.

B. Noninvasive Thermometry

The ideal temperature measurement for hyperthermia would be noninvasive. Four techniques are being pursued. The first is to detect the microwave radiation emitted from the human body (Edrich *et al.*, 1980). The second is to measure the velocity of ultrasound passing through the human body (Rajagopalan *et al.*, 1980). The third is to measure the change in the X-ray CT number (Fallone *et al.*, 1982). Another approach is to adapt nuclear magnetic resonance (NMR) (Tanaka *et al.*, 1981b; Kato *et al.*, 1983).

The magnetization derived from atomic nuclei can be measured by NMR. The magnetization (M_0) is inversely proportional to the absolute temperature (t) as follows (Hudson *et al.*, 1975):

$$M_0 = N_0 \frac{\mu^2 H_0}{kt} \frac{I + 1}{3I} \tag{7}$$

where N_0 is the number of nuclei in the nuclide of interest per unit volume, μ the nuclear magnetic moment, I nuclear spin, k Boltzmann's constant, and H_0 the intensity of the static magnetic field to the nuclei. The spin–lattice relaxation time (T_1) and the spin–spin relaxation time (T_2) are temperature dependent (Akitt, 1974) as is the magnetization, because they are relaxation processes due to collisions between atoms. As shown in NMR–CT, the magnetic spot can be made at any position in a human body by the magnetic-focusing method (Abe *et al.*, 1973), which induces the nuclear magnetic resonance. Thus the NMR signals can be measured in a noninvasive way, and the deep-body temperature can be measured outside the body.

Protons in the thigh muscle and the solid tumor of Jc1 : ICR mice were measured by a pulsed NMR method. Figures 18, 19, and 20 show the temperature dependencies of the T_1, T_2, and M_0, respectively. The open circles represent the thigh muscle as a normal tissue, and the closed circles the solid tumor of sarcoma A-180 transplanted on the thigh of the mice. The T_1, T_2, and M_0 are temperature dependent and are reduced with temperature.

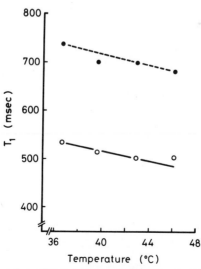

Fig. 18. Temperature dependency of the spin–lattice relaxation time T_1. (O) Normal tissue; (●) tumor.

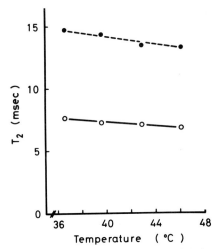

Fig. 19. Temperature dependency of the spin–spin relaxation time T_2. (○) Normal tissue; (●) tumor.

In low-temperature physics, the precision of the NMR thermometer is evaluated within a range of 0.1 to 1.0%. The noninvasive NMR thermometer would have less precision because the tissue volume to be measured is remarkably less than the volume of the receiver coil. Disturbance of

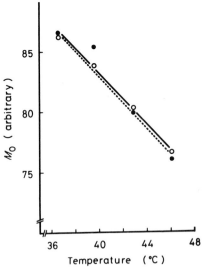

Fig. 20. Temperature dependency of M_0. The ordinate indicates the magnetization M_0 in arbitrary units. (○) Normal tissue; (●) tumor.

magnetic fields by blood flow, increment of blood flow with temperature, skin effect of oscillatory magnetic field, and movement of the region might affect the precision of the noninvasive NMR thermometer. The problem of simultaneous use of heating equipment and NMR thermometer awaits further investigation.

References

Abe, Z., Tanaka, K., Hotta, M., and Imai, M. (1974). Non-invasive measurements of biological information with application of nuclear magnetic resonance. In "Biologic and Clinical Effects of Low Frequency Magnetic and Electric Fields" (J. G. Llaurado, A. Sances, Jr., and J. H. Battoclatti, eds.), pp. 295–317. Thomas, Springfield, Illinois.

Akitt, J. W. (1973). "N.M.R. and Chemistry." Chapman & Hall, London.

Bowman, R. R. (1976). A probe for measuring temperature in radio-frequency-heated material. *IEEE MTT-S Int. Microwave Symp. Dig.* **24**, 43–45.

Cetas, T. C. (1975). Temperature measurement in microwave diathermy fields: principles and probes. *Proc. Int. Symp. Cancer Ther. Hyperthermia Radiat. April 28–30 Washington, D.C.,* pp. 193–203.

Cetas, T. C., Connor, W. G., and Boone, K. L. M. (1978). Thermal dosimetry: some biophysical considerations. In "Cancer Therapy by Hyperthermia and Radiation" (C. Streffer, D. von Beuninger, F. Dretzel, E. Röttinger, J. E. Robinson, E. Scherer, S. Seeber, and K.-R. Trott, Eds.), pp. 3–12. Urban & Schwarzenberg, Baltimore and Munich.

Chakrabarty, D. P., and Brezovich, I. A. (1980). Thermocouple errors in low frequency RF fields. *Int. Symp. Cancer Ther. Hyperthermia Drugs Radiat. 3rd,* p. 56.

Christensen, D. A. (1977). A new non-perturbing temperature probe using semiconductor band shift. *J. Bioeng.* **1**, 541–555.

Edrich, J., Jobe, W. E., Cacak, R. K., Hendee, W. R., Smyth, C. J., Gautherie, M., Gros, C., Zimmer, R., Robert, J., Thouvenot, P., Escanye, J. M., and Itty, C. (1980). Imaging thermograms at centimeter and millimeter wavelengths. *Ann. N.Y. Acad. Sci.* **335**, 456–471.

Eno, K., Kato, H., Nishida, T., Kano, E., Sugahara, T., Tanaka, H., and Ishida, T. (1981). Physical basis of RF hyperthermia for cancer therapy. III. A non-perturbed and non-perturbing thermometer at RF heating. *J. Radiat. Res.* **22**, 256–273.

Fallone, B. G., Moran, P. R., and Podgorsak, E. B. (1982). Noninvasive thermometry with a clinical x-ray CT scanner. *Med. Phys.* **9**, 715–721.

Feynman, R. P., Leighton, R. B., and Sands, M. (1971). "The Feynman Lectures on Physics." Addison-Wesley, Reading, Massachusetts.

Hahn, G. M., Kernahan, P., Martinez, A., Pounds, D., and Prionas, S. (1980). Some heat transfer problems associated with heating by ultrasound, microwaves or radio frequency. *Ann. N.Y. Acad. Sci.* **335**, 327–346.

Hudson, R. P., Marshak, H., Soulen, R. J., and Utton, D. B. (1975). Review paper: recent advances in thermometry below 300 mK. *J. Low Temp. Phys.* **20**, 1–102.

Ishida, T., Kato, H., Miyakoshi, J., Furukawa, M., Ohsaki, S., and Kano, E. (1980). Physical basis of RF hyperthermia for cancer therapy. I. Measurement for distribution in absorbed power from radiofrequency exposure in agar phantom. *J. Radiat. Res.* **21**, 180–189.

Johnson, C. C., and Guy, A. W. (1972). Nonionizing electromagnetic wave effects in biological materials and systems. *Proc. IEEE* **60,** 692–718.

Johnson, C. C., Durney, C. J., Lords, J. L., Rozzell, T. C., and Livingston, G. K. (1975). Fiberoptic liquid crystal probe for absorbed radio-frequency power and temperature measurement in tissue during irradiation. *Ann. N.Y. Acad. Sci.* **247,** 527–531.

Kato, H., and Ishida, T. (1982). Physical basis of RF hyperthermia for cancer therapy. IV. A device for non-invasive local deep heating in hyperthermia treatment. *J. Radiat. Res.* **23,** 228–233.

Kato, H., Kano, E., Sugahara, T., Ujeno, Y., Nishida, T., and Ishida, T. (1983). Possible application of non-invasive thermometry for hyperthermia using NMR. *In* "Fundamentals of Cancer Therapy by Hyperthermia, Radiation and Chemicals" (E. Kano, ed.), pp. 33–38. MAG Bros. Inc., Tokyo.

Lehmann, F. (1965). Diathermy. *In* "Handbook of Physical Medicine and Rehabilitation" (F. H. Krusen, ed.), pp. 273–345. Saunders, Philadelphia, Pennsylvania.

Moon, P., and Spencer, D. E. (1961). "Field Theory Handbook." Springer-Verlag, Berlin.

Rajagopalan, B., Greenleaf, J. F., Johnson, S. A., and Bahn, R. C. (1980). Variation of acoustic speed with temperature in various excised human tissues studied by ultrasound computerized tomography. *IEEE Trans. Sonics Ultrason.* **27,** 227–233.

Smythe, W. R. (1950). "Static and Dynamic Electricity." McGraw-Hill, New York.

Suggar, S., and LeVeen, H. H. (1979). A histopathologic study on the effects of radiofrequency thermotherapy on malignant tumor of the lung. *Cancer (Philadelphia)* **42,** 767–783.

Tanaka, H., Kato, H., Nishida, T., Kano, E., Sugahara, T., and Ishida, T. (1981a). Physical basis of RF hyperthermia for cancer therapy. II. Measurement of distribution of absorbed power from radiofrequency exposure in agar phantom. *J. Radiat. Res.* **22,** 101–108.

Tanaka, H., Kato, H., Ishida, T., and Kano, E. (1981b). Possible application of non-invasive thermometry for hyperthermia using NMR. *Nippon Igaku Hoshasen Gakkai Zasshi* **41,** 897–890.

Wickersheim, K. A., and Alves, R. B. (1979). Recent advances in optical temperature measurement. *Ind. Res. Dev.* **21,** 82–89.

18 Cellular Responses to Hyperthermia and Radiation in Chinese Hamster Cells

Junji Miyakoshi
Shin-ichiro Heki
Department of Radiation Biology
Kyoto College of Pharmacy
Kyoto 607, Japan

Eiichi Kano
Department of Experimental Radiology and Health Physics
Fukui Medical University School of Medicine
Fukui 910-11, Japan

I. Introduction

Hyperthermia, either alone or combined with radiation, has been considered as one form of cancer therapy. Results from *in vitro* studies provided evidence for the effectiveness of hyperthermia for treating cancer. Hyperthermia alone at temperatures over 41°C kills mammalian cells (Westra and Dewey, 1971; Palzer and Heidelberger, 1973; Robinson and Wizenberg, 1974; Gerner *et al.*, 1976a). In particular, the thermal cell

Modification of Radiosensitivity in Cancer Treatment

killing increases markedly at temperatures over 43°C. Step-down heating, such as severe hyperthermia (over 43°C) followed by moderate hyperthermia (under 42°C), enhances cell killing (Henle and Leeper, 1976a; Miyakoshi *et al.*, 1979; Henle, 1980; Jung and Kölling, 1980; Miyakoshi, 1981).

In addition, hyperthermia combined with ionizing radiation enhances cell killing (Ben-Hur *et al.*, 1972; Dewey *et al.*, 1977; Sapareto *et al.*, 1978). Thus hyperthermia selectively kills and radiosensitizes S-phase cells (cells in the DNA-synthetic phase), which are relatively resistant to ionizing radiation (Gerweck *et al.*, 1975; Kim *et al.*, 1976; Bhuyan *et al.*, 1977), and inhibits or reduces the repair from radiation damage, such as sublethal damage (Ben-Hur *et al.*, 1974; Harris *et al.*, 1977; Murthy *et al.*, 1977) and potentially lethal damage (Li *et al.*, 1976). Hyperthermia also enhances cell killing under conditions of low pH (Gerweck and Rottinger, 1976; Bichel and Overgaard, 1977; Freeman *et al.*, 1977; Gerweck, 1977). As the populations of tumor cells in the hypoxic or low-nutrient compartment are probably also at a low pH, they are relatively radioresistant; hence hyperthermia may selectively kill such tumor cells. Finally, hyperthermia enhances the toxicity of several chemotherapeutic agents (Hahn *et al.*, 1975, 1977). All these findings lead to the idea that hyperthermia may enhance the therapeutic efficacy of radio- and chemotherapeutic agents for treating clinical cancer.

However, fractionated hyperthermia leads to a thermotolerance, that is, a decreased sensitivity to heat killing (Gerner and Schneider, 1975; Gerner *et al.*, 1976a; Harisiadis *et al.*, 1977; Henle *et al.*, 1979a; Miyakoshi *et al.*, 1982b). Therefore, the establishment of clinical protocol for fractionation hyperthermia should be assessed with great caution.

This chapter reviews our findings concerning the cellular responses to hyperthermia, either alone or in combination with X irradiation, in Chinese hamster V-79 cells.

II. Materials and Methods

A. Cell Line, Media, and Culture Conditions

Chinese hamster V-79 cells were maintained in growth medium (MLN-15) consisting of modified Eagle's MEM supplemented with NCTC-109 medium (10% v/v), lactalbumin hydrolysate (25g/liter) solution (2% v/v), bovine serum (15% v/v), and antibiotics (Miyakoshi *et al.*, 1979; Miyakoshi, 1981). During hyperthermic exposure and X irradiation, these cells were suspended in MLN-3. During this time, progression in the cell cycle was reduced. (The numerals after MLN- indicate the serum volume percentage.) The cells in plastic plates were incubated at 37°C in a humidity-saturated condition with a mixture of 95% air and 5% CO_2. The pH of the culture medium was maintained at approximately 7.3.

B.   Hyperthermia and X Irradiation

A water bath (Toyo Seisakusho, Model ET-45P) was used for hyperthermic exposure. The temperatures, measured by an electrothermometer, were maintained within ±0.05°C. The physical conditions of X irradiation were 140 kVp, 5 mA, 2-mm Al filter, and at a dose rate of 0.3 Gy/min measured by a Radocon II dosimeter.

C.   Experimental Procedures

Details of the experimental procedures have been described elsewhere (Miyakoshi *et al.,* 1979; Miyakoshi, 1981). To summarize, exponentially growing cells in monolayers were put in 0.03% trypsin solution for about 3 min; then the trypsin solution was sucked off, and a single-cell suspension in MLN-3 medium was obtained. Cell concentrations were measured with a Coulter counter. The cells were serially diluted with MLN-3 for attainment of appropriate cell concentrations, after which 4 ml of each suspension were transferred into plastic tubes. These tubes were immersed in a water bath for 10 min at 37°C prior to hyperthermic treatment and/or X irradiation. In the control experiments, cells were immersed at 37°C for equivalent periods for exposure to hyperthermia and X irradiation. Under these conditions, the extracellular pH varied from 7.4 to 7.8 during hyperthermia.

After the treatments, cells were resuspended by pipeting into tubes. Finally, 1 ml of a single-cell suspension of 4 ml was seeded in plastic plates filled with fresh growth medium (MLN-15). By these methods, cell loss in the tubes was less than about 10% of the inoculated cell number, and the number of cells in MLN-3 did not increase up to 24 h after the initial treatments. In addition, the thermosensitivity was not significantly changed by the trypsinization.

D.   Criterion for Survival

After seeding, the cells were incubated for 6 to 8 days so that macroscopic colonies composed of 50 cells or more could be obtained. The colonies were stained with Giemsa solution, and the number of colonies per plate was counted. The cell survival fraction after each treatment was routinely estimated as the ratio between the number of colonies formed and the number of inoculated cells. The estimated fractions were normalized to the surviving fraction of the untreated control. Three replicate plates were used for each survival point, and the replicate experiments were repeated two to four times. The data point represents the mean of at least six plates, and the standard deviation is given for each survival point.

III.   Results and Discussion

A.   Hyperthermia Alone

Cells were exposed to hyperthermia alone at 42, 43, or 44°C for various periods. Figure 1 shows the hyperthermia treatment time–cell survival curves of cells exposed to 42, 43, or 44°C heating. Cell survival slowly decreased with increased exposure times at 42°C. Freeman et al. (1979) reported that the amount of lethality to Chinese hamster ovary (CHO) cells resulting from an increase in duration of heating reached a maximum for continuous heating at a relatively low temperature of 42°C. It is considered that cells exposed to 42°C hyperthermia may develop thermotolerance during heat exposure. In contrast, cell survival was exponentially

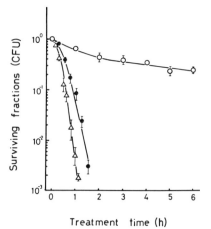

Treatment   time (h)

Fig. 1. Hyperthermia treatment time–cell survival curves at 42, 43, and 44°C. Hamster V-79 cells were exposed to 42°C (○), 43°C (●), or 44°C (△) hyperthermia for various periods. Vertical bars, ±SD.) Redrawn from Miyakoshi et al. (1982b).

reduced with increased exposure times at 43 and 44°C (Fig. 1). Thus, cellular thermotolerance would not develop during heat exposure at temperatures over 43°C.

As shown in Fig. 2, the data on survival obtained from various sources using Chinese hamster V-79 and CHO cells are compared, in an Arrhenius plot (Westra and Dewey, 1971; Bauer and Henle, 1979; Miyakoshi et al., 1982b). The abscissa of the plot is the reciprocal of the absolute temperature, and the ordinate is the reciprocal of the T_0 values, in which the T_0 is the slope of the exponential region of the survival curve, that is, the time at a given temperature that is required to reduce survival by a factor of $1/e$. The Arrhenius plot for hyperthermic cell killing shows an inflection point at approximately 43°C, which means that the inactivation energy is different above and below this temperature. The inactivation energy calculated from the slope indicates the chemical processes involved in the thermal cell killing. Change in the slope may reflect different mechanisms of thermal cell killing at different temperatures above and below 43°C. The inactivation energies calculated from these slopes are in the range of 150 kcal/mol at temperatures above 43°C. Dewey et al. (1977) suggested that the inactivation energies in this range correspond to the denaturation of critical protein(s) or enzyme(s) by hyperthermia.

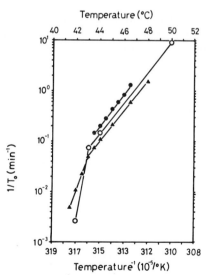

Fig. 2. An Arrhenius plot for thermal cell killing at various temperatures ranged from 41.5 to 50.0°C. The reciprocal of the T_0 values are plotted versus the reciprocal of the absolute temperature. The T_0 is the time required to reduce survival by a factor of $1/e$ in the exponential region of the survival curve. Cell lines and references are as follows: V-79, Miyakoshi *et al.* (1982b) (○); CHO, Westra and Dewey (1971) (●); and CHO, Bauer and Henle (1979) (▲).

B. Step-up and Step-down Heating

Cells were exposed to split-dose hyperthermia at 42 and 44°C. Immediately after a 2-h exposure at 42°C, the cells were further exposed to 44°C for various periods, that is, "step-up heating." The survival curves are shown in Fig. 3. When cells were exposed to step-up heating, the survival curve was more gently sloping than that for the nonpretreated control. At 44°C for 50 min treatment, survival of cells exposed to step-up heating was increased about 10-fold as compared to the control at 44°C. The thermotolerance against 44°C heating was induced by 42°C preheating. A similar effect was reported by Henle *et al.* (1978) and Jung and Kölling (1980), in which the thermotolerance of CHO cells was induced by both step-up heatings of 40 → 45°C and 40 → 43°C sequences, respectively. The cellular thermotolerance induced by 42°C pretreatment in the 42 → 44°C sequence began to decay at about 4-h intervals at 37°C and disappeared completely at 8-h intervals (Miyakoshi *et al.,* 1982b).

As the counterpart of this experiment, cells were exposed to 44°C for 15 min followed by exposure to 42°C for various periods, that is, "step-down heating." The curves are shown in Fig. 4. The survival of cells exposed to step-down heating was markedly decreased as compared with the control of 42°C alone. When cells were exposed to step-down heating, the effect of enhanced cell killing was evident in other cases of 45 → 40°C (Henle and Leeper, 1976a, 1977) and 43 → 40°C (Jung and Kölling, 1980). The Arrhenius analysis indicates that the inactivation energy is different in the different temperature ranges up to 43°C and above 43°C (Connor *et al.,*

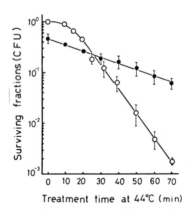

Fig. 3. Survival curves of cells exposed to 44°C hyperthermia alone and the step-up heating of 42 → 44°C sequence. Hamster V-79 cells were exposed to 42°C for 2 h and then further exposed to 44°C for various periods of time (●). As for the control experiment, cells were exposed to 44°C alone (○). Vertical bars, ±SD. Redrawn from Miyakoshi (1981).

1977; Dewey *et al.*, 1977; Bauer and Henle, 1979; Bhuyan, 1979; Ross-Riveros and Leith, 1979). These results suggest that hyperthermic damage produced by preexposure to high hyperthermia (43°C) may enhance cellular inactivation by low hyperthermia (43°C) and/or may inhibit the repair process from the damage by low hyperthermia.

C.   Thermotolerance Induction

Cells were exposed to split-dose hyperthermia at 44°C. Immediately after 25 min exposure at 44°C, the cells were maintained at 37°C for various intervals up to 72 h and then further exposed to 44°C for various periods. The survival curves are shown in Fig. 5. With over 3-h intervals, the survival of cells exposed to split-dose hyperthermia at 44°C was increased as compared with the single hyperthermic treatment. Thermotolerance against 44°C heating was induced by the first 44°C hyperthermic treatment. The survival level was retained at a maximum from 6- to 24-h intervals. Because cell survival nearly attained the independent level after a 48-h interval, thermotolerance induced by the first treatment at 44°C disappeared. A similar effect has been reported by Gerner and Schneider (1975) and Henle and Leeper (1976b). In addition, Gerner *et al.* (1976a) showed that the thermotolerance of HeLa cells exposed to 44°C for 1 h was rapidly increased and reached a maximum level after ~2- to 3-h intervals, at 37°C. Thus the development to thermotolerance may have already started when the cells were incubated at 37°C immediately after a 44°C hyperthermic exposure.

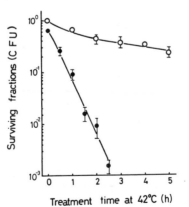

Fig. 4. Survival curves of cells exposed to 42°C hyperthermia alone and the step-down heating of 44 → 42°C sequence. Hamster V-79 cells were exposed to 44°C for 15 min and then further exposed to 42°C with various doses (●). Cells were exposed to 42°C alone for the control (○). Vertical bars, ±SD. Redrawn from Miyakoshi (1981).

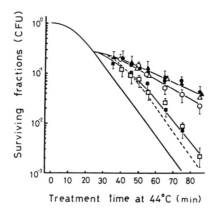

Fig. 5. Thermotolerance induction by split-dose hyperthermia at 44°C. Hamster V-79 cells were exposed to 44°C for 25 min, immediately followed by transfer to 37°C for various intervals up to 72 h, and then further exposed to 44°C for various periods. Each symbol represents the interval time at 37°C as follows: 3 h (○); 6 h (●); 18 h (△); 24 h (▲); 48 h (□); and 72 h (■). The control (——) and the independent (-----) curves represent 44°C hyperthermia alone. Vertical bars, ±SD. (Redrawn from Miyakoshi *et al.* (1982b).

When cells were kept at 0°C after the initial heating, the development of the thermotolerance was inhibited (Gerner and Schneider, 1975; Miyakoshi *et al.*, 1982b). However, the development of the thermotolerance proceeded when cells were exposed to temperatures of 37°C after being kept at 0°C between heatings. This indicates that development of the thermotolerance may depend on cellular metabolism.

The cellular thermotolerance was also induced by step-up heating (Fig. 3). In this case, however, the thermotolerance was induced and developed during preexposure to low hyperthermia at 42°C and decayed with increased intervals at 37°C (Miyakoshi *et al.*, 1982b). There may be differences in the time mode for development and decay of the thermotolerance between step-up heating of 42 → 44°C sequence and 44°C split-dose heating. Therefore, the mechanism(s) of thermotolerance induction against 44°C hyperthermia may differ somewhat between 42 and 44°C pretreatments. However, the thermotolerance induced by both the split treatments is transient. When hyperthermia is prescribed for cancer therapy, a time interval of more than 2–3 days is necessary in the hyperthermic fractionation schedule. Further research in this area is required before clinical hyperthermia protocols can be established.

D. Radioenhancement by Hyperthermia

Radiation combined with hyperthermia enhances radiation cell killing (Ben-Hur *et al.*, 1972; Dewey *et al.*, 1977; Henle *et al.*, 1979b). Change in

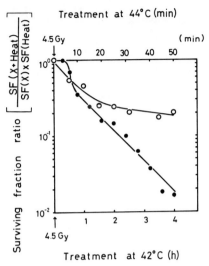

Fig. 6. The radioenhancing effect of the combined treatments of X irradiation (4.5 Gy) and hyperthermia at 42 or 44°C in V-79 cells. Cells were irradiated with the single dose of 4.5 Gy and then exposed to 42 or 44°C for various periods. Ordinate: Surviving fraction ratio, the denominator of which is the multiplication of two surviving fractions obtained from a single X irradiation (4.5 Gy) and hyperthermia alone, and the numerator the surviving fraction obtained from the combined treatment of X irradiation and hyperthermia. Less than 1.0 of the surviving fraction ratio means that the synergistic effect of the combined treatment of X irradiation and hyperthermia was observed. Upper abscissa: Treatment time at 44°C (●). Lower abscissa: Treatment time at 42°C (○). Redrawn from Miyakoshi (1981).

the radioenhancing effect is shown in Fig. 6. Cells were irradiated with a single dose of 4.5 Gy and then exposed to 42 or 44°C, for various periods. The extent of this effect was expressed in terms of surviving fraction ratio; the smaller the value of surviving fraction ratio, the larger the extent of the radioenhancing effect. The effect of 42°C hyperthermia increased gradually up to 2 h and then appeared to become saturated. In contrast, the effect of 44°C hyperthermia began to increase abruptly after about 7 min. The surviving fraction ratio at 44°C was exponentially decreased through 10 to 50 min exposure. As there are remarkable difference in thermal cell killing between 42 and 44°C (Fig. 1), the thermal radioenhancement may correlate with the cell killing by hyperthermia alone.

Cells were exposed to hyperthermia at 42°C for 2 h or 44°C for 15 min immediately after X irradiation with various doses, and the curves are shown in Fig. 7. The survival after both combined treatments was reduced in comparison with cells treated with X irradiation alone. The radiation responses enhanced by hyperthermia were expressed as decrements in both D_q and D_0 values. Thermal enhancement ratio (TER) was

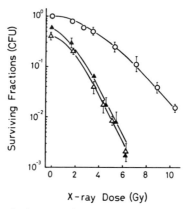

Fig. 7. X-Ray dose–survival curves of V-79 cells treated with X irradiation, alone and in combination with hyperthermia at 42 or 44°C. Cells were exposed to 42°C for 2 hr (△) or 44°C for 15 min (▲) immediately after X irradiation with various doses. For the control, cells were treated with X irradiation alone (○). Vertical bars, ±SD. Redrawn from Miyakoshi (1981).

calculated as a criterion to show the degree of the enhancing effect (Ben-Hur *et al.*, 1974). The TER value was estimated as the ratio of the D_0 for X irradiation alone to the D_0 for the combined treatment. A similar TER value, such as approximately 2.0, was obtained in both 42 and 44°C hyperthermia combined with X irradiation. These radioenhancing effects of hyperthermia were deduced from the evidence that (*a*) hyperthermia selectively kills and radiosensitizes S-phase cells, which are relatively resistant to ionizing radiation (Gerweck *et al.*, 1975; Kim *et al.*, 1976; Bhuyan *et al.*, 1977), (*b*) hyperthermic radiosensitization is much greater for cells irradiated with low-LET radiation than with high-LET radiation (Gerner *et al.*, 1976b; Gerner and Leith, 1977), and (*c*) hyperthermia eliminates or reduces recovery from sublethal (Ben-Hur *et al.*, 1974; Harris *et al.*, 1977; Murthy *et al.*, 1977) and potentially lethal (Li *et al.*, 1976) radiation damage.

E. Radiation in Combination with Step-up and Step-down Heating

Two hyperthermic exposures (42°C for 60 min and 44°C for 15 min) were chosen, and these had much the same effect on cell killing. X-irradiation with various doses was combined with either step-up or step-down heating by using 42 and 44°C hyperthermic exposures. Figure 8 shows the X-ray dose–cell survival curves for the combined treatments of

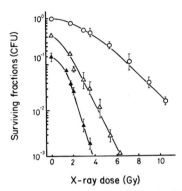

Fig. 8. X-Ray dose–survival curve of V-79 cells treated with X irradiation alone or in combination with 42 and 44°C hyperthermia. Each hyperthermic treatment time is fixed at 42°C for 60 min and 44°C for 15 min. Cells were exposed to step-up heating of 42 → 44°C sequence (△) or step-down heating of 44 → 42°C (▲), followed by X irradiation with various doses. For the control, cells were treated with X irradiation alone (○). Vertical bars, ±SD. Redrawn from Miyakoshi *et al.* (1979).

42 → 44°C → X and 44 → 42°C → X sequences, and for the control of X irradiation alone. Enhanced cell killing was observed with both combined treatments. The extent of this enhancing effect was greater in the 44 → 42°C → X sequence than in 42 → 44°C → X. Such radioenhancing effects were observed in all of the six sequential combined treatments (Miyakoshi *et al.*, 1979). The D_0 and the TER values, which were estimated from the survival curves of cells exposed to these treatments, are summarized in Table I. The TER value was calculated from the D_0 ratio as mentioned previously. These combined treatments could be classified into two groups based on the extent of the enhanced cell killing effect. The first group, which shows a relatively smaller radioenhancing effect by hyperthermia, consists of X → 42 → 44°C, 42 → X → 44°C, and 42 → 44°C → X sequential treatments. The second group, which shows a more marked radioenhancing effect, is represented by X → 44 → 42°C, 44 → X → 42°C, and 44 → 42°C → X treatments. The TER value ranged from 1.81 to 2.07 in the first group and from 2.87 to 3.58 in the second group. These results indicate that, regardless of the position of X irradiation in the sequence, the magnitude of radioenhancing effect by these combined treatments is greater in combination with step-down heating than with step-up heating.

Recovery kinetics from the synergistic damage resulting from the combination treatments of X irradiation and 42 and 44°C hyperthermia were analyzed. X-ray and heat doses were fixed at 3 Gy, and 42°C for 60 min and 44°C for 15 min, respectively. Cells were exposed to the split treat-

TABLE I

D_0 Value and TER for Survival Curves of
V-79 Cells Subjected to Combined
Treatments with X Irradiation, and 42 and
44°C Hyperthermia[a]

Sequence[b]	D_0(Gy)[c]	TER[d]
X alone	1.72	(1.00)
X → 42 → 44°C	0.95	1.81
42 → X → 44°C	0.83	2.07
42 → 44°C → X	0.88	1.95
X → 44 → 42°C	0.60	2.87
44 → X → 42°C	0.48	3.58
44 → 42°C → X	0.55	3.13

[a] Data from Miyakoshi et al. (1979).
[b] Hyperthermia was applied for 60 min at 42°C
and 15 min at 44°C.
[c] The D_0 is the dose required to reduce survival
by a factor of $1/e$ in the exponential region of the
survival curve.
[d] TER is calculated as the ratio of the D_0 for X
irradiation alone to the D_0 for the combined treatment without the 37°C interval.

ments of X irradiation and step-up heating (42°C + 44°C), and X irradiation and step-down heating (44°C + 42°C) with 37°C intervals of differing
lengths. Recovery curves are shown in Fig. 9. Survival of cells irradiated
with X irradiation alone for the first treatment was rapidly increased with
extended intervals. Cell survival recovered to the additive level when the
interval was about 1 to 2 h and 4 to 5 h, for X $\xrightarrow{37°C(t)}$ 42°C + 44°C and X
$\xrightarrow{37°C(t)}$ 44°C + 42°C treatments, respectively. No further recovery was
seen up to a 24-h interval, for both treatments. In the case of 42°C + 44°C
$\xrightarrow{37°C(t)}$ X treatment, cell survival was slowly increased with increased
intervals, and then all but recovered to the additive level seen at about 8-h
intervals. For the other group of 44°C + 42°C $\xrightarrow{37°C(t)}$ X treatment, cell
survival was slightly increased with longer intervals and did not recover
to the additive level up to 24-h intervals. The radioenhancing effect on the
step-down heating of 44°C + 42°C was observed even after a 24-h interval.
Data from other cases of the split treatments indicated that the recovery
time was less than about 7 h when the first treatment was both hyperthermia (42 or 44°C) alone and combinations with X irradiation (Miyakoshi et
al., 1982a). When the step-down heating was given as the first treatment,
cells did not fully recover within a 24-h interval (Fig. 9). An interpretation

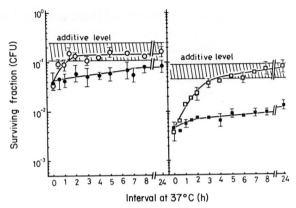

Fig. 9. Recovery kinetics of V-79 cells exposed to the combined treatments of X irradiation alone, and step-up and step-down heating. The sequences of these combined treatments are as follows: X $\xrightarrow{37°C(t)}$ 42°C + 44°C (○); 42°C + 44°C $\xrightarrow{37°C(t)}$ X (●); X $\xrightarrow{37°C(t)}$ 44°C + 42°C (□); and 44°C + 42°C $\xrightarrow{37°C(t)}$ X (■). X-Ray dose and hyperthermia time are fixed as 3 Gy, 42°C for 60 min, and 44°C for 15 min, respectively. The arrow ($\xrightarrow{37°C(t)}$) represents the interpolated interval at 37°C. The additive level (shown by the slanting lines), is estimated by multiplying the independent survival values obtained from the two components prior to and followed by the interval time in a fractionation treatment. Vertical bars, ±SD. Redrawn from Miyakoshi *et al.* (1982a).

of this finding is that the step-down heating may have a destructive effect on the repair process from the damage induced by the subsequent X irradiation. The recovery time may be longer in the conditioning treatments with step-up and step-down heating than in those with X irradiation and/or hyperthermia (42 or 44°C) alone.

For the application of hyperthermia to radiotherapy, two important points are suggested by the present investigation. First, because the cell killing effect was markedly different between step-up and step-down heating (Figs. 3 and 4), the temperature of the tissues in question should be assessed with great caution and of course be accurately measured. Second, because a greater radioenhancement and a lower recovery from the synergistic damage were obtained by the combination of step-down heating and X irradiation (Figs. 8 and 9), the step-down heating followed by X irradiation may be an effective protocol.

IV. Summary

Cellular responses to hyperthermia (42–44°C), alone and in combination with X irradiation, were assessed using Chinese hamster V-79 cells. Thermal cell killing was greater at temperatures over 43°C. An Arrhenius plot for hyperthermic cell killing showed an inflection point at approximately 43°C, which means that the inactivation energy is different above and below this temperature. Preheating at 42°C for 2 h decreased the cellular sensitivity to the subsequent exposure to 44°C (step-up heating), whereas an exposure to 44°C for 15 min markedly increased the cellular sensitivity to 42°C (step-down heating). The cellular thermotolerance was induced by the split-dose hyperthermia at 44°C. The magnitude of the thermotolerance reached a maximum at 6- to 24-h intervals, and the thermotolerance completely decayed after a 48-h interval.

Hyperthermia at 42 and 44°C combined with X irradiation enhanced cell killing. The radioenhancement by hyperthermia was expressed as decrements in both D_q and D_0 values. For X irradiation in combination with step-up and step-down heating, the magnitude of radioenhancing effect is greater in case of the step-down heating, regardless of the position of X irradiation in the sequence. The synergistic damage resulting from those combination treatments was repaired in less than about 8-h intervals when the conditioning treatment was X irradiation alone and step-up heating. However, when the step-down heating was given as the conditioning treatment, the synergistic damage was not fully repaired within a 24-h interval. These results suggest that step-down heating followed by X irradiation may be an effective protocol for the application of hyperthermia to radiotherapy.

Acknowledgments

We are grateful to Dr. T. Sugahara (Kyoto National Hospital), for advice and encouragement. This research was supported in part by a grant from the Ministry of Education, Science and Culture, Japan.

References

Bauer, K. D., and Henle, K. J. (1979). Arrhenius analysis of heat survival curves from normal and thermotolerant CHO cells. *Radiat. Res.* **78,** 251–263.

Ben-Hur, E., Bronk, B. V., and Elkind, M. M. (1972). Thermally enhanced radiosensitivity of cultured Chinese hamster cells. *Nature New Biol.* **238,** 209–210.

Ben-Hur, E., Elkind, M. M., and Bronk, B. V. (1974). Thermally enhanced radioresponse of cultured Chinese hamster cells: inhibition of repair of sublethal damage and enhancement of lethal damage. *Radiat. Res.* **58,** 35–51.

Bhuyan, B. K. (1979). Kinetics of cell kill by hyperthermia. *Cancer Res.* **39,** 2277–2284.

Bhuyan, B. K., Day, K. J., Edgerton, C. E., and Ogunbase, O. (1977). Sensitivity of different cell lines and different phases in the cell cycle to hyperthermia. *Cancer Res.* **37,** 3780–3784.

Bichel, P., and Overgaard, J. (1977). Hyperthermic effect on exponential and plateau ascites tumor cells *in vitro* dependent on environmental pH. *Radiat. Res.* **70**, 449–454.

Connor, W. G., Gerner, E. W., Miller, R. C., and Boone, M. L. M. (1977). Prospects for hyperthermia in human cancer therapy. II. Implications of biological and physical data for applications of hyperthermia to man. *Radiology (Easton, Pa.)* **123**, 497–503.

Dewey, W. C., Hopwood, L. E., Sapareto, S. A., and Gerweck, L. E. (1977). Cellular responses to combinations of hyperthermia and radiation. *Radiology (Easton, Pa.)* **123**, 463–474.

Freeman, M. L., Dewey, W. C., and Hopwood, L. E. (1977). Effect of pH on hyperthermic cell survival: brief communication. *J. Natl. Cancer Inst. (US)* **58**, 1837–1839.

Freeman, M. L., Raaphorst, G. P., and Dewey, W. C. (1979). The relationship of heat killing and thermal radiosensitization to the duration of heating at 42°C. *Radiat. Res.* **78**, 172–175.

Gerner, E. W., and Leith, J. T. (1977). Interaction of hyperthermia with radiations of different linear energy transfer. *Int. J. Radiat. Biol.* **31**, 283–288.

Gerner, E. W., and Schneider, M. J. (1975). Induced thermal resistance in HeLa cells. *Nature (London)* **256**, 500–502.

Gerner, E. W., Boone, R., Connor, W. G., Hicks, J. A., and Boone, M. L. M. (1976a). A transient thermotolerant survival response produced by single thermal doses in HeLa cells. *Cancer Res.* **36**, 1035–1040.

Gerner, E. W., Leith, J. T., and Boone, M. L. M. (1976b). Mammalian cell survival response following irradiation with 4 MeV X-ray or accelerated helium ions combined hyperthermia. *Radiology (Easton, Pa.)* **119**, 715–720.

Gerweck, L. E. (1977). Modification of cell lethality at elevated temperatures. The pH effect. *Radiat. Res.* **70**, 224–235.

Gerweck, L. E., and Rottinger, E. (1976). Enhancement of mammalian cell sensitivity to hyperthermia by pH alteration. *Radiat. Res.* **67**, 508–511.

Gerweck, L. E., Gillette, E. L., and Dewey, W. C. (1975). Effect of heat and radiation on synchronous Chinese hamster cells: killing and repair. *Radiat. Res.* **64**, 611–623.

Hahn, G. M., Braun, J., and Har-Keder, L. (1975). Thermochemotherapy: synergism between hyperthermia (42–43°) and adriamycin (or bleomycin) in mammalian cell inactivation. *Proc. Natl. Acad. Sci. USA* **72**, 937–940.

Hahn, G. M., Li, G. C., and Shiu, E. (1977). Interaction of amphotericin B and 43° hyperthermia. *Cancer Res.* **37**, 761–764.

Harisiadis, L., Sung, D., II, and Hall, E. J. (1977). Thermal tolerance and repair of thermal damage by cultured cells. *Radiology (Easton, Pa.)* **123**, 505–509.

Harris, J. R., Murthy, A. K., and Belli, J. A. (1977). Repair following combined X-ray and heat at 41° in plateau-phase mammalian cells. *Cancer Res.* **37**, 3374–3378.

Henle, K. J. (1980). Sensitization to hyperthermia below 43°C induced in Chinese hamster ovary cells by step-down heating. *J. Natl. Cancer Inst. (US)* **64**, 1479–1483.

Henle, K. J., and Leeper, D. B. (1976a). Combinations of hyperthermia (40°,45°C) with radiation. *Radiology (Easton, Pa.)* **121**, 451–454.

Henle, K. J., and Leeper, D. B. (1976b). Interaction of hyperthermia and radiation in CHO cells: recovery kinetics. *Radiat. Res.* **66**, 505–518.

Henle, K. J., and Leeper, D. B. (1977). The modification of radiation damage in CHO cells by hyperthermia at 40 and 45°C. *Radiat. Res.* **70**, 415–424.

Henle, K. J., Karamuz, J. E., and Leeper, D. B. (1978). Induction of thermotolerance in Chinese hamster ovary cells by high (45°) or low (40°) hyperthermia. *Cancer Res.* **38**, 570–574.

Henle, K. J., Tomasovic, S. P., and Dethlefsen, L. A. (1979b). Fractionation of combined heat and radiation in asynchronous CHO cells. I. Effects on radiation sensitivity. *Radiat. Res.* **80,** 369–377.

Jung, H., and Kölling, H. (1980). Induction of thermotolerance and sensitization in CHO cells by combined hyperthermic treatments at 40 and 43°C. *Eur. J. Cancer* **16,** 1523–1528.

Kim, S. H., Kim, J. H., and Hahn, E. W. (1976). The enhanced killing of irradiated HeLa cells in synchronous culture by hyperthermia. *Radiat. Res.* **66,** 337–345.

Li, G. C., Evans, R. G., and Hahn, G. M. (1976). Modification and inhibition of repair of potentially lethal X-ray damage by hyperthermia. *Radiat. Res.* **67,** 491–501.

Miyakoshi, J. (1981). Responses to hyperthermia (42°,44°) and/or radiation in four mammalian cell lines *in vitro*. *J. Radiat. Res.* **22,** 352–366.

Miyakoshi, J., Ikebuchi, M., Furukawa, M., Yamagata, K., Sugahara, T., and Kano, E. (1979). Combined effects of X-irradiation and hyperthermia (42 and 44°C) on Chinese hamster V-79 cells *in vitro*. *Radiat. Res.* **79,** 77–88.

Miyakoshi, J., Heki, S., Furukawa, M., and Kano, E. (1982a). Recovery kinetics from the damage by step-up and step-down heatings in combination with radiation in Chinese hamster cells. *J. Radiat. Res.* **23,** 187–197.

Miyakoshi, J., Heki, S., Yamagata, K., Furukawa, M., and Kano, E. (1982b). Induction of thermotolerance by two different temperatures of hyperthermia (42°,44°) in Chinese hamster cells. *In* "Fundamentals of Cancer Therapy by Hyperthermia, Radiation and Chemicals" (E. Kano, J. Egawa, Y. Onoyama and R. U, eds.), pp. 135–137. MAG Bros. Inc., Tokyo.

Murthy, A. K., Harris, J. R., and Belli, J. A. (1977). Hyperthermia and radiation response of plateau phase cells: potentiation and radiation damage repair. *Radiat. Res.* **70,** 241–247.

Palzer, R. J., and Heidelberger, C. (1973). Studies on the quantitative biology of hyperthermic killing of HeLa cells. *Cancer Res.* **33,** 415–421.

Robinson, J. E., and Wizenberg, M. J. (1974). Thermal sensitivity and the effect of elevated temperatures on the radiation sensitivity of Chinese hamster cells. *Acta Radiol. Ther. Phys. Biol.* **13,** 241–248.

Ross-Riveros, P., and Leith, J. T. (1979). Response of 9L tumor cells to hyperthermia and X irradiation. *Radiat. Res.* **78,** 296–311.

Sapareto, S. A., Hopwood, L. E., and Dewey, W. C. (1978). Combined effects of X-irradiation and hyperthermia on CHO cells for various temperatures and orders of application. *Radiat. Res.* **73,** 221–233.

Westra, A., and Dewey, W. C. (1971). Variation in sensitivity to heat shock during the cell-cycle of Chinese hamster cells *in vitro*. *Int. J. Radiat. Biol.* **19,** 467–477.

19 Cellular Transformation and Intracellular Targets of Hyperthermia

Masami Watanabe
Osamu Nikaido

Division of Radiation Biology
Faculty of Pharmaceutical Sciences
Kanazawa University
Kanazawa 920, Japan

Tsutomu Sugahara

Kyoto National Hospital
Kyoto 612, Japan

I. Introduction

Clinical applications of hyperthermia have produced promising results, and improvement of instruments used for hyperthermic therapy for patients with a malignancy is under way. The effectiveness of hyperthermia

Modification of Radiosensitivity in Cancer Treatment
Copyright © 1984 by Academic Press Japan, Inc.
All rights of reproduction in any form reserved.
ISBN 0-12-676020-9

applied in combination with radiation or chemicals seems related to an enhancement of cell killing effects by these damaging agents (Henle and Leeper, 1976; Li *et al.*, 1976; Li and Kal, 1977; Sapareto *et al.*, 1978).

Although the current and major therapy for cancer includes radiotherapy and chemotherapy, both have the potential to produce carcinogenesis. Therefore, it has to be determined whether or not hyperthermia itself or in combination with radiation or chemicals would induce cancer.

Discussed in several reviews were the effect of elevated temperatures on biological systems. Hyperthermia has been shown to inhibit the synthesis of macromolecules, that is, DNA, RNA, and protein (Mondovi *et al.*, 1969; Dickson and Shaw, 1972; Roti-Roti and Winward, 1978; Tomasovic *et al.*, 1978; Henle and Leeper, 1979). The activation energy for cell killing corresponds to protein denaturation (Dewey *et al.*, 1977; Connor *et al.*, 1977), so the inhibition of macromolecule synthesis may be due to the functional inability of enzymes such as polymerases. Other evidence also indicates that hyperthermia produces cell membrane changes (Dickson, 1976). The frequency of sister chromatid exchange increases fivefold when the incubation temperature is raised from 31 to 42°C, and this increase was temperature dependent (Kato, 1980). Furthermore, hyperthermia alters the capacity of cells to repair sublethal and/or potentially lethal radiation damage in addition to sensitizing cells to radiation (Ben-Hur *et al.*, 1974; Sapareto *et al.*, 1978). However, mechanisms underlying the interaction of hyperthermic damage and radiation damage are unknown.

The effects of hyperthermia alone or in combination with X rays were studied with regard to malignant transformation in GHE cells. Dynamics of DNA single-strand breaks (ssb) induced by hyperthermia were also investigated using the alkaline elution method.

II. Materials and Methods

A. Cells

Primary or secondary GHE cells were used. The tissue culture techniques used to obtain the GHE cells have been described in detail (Watanabe *et al.*, 1982). Cells were grown in Dulbecco's modified MEM (DMEM, Nissui Seiyaku Co. Ltd., Tokyo) supplemented with 10% fetal bovine serum (Microbiological Associates, Maryland, Lot No. 99268), penicillin (50 units/ml; Meiji Seika Co. Ltd., Tokyo), and kanamycin (50 μg/ml; Takeda Chemical Industries Ltd., Osaka).

B. Transformation Assay

For transformation studies, 10^6 cells were inoculated into 75-cm^2 culture bottles and incubated at 37°C. The cells were harvested 48 h later by trypsinization, and 1000 cells suspended in 5 ml of DMEM were transferred into a test tube. Hyperthermia treatments consisted of immersing the tubes in a water bath with a temperature between 39 and 45°C, according to the plan of particular experiments. Temperature variation was within ±0.1°C. Irradiation was carried out using a Shimadzu X-ray generator operating at 182 kVp and 15 mA with a 0.9-mm Cu plus 0.5-mm Al filter, yielding a dose of 0.5 Gy/min. Following the completion of heat and radiation exposure, each 1 ml of cell suspension was inoculated into a 60-mm plastic dish, and to each dish were added 4 ml of fresh medium. After 7 to 10 days, colonies were fixed with ethanol and stained with Giemsa. Transformed colonies were readily identified by their altered morphology, as the cells in the transformed colony piled up to form densely stained colonies with a characteristic crisscross pattern at the periphery, indicated previously as type B colony (Watanabe *et al.*, 1982). In parallel with the transformation study, a survival study was done using the colony-forming method. The transformation frequency (TF) was determined by dividing the number of transformed colonies by the number of surviving colonies.

C. Method for DNA Alkaline Elution

The DNA alkaline elution method we used was a slight modification of that described by Kohn *et al.* (1974). Exponentially growing cells were cultured for 20 h in medium containing 0.02 μCi/ml of [*methyl*-^{14}C]TdR (50–60 Ci/mmol: Amersham International Ltd., United Kingdom). After cultivation for over 6 h in fresh medium, the cells were harvested and washed with PBS (−). Each batch of 10^6 labeled cells was suspended in 5 ml of culture medium, and the cells were treated with heat and/or X rays.

Immediately after treatments or at various intervals of incubation after the treatments, the cells were trapped on a polyvinyl chloride filter (25 mm diameter, 2-μm pore size; Millipore Corp., Bedford, Massachusetts). These cells were washed three times with 5 ml of ice-cold PBS (−) and then lysed at 30°C with 4 ml of lysis solution (2 M NaCl, 0.02 M Na$_3$EDTA, 0.2% Sarcosyl, pH 10.2), which was allowed to flow by gravity and collected in a test tube. After removal of lysis solution by washing with 4 ml of 0.02 M Na$_3$EDTA (pH 10.2), DNA was eluted with alkaline solution [0.1 M tetrapropylammonium hydroxide (Pr$_4$NOH), 0.02 M H$_4$EDTA; pH 12.2] in the dark, at a pump speed of 0.07 ml/min.

Ten fractions were collected at 60-min intervals, and each eluted solution was neutralized by adding 2 N HCl. Then 1 ml of each fraction was mixed with 4 ml of a Triton X-100 toluene scintillant, and radioactivity of each fraction was counted in a liquid scintillation counter. Radioactivity remaining on the filter was determined by soaking the filters in 5 ml of the scintillant and counting in a scintillation counter. Radioactivity remaining on the filter after various lengths of time of elution was estimated by subtracting the radioactivity of each eluted fraction from the radioactivity remaining on the filters before the elution.

D. Detection of DNA and Protein Degradation

Exponentially growing cells were cultured in medium containing 0.02 μCi/ml of [U-^{14}C]lysine (10 mCi/mmol; Amersham International Ltd., United Kingdom) and 0.5 μCi/ml of [*methyl*-^{3}H]TdR (40–60 Ci/mmol; Amersham International Ltd., United Kingdom) for 16 h, and the cells were cultured for another 12 h in fresh medium. The cells were then harvested and washed with PBS ($-$), and each batch of 10^6 labeled cells was suspended in 5 ml of culture medium and treated with heat (43°C) for various periods of time. After heat treatment, the cells were centrifuged at 10,000 rpm for 10 min at 4°C. The resulting pellet was washed three times in 5 ml of cold 5% PCA, then was lysed by adding 0.5 ml of NaOH and the cell lysate diluted by addition of 4 ml of distilled water. Then 1 ml of the lysate was mixed with 4 ml of Triton X-100 toluene scintillant, and radioactivity was counted in a liquid scintillation counter. Degradation rates of DNA and protein were calculated by dividing the remaining radioactivity, ^{3}H for DNA and ^{14}C for protein, in 10^6 heat-treated cells by the total radioactivity in 10^6 cells at initiation of the heat treatment.

III. Results

A. Heat Sensitivity of GHE Cells

The kinetics of the heat inactivation curve was determined for asynchronous cell populations for different time intervals and for temperatures ranging from 39 to 45°C. The resulting survival curves indicate that the inactivation was sigmoidal in response, that is, a shoulder followed by a exponential decrease (Fig. 1).

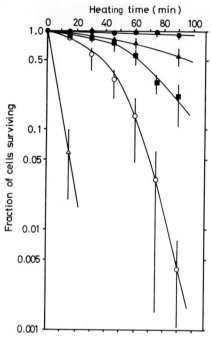

Fig. 1. Killing effect of hyperthermia on GHE cells. Heating temperatures: 37°C (●), 39°C (▲), 41°C (■), 43°C (○), and 45°C (△). Vertical bar is standard deviation.

The relationship between inactivation rate and temperature was analyzed by an Arrhenius plot, in which the logarithm of the inactivation rate ($1/D_{37}$) was plotted as a function of the inverse of absolute temperature, $1/T$ (Fig. 2). The activation energy is about 140 kcal/mol for a temperature below 43°C.

B. Effects of Hyperthermia on GHE Cells Irradiated with X Rays

The effects of hyperthermia on GHE cells irradiated with X rays are shown in Figs. 3 and 4. To obtain information on changes in survival, as related to the sequence of heat and radiation, the cells were exposed to a temperature of 43°C for 30 min in combination with 2 Gy given before, during, or after the heating. The most extensive radiosensitizing effect of hyperthermia was observed when X irradiation was given simultaneously with heating, as shown in Fig. 3. When radiation was given more than 90 min before heating, the cells showed a higher fraction of survival than

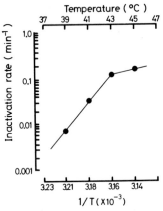

Fig. 2. Arrhenius plot for cell killing at various temperatures.

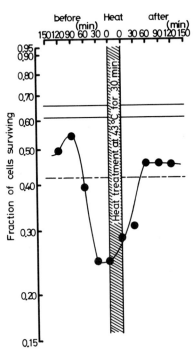

Fig. 3. Effect on the thermal enhancement of lethality when the sequence between heat (43°C for 30 min) and radiation dose of 2 Gy is varied.

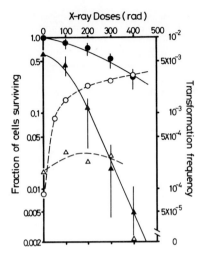

Fig. 4. Survival (closed symbols) and transformation frequency (open symbols) in GHE cells irradiated with various doses of X rays, with (△,▲) or without (○,●) hyperthermia at 43°C for 30 min. Vertical bar is standard deviation.

expected (the dotted line was theoretically obtained assuming that radiation and heat act independently on cells). When radiation was delivered to the cells more than 60 min after heating, the surviving fractions were slightly higher than expected. Radiosensitizing effects of hyperthermia were observed over a wide dose range of X rays, as shown in Fig. 4.

C. Transforming Ability of Hyperthermia in Combination with X Rays

Transformations of the cells exposed to a temperature of 43°C are summarized in Table I. Hyperthermia alone had a very low activity with regard to induction of transformation. The frequency of transformation by heat alone did not vary much with increasing doses of heat treatment, while the surviving fraction of the cells decreased rapidly. This indicates that the hyperthermic damage is lethal to the cells but does not lead to their transformation. The transformation following X irradiation alone increased with dose, as shown in Fig. 4. When hyperthermia (43°C for 30 min) was combined with X irradiation, a substantial reduction in the transformation for given doses was observed. The reduction of X-ray-induced transformation by hyperthermia was independent of the cell killing (Fig. 4).

TABLE I

Malignant Transformation in Golden Hamster Embryo Cells
Exposed to 43°C

Heat time (min)	Surviving fraction	Number of colonies counted (A)	Number of transformed colonies (B)	Transformation frequency (B/A) ($\times 10^4$)
0	1.00	3603	0	<2.78
15	0.837	3390	1	2.95
30	0.561	3062	1	3.27
45	0.318	3820	1	2.61
60	0.137	3839	1	2.60
75	0.031	1890	0	<5.29
90	0.004	1990	0	<5.03

D. Induction of DNA Single-Strand Breaks (ssb) by X Rays and Heat Treatment

Figure 5A shows the alkaline elution patterns of DNA from X-irradiated cells. At higher doses of X ray, the biphasic elution curves consisting of an initial steep and shallow phases were obtained. At lower doses, elution curves consisted of a straight line on a logarithm plot, and the speed of elution was slow compared with findings in the case of higher doses.

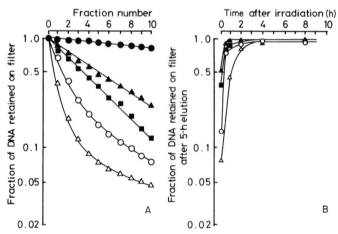

Fig. 5. DNA ssb induced by X irradiation (A), and its rejoining (B). (●) 0 Gy, (▲) 2 Gy, (■) 4 Gy, (○) 8 Gy, and (△) 12 Gy.

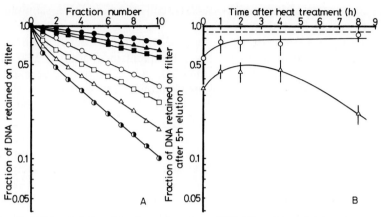

Fig. 6. DNA ssb induced by hyperthermia at 43°C (A) and its rejoining (B). Heating times: (●) 0 min, (▲) 30 min, (■) 60 min, (○) 90 min, (□) 120 min, (△) 180 min, and (◑) 240 min. Dashed line in (B) represents control level. Vertical bar is standard deviation.

Figure 6A shows alkaline elution patterns of DNA from heat-treated GHE cells. Shapes of the elution patterns obtained by heat-treated GHE cells are nearly the same as in the case of X-irradiated GHE cells. However, all curves were biphasic, regardless of the heat temperatures. We examined the relationship between the surviving fraction and DNA ssb induced by X rays and heat, and the results are shown in Fig. 7. At the same levels of survival, the DNA ssb in the cells irradiated with X rays were 10-fold higher than in the cells treated with hyperthermia (43°C).

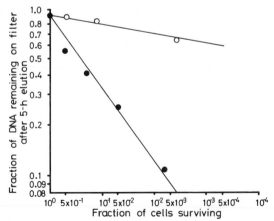

Fig. 7. Relationship between surviving fraction and DNA ssb induced by X rays (●) or hyperthermia at 43°C (○).

We next examined the ability of GHE cells to rejoin DNA ssb induced by X rays and heat. Figure 5B shows the changes in alkaline elution patterns of DNA from GHE cells, immediately after irradiation with various doses of X rays and during the subsequent incubation at 37°C after irradiation. In this figure, the fraction of DNA retained on the filter after 5 h of elution was plotted against incubation time. Maximum DNA elution reverted to levels in the nonirradiated controls within 1 to 2 h, when the cells were kept at 37°C after irradiation.

DNA ssb induced by heat treatment at 43°C for 90 min were rejoined completely within 1 to 2 h after heat treatment (Fig. 6B). In contrast, when the cells were treated with heat under severe conditions, such as at 43°C for 180 min, DNA ssb induced with heat were not rejoined. On the contrary, DNA began to degrade after 4 h of posttreatment incubation. Heat treatment did not inhibit the rejoining of DNA ssb induced by X rays (data not shown).

E.   Degradation of DNA and Protein from Heat-Treated GHE Cells

We examined the degradation of DNA and protein from heat-treated GHE cells. As shown in Fig. 8, there was no evidence of release of ^{3}H

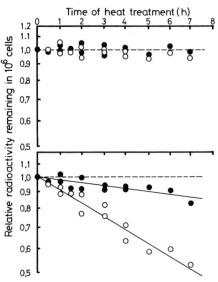

Fig. 8. Degradation of DNA ([^{3}H]TdR) and protein ([^{14}C]lysine) induced by hyperthermia at 43°C (O). Control (●).

radioactivity from DNA in GHE cells during heat treatment at 43°C. However, ^{14}C radioactivity from protein was released from both untreated and treated cells. The release of ^{14}C radioactivity from cells incubated at 43°C was about fourfold higher than that in untreated cells.

IV. Discussion

We found that hyperthermia alone did not induce a malignant transformation (Table I). When hyperthermia was combined simultaneously with X irradiation, a substantial reduction in the transformation for a given dose of X rays was observed (Fig. 4). Transformation was independent of cell killing when cells were treated with hyperthermia alone (Table I). Furthermore, cells treated with hyperthermia became refractory to X-ray induction of transformation. Similar results were reported by Harisiadis *et al.* (1980), who studied hyperthermia, alone or in combination with X ray, with regard to induction of malignant transformation in C3H/10T1/2 cells. They reported that hyperthermia (41.5°C) alone did not induce malignant transformation and that hyperthermia at 41.5°C for 2 h reduced the frequency of malignant transformation induced by X rays. In contrast, Marcznska *et al.* (1980) found that rat embryo cells exposed *in vitro* to an elevated temperature (39°C) were transformed and that this transformation correlated with the occurrence of karyotypic changes that appeared long after the treatment of cells at 39°C. As there is still some discrepancy with regard to the induction of malignant transformation by hyperthermia, mechanisms of cell killing by hyperthermia and the interaction between damage induced by heat and X rays require further investigation.

Cell lethality and DNA ssb induced by hyperthermia were discussed by Corry *et al.* (1977) and Ben-Hur and Elkind (1974). We also detected heat-induced DNA ssb using the alkaline elution method (Fig. 6). Heat treatment did induce DNA ssb; however, the number of ssb induced by hyperthermia was one-tenth less than that induced by X rays, at the same survival levels (Fig. 7). In addition, the activation energy for DNA damage was as follows: 28 kcal/mol for depurination, 25 kcal/mol for DNA ssb, and 34 kcal/mol for loss of transforming activity in viral DNA (Wasta and Dewey, 1971). However, when cells were exposed to 43°C, the protein gradually degraded with increasing exposure (Fig. 8), but DNA did not degrade with continuing heat exposure up to 8 h (Fig. 8). Analyses by Arrhenius plots indicated that the activation energy for cell killing by heat is about 140 kcal/mol at a temperature below 43°C, in our experiments (Fig. 2). This inactivation energy of 125 to 140 kcal/mol has been observed in various mammalian cells (Johnson *et al.*, 1954). These values are much the same as the activation energy for protein denaturation (Johnson *et al.*, 1954; Dewey *et al.* 1977; Connor *et al.*, 1977) but differed greatly from the activation energy for heat-induced damage to DNA, as discussed previously. Therefore, mammalian cells may be inactivated because of denaturation of critical protein by hyperthermia (Dewey *et al.*, 1977; Connor *et al.*, 1977).

As to why hyperthermia reduces transformation induced by X rays, the sequence in which the hyperthermic and X-ray treatments were applied is of some importance. We investigated the effects of heat treatments at 43°C for 30 min on the sensitization of GHE cells irradiated with Gy. The radiosensitizing effects of hyperthermia were the most extensive when X irradiation was given during heating (Fig. 3). We also investigated the potency of hyperthermia (43°C for 30 min) in combination with X rays in doses that would induce malignant transformation. Under such conditions, there was a substantial reduction in transformation for given doses (Fig. 4). This finding differs from earlier reports on the interactions between X irradiation and hyperthermia (Clark *et al.*, 1981). In their study, combined treatment led to a four- to fivefold increase in the transformation. This difference may be accounted for by two factors. First, they used established C3H/10T1/2 cells, whereas we used primary GHE cells. There are great differences in biological responses between established and primary cells. Second, head exposure was carried out on plateau phase culture, as opposed to the cell suspensions used in our study.

We found that heat treatment plus irradiation did not enhance X-ray-induced DNA ssb and did not inhibit the rejoining of DNA ssb induced by X rays (data not shown), as was also found by Ben-Hur and Elkind (1974) and Corry *et al.* (1977). Kato (1980) found an abrupt increase in the frequencies of chromosome aberrations and sister chromatid exchanges in Chinese hamster (D-6) cells incubated at a temperature over 39°C. These phenomena may be due to a disturbance in the semiconservative DNA synthesis and may bring about the enhancement of cell killing and the reduction of malignant transformation induced by X rays. However, Tomasovic *et al.* (1978) showed that hyperthermic radiosensitization may not be associated with increase in chromosome aberrations, in studies using synchronous CHO cells.

Transformation induced by unit doses of X rays is higher in cells irradiated with doses below Gy than when doses over Gy are applied (Fig. 4; Borek and Hall, 1974; Miller and Hall, 1978; Little, 1979; Watanabe *et al.*, 1982). Thus, mechanisms related to transformation seem to correlate with repair of lethal damage, that is, sublethal damage (Borek and Hall, 1974; Miller and Hall, 1978; Little, 1979; Watanabe *et al.*, 1982) and potentially lethal damage (Terzaghi and Little, 1975), which occurs in the cells irradiated with low doses of X rays. These repair processes (or repair enzymes) may be sensitive to heat treatment. Li *et al.* (1976) proposed that the enhancement of radiosensitization of Chinese hamster HA-1 cells by heat treatment is due to the heat potentiation of fixation of potentially lethal X-ray damage. Ben-Hur *et al.* (1974) found an inhibition of repair of sublethal damage and an enhancement of lethal damage in heated Chinese hamster cells. This disturbance of repair mechanisms may induce dynamic changes in structure of chromatin (Dewey *et al.*, 1972); moreover this may induce disorder in DNA synthesis (Schlag and Lücke-Huhle, 1981) in the irradiated cells. Kato (1980) found an abrupt increase in the frequencies of chromosome aberrations and sister chromatid exchanges in Chinese hamster (D-6) cells incubated at temperatures over 39°C. These phenomena may bring about the enhancement of cell killing and the reduction of malignant transformation induced by X-rays.

In conclusion, hyperthermia alone did not transform cells, and hyperthermia in combination with X ray reduced the transformation by X rays. Thus, the target of hyperthermia may be the protein rather than the DNA. Hyperthermia, alone or in combination with X rays, may prove to be effective for anticancer therapy.

Acknowledgments

This work was supported in part by a Grant-in-Aid for Cancer Research from the Ministry of Education, Science and Culture, Japan.

References

Ben-Hur, E., and Elkind, M. M. (1974). Thermally enhanced radioresponse of cultured Chinese hamster cells: damage and repair of single-stranded DNA and a DNA complex. *Radiat. Res.* **59**, 484–495.

Ben-Hur, E., Elkind, M. M., and Bronk, B. V. (1974). Thermally enhanced radioresponse of cultured Chinese hamster cells: inhibition of repair of sublethal damage and enhancement of lethal damage. *Radiat. Res.* **58**, 38–51.

Borek, C., and Hall, E. J. (1974). Effect of split doses of X-rays on neoplastic transformation of single cell. *Nature (London)* **252**, 499–501.

Clark, E. P., Hann, G. M., and Little, J. B. (1981). Hyperthermic modulation of X-ray-induced oncogenic transformation in C3H 10T1/2 cells. *Radiat. Res.* **88**, 619–622.

Connor, W. G., Gerner, E. W., Miller, R. C., and Boone, M. L. M. (1977). Prospects for hyperthermia in human cancer therapy. *Radiology (Easton, Pa.)* **123**, 497–503.

Corry, P. M., Robinson, S., and Getz, S. (1977). Hyperthermic effects on DNA repair mechanisms. *Radiology (Easton, Pa.)* **123**, 475–482.

Dewey, W. C., Noel, J. S., and Dottor, C. M. (1972). Changes in radiosensitivity and dispersion of chromatin during the cell cycle of synchronous Chinese hamster cells. *Radiat. Res.* **52**, 373–394.

Dewey, W. C., Hopwood, L. H., Sapareto, S. A., and Gerweck, L. E. (1977). Cellular response to combination of hyperthermia and radiation. *Radiology (Easton, Pa.)* **123**, 463–474.

Dickson, J. A. (1976). Hazards and potentiators of hyperthermia. *Proc. Int. Symp. Cancer Ther. Hyperthermia Radiat. Washington, D.C. Apr. 28–30, 1975*, pp. 134–150.

Dickson, J. A., and Shaw, D. M. (1972). The effects of hyperthermia (42°C) on the biochemistry and growth of malignant cell line. *Eur. J. Cancer* **8**, 561–571.

Harisiadis, L., Miller, R. C., Harisiadis, S., and Hall, E. J. (1980). Oncogenic transformation and hyperthermia. *Br. J. Radiol.* **53**, 479–482.

Henle, K. J., and Leeper, D. B. (1976). Interaction of hyperthermia and radiation in CHO cells: recovery kinetics. *Radiat. Res.* **66**, 505–518.

Henle, K. J., and Leeper, D. B. (1979). Effect of hyperthermia (45°C) on macromolecular synthesis in Chinese hamster ovary cells. *Cancer Res.* **39**, 2665–2674.

Johnson, F. H., Eyring, H., and Polissar, M. J. (1954). "The Kinetic Basis of Molecular Biology." Wiley, New York.

Kato, H. (1980). Temperature-dependence of sister chromatid exchange: an implication for its mechanism. *Cancer Genet. Cytogenet.* **2**, 61–67.

Kohn, K. W., Friedman, C. A., Ewig, R. A. G., and Iqbal, Z. M. (1974). DNA chain growth during replication of asynchronous L1210 cells. Alkaline elution of large DNA segments from cell lysed on filters. *Biochemistry* **13**, 4134–4139.

Li, G. C., and Kal, H. B. (1977). Effect of hyperthermia on the radiation response of two mammalian cell lines. *Eur. J. Cancer* **13**, 65–69.

Li, G. C., Evans, R. G., and Hahn, G. M. (1976). Modification and inhibition of repair of potentially lethal X-ray damage by hyperthermia. *Radiat. Res.* **67**, 491–501.

Little, J. B. (1979). Quantitative studies of radiation transformation with A31-11 mouse BALB/3T3 cell line. *Cancer Res.* **39**, 1474–1480.

Marcznska, B., Berghikz, C. M., and Wolfe, L. G. (1980). Role of elevated temperature in malignant transformation of mammalian cells *in vitro. Int. J. Cancer* **25**, 813–818.

Miller, R., and Hall, E. J. (1978). X-ray dose fractionation and oncogenic transformation in cultured mouse embryo cells. *Nature (London)* **272**, 58–60.

Mondovi, B., Agro, A. F., Rotilio, G., Strom, R., Moricca, G., and Fanelli, A. R. (1969). The biochemical mechanism of selective heat sensitivity of cancer cells. II. Studies on nucleic acids and protein synthesis. *Eur. J. Cancer* **5**, 137–146.

Roti-Roti, J. L., and Winward, R. T. (1978). The effects of hyperthermia on the protein to DNA ratio of isolated HeLa cell chromatin. *Radiat. Res.* **74**, 159–169.

Sapareto, S. A., Hopwood, L. E., and Dewey, W. C. (1978). Combined effects of X-irradiation and hyperthermia on CHO cells for various temperatures and orders of application. *Radiat. Res.* **73**, 221–233.

Schlag, H., and Lücke-Huhle, C. (1981). The influence of ionization density on the DNA synthetic phase and survival of irradiated mammalian cells. *Int. J. Radiat. Biol.* **40**, 75–85.

Terzaghi, M., and Little, J. B. (1975). Repair of potentially lethal radiation damage in mammalian cells is associated with enhancement of malignant transformation. *Nature (London)* **253**, 548–549.

Tomasovic, S. P., Turner, G. N., and Dewey, W. C. (1978). Effect of hyperthermia on nonhistone proteins isolated with DNA. *Radiat. Res.* **73**, 535–552.

Wasta, A., and Dewey, W. C. (1971). Variation in sensitivity to heat shock during the cell-cycle of Chinese hamster cells *in vitro. Int. J. Radiat. Biol.* **19**, 467–477.

Watanabe, M., Suzuki, N., and Nikaido, O. (1982). Transformation and mutation of golden hamster embryo cells induced by low doses of X-rays. *Proc. Tritium Radiobiol. Health Phys.*, pp. 46–59.

20 *Clinical Studies on Radiothermotherapy in Cancer Treatment*

Masahiro Hiraoka
Mitsuyuki Abe

Department of Radiology
Faculty of Medicine
Kyoto University
Kyoto 606, Japan

I. Introduction

Biological investigations reveal that hyperthermia alone or in combination with radiation has remarkable effects. Thus there is increasing interest in using hyperthermia as a clinical modality for treating human cancers. The biological rationale for combining hyperthermia and radiation is based on the following experimental findings:

1. Hyperthermia and radiation interact synergistically.
2. Cells in the late S phase, known to be radioresistant, are sensitive to heat.
3. Hypoxic cells are at least as sensitive to heat as oxic cells.
4. Heat inhibits the repair of both sublethal and potentially lethal damage by radiation.

5. Tumors with a poor blood supply may retain a higher temperature than normal tissues in cases of localized heating with ultrasound or electromagnetic waves, and this effect will have a differential effect on tumors.

In contrast with these biological results, physical techniques for inducing hyperthermia in the human body have not been fully developed.

Clinically, hyperthermia is divided into two categories: whole-body and localized hyperthermia. Among the methods available for localized hyperthermia, ultrasound and electromagnetic waves including microwaves and radiofrequency (RF) are considered to be most promising. Ultrasound has been used successfully in the treatment of superficial tumors (Marmor *et al.*, 1979). The ultrasound equipment for heating deep-seated tumors has now been developed, and the clinical studies are under way. Microwave hyperthermia combined with radiation has been applied (U *et al.*, 1980; Arcangeli *et al.*, 1980) mainly for the treatment of superficial tumors, with encouraging results. The principal advantage of RF hyperthermia is that it is suitable for heating tumors in deep locations. There are two methods for RF heating: inductive and capacitive. Inductive heating has been discussed by Storm *et al.* (1979), who reported a selective heating of tumors in the thorax and abdomen. LeVeen *et al.* (1976) reported encouraging results with RF capacitive heating.

In 1978 we initiated clinical application of hyperthermia combined with radiation in an attempt to determine the effectiveness and safety of this modality for the treatment of refractory cancers. This chapter concerns our clinical results obtained in the case of 2450-MHz microwave or 13.56-MHz RF hyperthermia, in combination with radiotherapy.

II. Methods

A. Heating Method

Hyperthermia was administered by microwave (2450 MHz) or RF (13.56 MHz), according to size and location of the tumors.

1. *Microwave (2450 MHz) Heating Equipment*

Initially, we used a commercially available microwave unit developed for physiotherapy. However, we found that a noncontact horn-type applicator supplied with this unit was not suitable for hyperthermic treatment because of difficulties in adjusting the applicator precisely toward the lesion and the reflected radiation from the skin surface. Therefore, we designed a contact applicator with a surface-cooling device. This applicator is filled with a low-loss dielectric constant material that minimizes the diameter (6.5 cm). Within the end of the applicator, temperature-controlled water circulates to avoid excessive heating of the skin. Figure 1 shows a microwave generator equipped with this contact applicator.

2. *Equipment for RF Heating*

The RF capacitive heating equipment we developed is shown in Fig. 2. It has a maximal output of 600 W and operates at a frequency of 13.56 MHz. The RF energy is transmitted from the generator by two coaxial

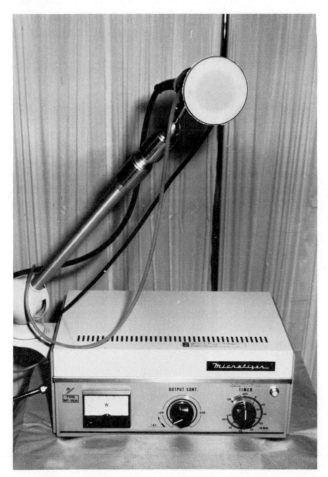

Fig. 1. Microwave heating equipment (2450 MHz).

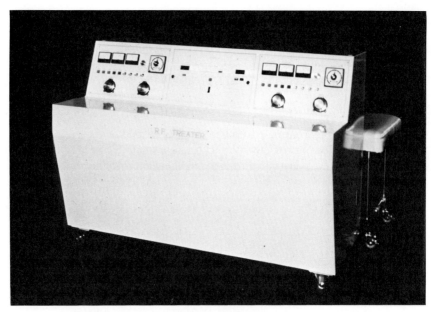

Fig. 2. Radiofrequency capacitive heating equipment (13.56 MHz).

cables to two disk electrodes of varying sizes. The alternating current generated between parallel opposing electrodes produces heat in the body. Within the electrodes, temperature-controlled water circulates to avoid excessive heating of the skin and subcutaneous fat. The electrodes can be made to adhere to the skin by using a flexible water pad containing salt solution. Electrodes in sizes ranging from 4 to 30 cm in diameter were designed and were selected for use according to the size and location of the particular lesion. Figure 3 demonstrates the arrangement used when treating metastatic neck tumors.

B. Temperature Measurements

Temperatures were monitored in most patients only in the tumor center, whereas those of the adjacent normal tissues were measured occasionally. In the case of microwave heating, temperatures were continuously measured during treatments with thermocouples or thermistors embedded in 29-gauge needles and monitored with a Bailey Model BA-8 electric thermometer. Both needles and thermometer were shielded with copper mesh to avoid interference by the electromagnetic field. We have since used Teflon-coated thin thermocouples (Bailey Instruments Inc., Type IT-18) and a digital temperature recorder (YEW Co., Type 3874).

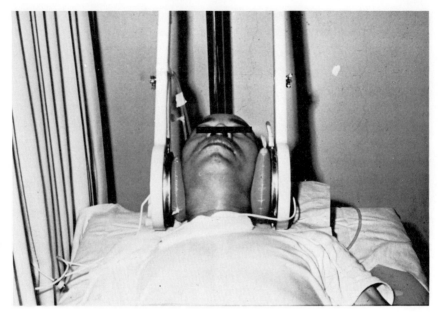

Fig. 3. Arrangement of electrodes when treating metastatic neck tumors.

The sensors were inserted into the tumor through 21-gauge angiocatheters. In the case of RF heating, continuous temperature measurement was impossible because of interference by the electromagnetic field. Therefore, temperatures were measured during brief periods of wave cessation, using Teflon-coated thin thermocouples.

C.   Patient Selection

1. Patients were selected whose tumors were radioresistant, including malignant melanoma, locally advanced tumors considered to be refractory to conventional treatment, and tumors that recurred after definitive radiotherapy.
2. Tumors were selected in which intratumor temperature could be measured.
3. Tumors were selected in which the response to heat could be assessed objectively.

D.   Assessment of Tumor Response

Size of the treated lesions was measured by palpation, ultrasound, and radiographic studies including CT scan. Tumor response was graded as complete, partial, or no response. A decrease in tumor volume of more than 50% signified a partial response; less than a 50% decrease signified no response.

III. Results

A. Thermal Distribution

1. *Thermal Distribution by Microwave Heating*

Thermometry in agar phantom was performed using a thermography unit (Thermoviewer JTG-MD). Figure 4 shows the isothermal distributions in the central plane of agar phantoms after heating with a contact applicator. This figure suggests that the effective thermal depth is less than 3 cm without surface cooling and up to 3 cm with surface cooling.

2. *Thermal Distribution by RF Heating*

The thermal distribution after RF heating in the muscle-equivalent agar phantom developed by Ishida and Kato (1980) was determined using a thermography unit (Fig. 5). Homogeneous thermal distribution was obtained in the central region of the phantom when large electrodes of the same size were placed on the top and the bottom of a phantom (Fig. 5A). When different-sized electrodes were paired, a high-thermal region shifted to the side of the smaller electrode (Fig. 5B). In the presence of a

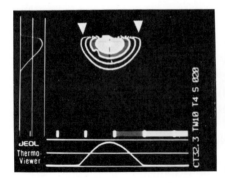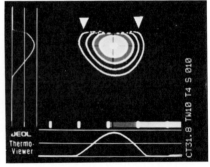

cooling (−)   cooling (+)

Fig. 4. Thermogram taken after 2450-MHz microwave heating, with or without surface cooling. The graphs at the left and the lower sides represent temperature profiles along the vertical and the horizontal lines indicated in the picture, respectively. Space between small arrows is 5 cm.

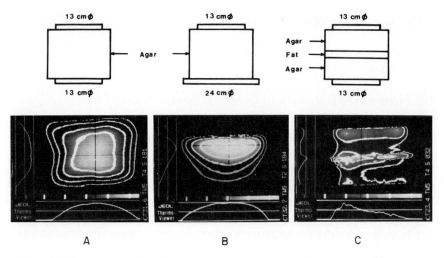

Fig. 5. Thermogram taken after 13.56-MHz RF heating (∅, diameter). See text for details.

fat layer 2 cm in thickness between the top and bottom agar phantoms, a hot spot was observed in this layer (Fig. 5C). These experiments demonstrate that a high-thermal region suitable for the size and location of the tumor can be obtained by changing the size of the electrodes and that temperatures in a tumor surrounded by thick fat will be little increased using this equipment.

Figure 6 shows the temperature profile of a metastatic neck tumor. Selective tumor heating up to 43°C was obtained.

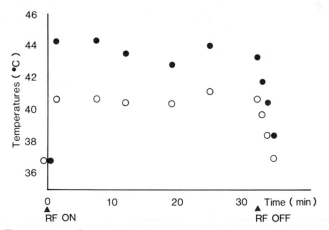

Fig. 6. Temperatures of tumor (●) and normal tissue (○) during RF heating, metastatic neck tumor.

B. Clinical Results

Between September 1978 and June 1982, 51 patients with 54 lesions were studied.

1. Microwave Hyperthermia Combined with Radiation

A total of 29 lesions were treated with microwave hyperthermia plus radiation. Of 29 superficial tumors treated, 16 were metastatic neck tumors, 3 metastatic tumors of the chest wall, 2 breast cancer, and 8 other various tumors. In the initial clinical trial, 3 lesions were treated with hyperthermia, before and after irradiation five times a week. The remaining 26 lesions were heated one to three times a week immediately after irradiation with doses ranging from 3 to 6 Gy. Intratumor temperatures of 41 to 43.5°C were maintained for 20 to 30 min/session. Total radiation doses varied from 12 to 70 Gy, according to the lesion. Most lesions not

TABLE I

Local Tumor Response following Microwave Hyperthermia plus Radiotherapy

Area treated	Primary site	Histology	No. of treated sites	Tumor response		
				CR	PR	NR
Neck node	Head and neck	SCC[a]	10	6	2	2
	Parotid gland	Adenocarcinoma	1	1	0	0
	Skin	Myoblastoma	1	1	0	0
	Skin	Malignant melanoma	1	0	0	1
	Breast	Adenocarcinoma	1	1	0	0
	Unknown	Adenocarcinoma	1	1	0	0
	Ovary	Adenocarcinoma	1	0	1	0
Chest wall	Breast	Adenocarcinoma	2	2	0	0
	Skin	Malignant melanoma	1	0	1	0
Breast	Breast	Adenocarcinoma	2	2	0	0
Cheek	Maxillary sinus	SCC	1	1	0	0
Face	Parotid gland	Adenocarcinoma	1	1	0	0
Leg	Foot	Malignant schwannoma	1	1	0	0
Anus	Rectum	Adenocarcinoma	1	1	0	0
Back	Skin	Myoblastoma	1	1	0	0
Scalp	Skin	SCC	1	0	1	0
Wrist	Skin	SCC	1	0	1	0
Lip	Lip	SCC	1	0	0	1
			29	19 (66%)	6 (20%)	4 (14%)

[a] SCC, Squamous cell carcinoma.

given previous radiotherapy received cumulative doses of 40 to 50 Gy, whereas those that had had previous radiotherapy received less than 40 Gy.

The results are summarized in Table I. In 19 of the 29 lesions, there was a complete response (CR); partial response (PR) was noted in 6 and no response (NR) in 4 lesions. Skin burn in three patients healed completely within 2 weeks.

The following example shows the effect of this combined treatment. Figure 7A illustrates a 61-year-old patient with left extensive breast cancer with an ulceration measuring approximately 6 cm in diameter. The tumor was irradiated with a cumulative dose of 50 Gy in 15 fractions over 42 days through an opposed tangential field. Microwave hyperthermia was given after irradiation twice weekly for 10 sessions, with a tumor temperature of 43°C for 20 min/session. Complete response was obtained at the completion of this combined treatment (Fig. 7B).

2.   Radiofrequency Hyperthermia Combined with Radiation

Twenty-four patients with 25 lesions were treated by RF hyperthermia plus radiation. Most patients had locally advanced bulky tumors, many of

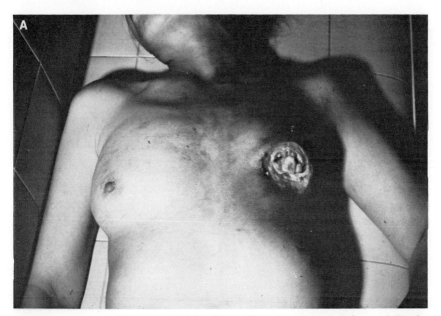

Fig. 7. A 61-year-old patient with left advanced breast cancer, (A) before and (B) after treatment.

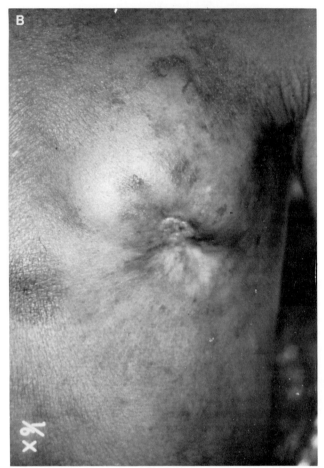

Fig. 7B.

which reached over 10 cm in diameter. Treated by this method were tumors of the head and neck, metastatic tumors in the chest and abdominal walls and in the inguinal region, carcinomas of the breast and the lung, and soft tissue sarcomas.

Intratumor temperatures of 41 to 44°C (mostly 43°C) were maintained for 30 to 60 min twice weekly. Radiotherapy was given in two fractions/week with 4 Gy/fraction. However, for tumors in which delivery of radiation with 4 Gy was difficult because of the intolerance of adjacent normal tissues, 2 Gy/session five times a week were given.

The results obtained with this combined modality are shown in Table II.

TABLE II

Local Tumor Response following RF Hyperthermia plus Radiotherapy

Area treated	Primary site	Histology[a]	No. of treated sites	Tumor response CR	PR	NR
Neck node	Head and neck	SCC	3	0	3	0
	Parotid gland	Adenocarcinoma	1	1	0	0
	Esophagus	SCC	1	1	0	0
	Uterine cervix	SCC	1	1	0	0
	Shoulder	Rhabdomyosarcoma	1	1	0	0
	Unknown	Adenocarcinoma	1	1	0	0
Chest wall	Skin	Malignant melanoma	1	1	0	0
	Pleura	Fibrosarcoma	1	1	0	0
	Bone marrow	Myeloma	1	1	0	0
	Lung	Adenocarcinoma	1	0	1	0
Abdominal wall	Stomach	Adenocarcinoma	2	0	2	0
	Ureter	TCC	1	1	0	0
Inguinal node	Skin	SCC	1	1	0	0
	Penis	SCC	1	0	0	1
Buccal mucosa	Buccal mucosa	SCC	2	0	1	1
Pharynx	Pharynx	SCC	1	1	0	0
Breast	Breast	Adenocarcinoma	1	1	0	0
Shoulder	Shoulder	Rhabdomyosarcoma	1	0	1	0
Leg	Leg	MFH	1	0	1	0
Tongue	Tongue	SCC	1	0	1	0
Lung	Lung	Giant cell carcinoma	1	0	1	0
			25	12 (48%)	11 (44%)	2 (8%)

[a] MFH, Malignant fibrous histiocytoma; SCC, squamous cell carcinoma; TCC, transitional cell carcinoma.

Of 25 lesions treated, 12 showed complete response, 11 partial response, and 2 no response.

In the two patients described next, the effects of combined treatment with RF hyperthermia and irradiation were remarkable. Figure 8A concerns a 62-year-old patient with an ulcerated tumor of the pharynx that had recurred after a full course of radiotherapy. This patient received nine treatments of RF hyperthermia at 43°C for 30 min, with a cumulative dose of 36 Gy. Complete response was achieved, as shown in Fig. 8B. Both CT and fiberscopic examinations revealed complete disappearance of the lesion. Figure 9 demonstrates a supraclavicular metastasis of uterine cancer, before (Fig. 9A) and after treatment with hyperthermia plus radiation (Fig. 9B). The bulky tumor, reaching 8 × 6 × 6 cm, completely regressed

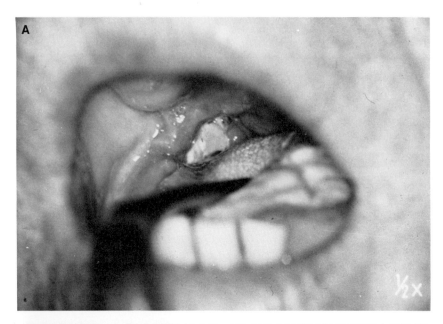

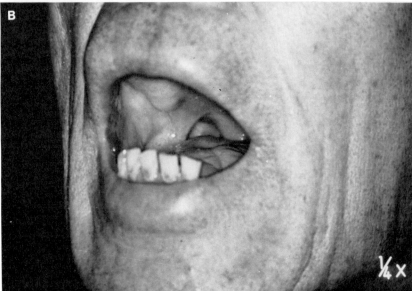

Fig. 8. A 62-year-old patient with recurrent pharyngeal tumor, (A) before and (B) after treatment.

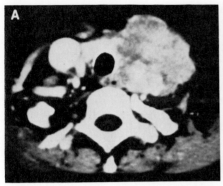
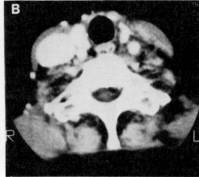

Fig. 9. Computer tomographic (CT) scans of a metastatic supraclavicular tumor from uterine cancer, (A) before and (B) after treatment.

when a total dose of 60 Gy in 30 fractions was delivered, in combination with 11 sessions of RF hyperthermia in which the intratumor temperature of approximately 43°C was maintained for 60 min.

With regard to complications, biochemical and hematological data revealed no significant abnormality. The only systemic symptoms were sweating and general malaise. The skin was burned in one patient, as fixation of the electrodes was poor. In one patient with a metastatic submandibular tumor, severe stomatitis appeared in the heated area. Both injuries healed completely.

3. Effects of Radiothermotherapy on Previously Irradiated and Nonirradiated Tumors

Of 54 lesions that were treated with RF or microwave hyperthermia in combination with radiotherapy, 17 had been previously treated with definitive radiotherapy. The tumor control effect of radiothermotherapy on these recurring lesions after radiotherapy is shown in Table III. A 70% complete response was obtained, even in cases of recurrences of previously irradiated tumors.

TABLE III

Comparison of Response Rate between Lesions with
(+) and without (−) Previous Radiotherapy

Previous radiotherapy	CR (%)	PR (%)	NR (%)	Total
−	19 (51)	15 (41)	3 (8)	37
+	12 (70)	2 (12)	3 (18)	17

TABLE IV

Tumor Response Rate to Radiothermotherapy according to
Histology

Histology[a]	No. of treated sites	Tumor response CR (%)	PR (%)	NR (%)
SCC	25	11 (44)	9 (36)	5 (20)
Adenocarcinoma				
All except breast cancer	10	7 (70)	3 (30)	0
Breast cancer	6	6 (100)	0	0
Malignant melanoma	3	1 (33)	1 (33)	1 (33)
Others				
Myoblastoma	2	2 (100)	0	0
Rhabdomyosarcoma	2	1 (50)	1 (50)	0
Malignant schwannoma	1	1 (100)	0	0
Fibrosarcoma	1	1 (100)	0	0
Myeloma	1	1 (100)	0	0
TCC	1	1 (100)	0	0
MFH	1	0	1 (100)	0
Giant cell carcinoma	1	0	1 (100)	0
	54	32 (59)	16 (30)	6 (11)

[a] Abbreviations are as in Table II.

4. Effects of Radiothermotherapy according to Histology

Table IV summarizes the results of radiothermotherapy, assessed histologically. A higher incidence of complete response was obtained in those with adenocarcinoma than in cases of squamous cell carcinoma. In three patients with malignant melanoma, complete response occurred in one, partial response in one, and no response in the third patient.

IV. Discussion

One of the most important problems in cancer treatment is achieving hyperthermia in the human body. Our phantom and clinical studies have shown that superficial tumors can be heated to more than 41°C using 2450-MHz microwave heating equipment. This finding plus the few complications demonstrates that the 2450-MHz microwave treatment is useful for heating of superficial tumors. We designed 13.56-MHz RF capacitive heating equipment and treated various nonsuperficial tumors. Our phantom studies as well as the findings of other investigators (Guy *et al.*, 1974; Hahn *et al.*, 1980) showed that fat tissue can be selectively heated with this method. However, with the surface-cooling device, the intratumor temperatures could be elevated to 43°C in most cases without serious skin damage. Thus, the capacitive heating appears to be a promising approach to treatment of more deeply seated tumors.

Two new approaches to RF hyperthermia have been attempted. Manning *et al.* (1982) described the interstitial hyperthermia method. Electrical currents of 500 KHz were passed through by needle electrodes inserted around the tumor. They combined this technique with interstitial brachytherapy. Some kinds of metal are known to be selectively heated when exposed to a magnetic field. Stauffer *et al.* (1982) implanted ferromagnetic agents into the region and exposed the region to an external RF electromagnetic field. Both methods selectively heated the localized area. However, there were disadvantages, in that surgical procedures were required to insert the electrodes or metals into or around a tumor. Ideal placement to obtain uniform localized heating is considerably difficult in clinical practice.

In *in vitro* studies, Dewey *et al.* (1977) found that heat sensitivity is considerably different between cell lines. Specific heat-sensitive histology has not been clearly defined. Kim *et al.* (1978) and Stehlin *et al.* (1975) reported that radioresistant malignant melanoma is most sensitive to heat, yet only one of three lesions showed a complete response in our studies.

Radiothermotherapy is a promising treatment for a variety of cases. A large-scale study is under way in Japan to assess the effectiveness of RF hyperthermia combined with radiotherapy.

References

Arcangeli, G., Barni, E., Cividalli, A., Mauro, F., Morelli, A., Nervi, C., Spano, M., and Tabocchini, A. (1980). Effectiveness of microwave hyperthermia combined with ionizing radiation: clinical results on neck node metastases. *Int. J. Radiat. Oncol. Biol. Phys.* **6,** 143–148.

Dewey, W. C., Hopwood, L. E., Sapareto, S. A., and Gerweck, L. E. (1977). Cellular responses to combinations of hyperthermia and radiation. *Radiology (Easton, Pa.)* **123,** 463–474.

Guy, A. W., Lehmann, J. F., and Stonebridge, J. B. (1974). Therapeutic applications of electromagnetic power. *Proc. IEEE.* **62,** 55–75.

Hahn, G. M., Kernahan, P., Martinez, A., Pounds, D., Prionas, S., Anderson, T., and Justice, G. (1980). Some heat transfer problems associated with heating by ultrasound, microwaves, or radio frequency. *Ann. N.Y. Acad. Sci.* **335,** 327–335.

Ishida, T., and Kato, H. (1980). Muscle equivalent agar phantom for 13.56 MHz RF-induced hyperthermia. *Shimane J. Med. Sci.* **4,** 134–140.

Kim, J. H., Hahn, E. W., and Tokita, N. (1978). Combined hyperthermia and radiation therapy for cutaneous malignant melanoma. *Cancer (Philadelphia)* **41,** 2143–2148.

LeVeen, H. H., Wapnik, S., Piccone, V., Falk, G., and Ahmed, N. (1976). Tumor eradication by radiofrequency therapy: response in 21 patients. *JAMA J. Am. Med. Assoc.* **235,** 2198–2290.

Manning, M. R., Cetas, T. C., Miller, R. C., Oleson, J. R., Connor, W. G., and Gerner, E. W. (1982). Clinical hyperthermia: results of a phase I trial employing hyperthermia alone or in combination with external beam or interstitial radiotherapy. *Cancer (Philadelphia)* **49,** 205–216.

Marmor, J. B., Pounds, D., Postec, T. B., and Hahn, G. M. (1979). Treatment of superficial human neoplasms by local hyperthermia induced by ultrasound. *Cancer (Philadelphia)* **43,** 188–197.

Stauffer, P. R., Cetas, T. C., and Jones, R. (1982). System for producing localized hyperthermia in tumors through magnetic induction heating of ferromagnetic implants. *Natl. Cancer Inst. Monogr.* **61,** 483–487.

Stehlin, J. S., Giovanella, B. C., Ipolyi, P. D., Muenz, L. R., and Anderson, R. T. (1975). Results of hyperthermic perfusion for melanoma of the extremities. *Surg. Gynecol. Obstet.* **140,** 339–348.

Storm, F. K., Elliot, R. S., Harrison, W. H., and Morton, D. L. (1979). Normal tissue and solid tumor effects of hyperthermia in animal models and clinical trials. *Cancer Res.* **39,** 2245–2251.

U, R., Noell, K. T., Woodward, K. T., Worde, B. T., Fishburn, R. I., and Miller, L. S. (1980). Microwave induced local hyperthermia in combination with radiotherapy of human malignant tumors. *Cancer (Philadelphia)* **45,** 638–646.

21 Clinical Experience with Hyperthermia in Cancer Radiotherapy: Special Reference to in Vivo Thermometry

Toshifumi Nakajima
Masashi Tsumura
Yasuto Onoyama

Department of Radiology
Osaka City University Medical School
Osaka 545, Japan

I. Introduction

Combined use of heat and ionizing radiation is a promising treatment for radioresistant tumors, because the two modalities act complementarily for cell killing *in vitro*. Cells in S phase and chronically hypoxic cells, which as a consequence have a low pH, are vulnerable to heat (Gerweck *et al.*, 1975; Kim *et al.* 1975, 1976; Dewey *et al.*, 1977; Overgaard and

Bichel, 1977; Suit, 1977; Overgaard, 1981). For solid tumors *in vivo*, localized application of heat improves the effects of cancer radiotherapy, as preferential heating of the tumor will occur with the low net blood flow in large tumors (LeVeen *et al.*, 1976; Kim *et al.*, 1978; Storm *et al.*, 1976b; Hahn and Kim, 1980; Jain, 1980; Song *et al.*, 1980). The results of localized hyperthermia in cases of human cancer therapy, in particular electromagnetic heating with radiation, are encouraging (Kim *et al.*, 1978; Storm *et al.*, 1979a; Arcangelli *et al.*, 1980; Bicher *et al.*, 1980; LeVeen *et al.*, 1980; U *et al.*, 1980). However, problems such as measurement and control of temperature at depth, the optimal temperature and duration of the heat treatment, and the adequate sequence and interval of both modalities require further study.

A clinical pilot study of localized hyperthermia in combination with radiotherapy was initiated in early 1980 in the Department of Radiology at Osaka City University Medical School. Two types of heating equipment are available. One is a microwave unit, MT 300 (Minato Medical Science Ltd.), which generates 2450-MHz microwave with a power output of 300 W and was clinically used for superficial lesions. The microwave is transmitted from the generator to the helical antenna through a coaxial cable. The second generator is a RF hyperthermia unit (Yamamoto Vinyter Ltd.) with a power output of 900 W at dual frequencies of 6 and 13.56 MHz. A pair of circular water-cooled electrodes of various sizes are placed on opposite sides of the patient's body for capacitive heating to the relatively deep-seated lesions. A total of 248 sessions of heat treatment in 36 patients had been performed as of April 1982, and various technical difficulties, in particular thermometry *in vitro*, were overcome with improvement of the equipment.

This chapter describes our clinical experiences of combined localized hyperthermia in cancer radiotherapy and discusses mainly problems associated with temperature measurement and its evaluation, including the effects of electromagnetic waves on the thermometer system, the difference of temperature distribution in static phantom and *in vivo*, and the method for evaluating the heat dose, administered under conditions of various temperatures.

II. Temperature Measurement in the Electromagnetic Field

Influence of the electromagnetic field on thermometric devices sometimes causes difficulties in temperature measurement, and it is essential to know exact temperatures in order to evaluate quantitatively the effect of hyperthermia in cancer therapy. Various components of the thermometer are influenced; however, the effect on the thermometer probe, which is inevitably exposed to the direct electromagnetic field, is considered the most important. Erroneous behavior of the thermometer and development of hot spots have been reported in temperature measurement using metallic probes such as thermocouples (Dickson *et al.*, 1977; Cetas *et al.*, 1978; Cetas and Connor, 1978; Christensen, 1979). Temperature measurement has most often been made only intermittently after the cessation of electromagnetic power (Dickson *et al.*, 1977; Kim *et al.*, 1978; Storm *et al.*, 1979a,b; Arcangelli *et al.*, 1980; U *et al.*, 1980).

These time delays may lead to inaccuracies in the recorded temperature, particularly *in vivo*, because of the rapid cooling effect of blood circulation. Moreover, power control of the heating machine under continuous temperature monitoring is desirable for accurate and safe application of hyperthermia. Nonperturbing probes, which involve the use of high-impedance leads or optical fiber, have been developed (Larsen *et al.*, 1974; Bowman, 1976; Christensen, 1977); however, these measures are not so reliable as and are more expensive than conventional thermocouples. We designed several types of thermocouple probes and studied the response in electromagnetic fields of various frequencies. Our objective was to determine the applicability of thermocouple probes for temperature measurement, in cases of hyperthermic treatment induced by electromagnetic waves.

A.   Thermometric Device

Our thermometric system was composed of a thermocouple probe, a cold junction compensator, and a three-channel chart recorder (Fig. 1). A cold junction compensator of the ice water type was used, as this type was less sensitive to the electromagnetic field, as compared to the electronic type. The chart recorder and control unit of the heating machines were installed in an operating room with a 300-kV deep-therapy machine shielded by 3-mm thick lead from the treatment room. The control unit

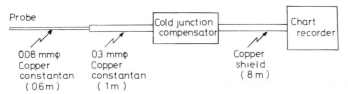

Fig. 1. Block diagram of the thermometric system. For all figures, the symbol $\emptyset$ represents diameter.

and the recorder were separated, as electromagnetic power can sometimes leak out from the control unit itself. Lead lines of the thermometer
and those of the heating machine were placed as distant as possible to
avoid effects of interference. Four types of thermocouple probes were
made by putting a thin Teflon- (polytetrafluoroethylene) covered copper
constantan thermocouple (0.08 mm in diameter) into a 21-gauge metallic
needle, polyethylene catheter for angiography (Becton Dickinson Formo-
cath Polyethylene Tubing No. 7620), or Teflon tube (Makiguchi Rubber
Corp. Teflon Tube AWG 24). The wires of a thermocouple were insulated
by epoxy resins (Konishi Corp., Mender) or heat-melted Teflon (Fig. 2).
The latter three flexible probes were introduced to the desired depth,
through an 18-gauge Teflon catheter.

B. Response of Probes in the Electromagnetic Field

Temperatures indicated by each type of probe during irradiation of
2450-MHz microwave and 6- or 13.56-MHz radiofrequency were continuously recorded to examine the effect of the electromagnetic field on the
prepared thermocouple probes.

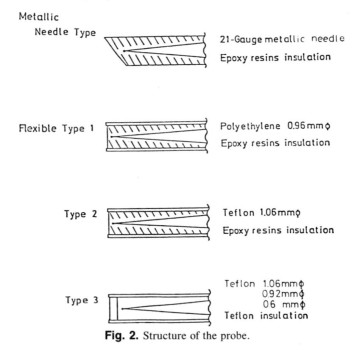

Fig. 2. Structure of the probe.

1.   Microwaves, 2450 MHz

Figure 3 shows the temperature record measured by metallic needle probe and flexible type 1 probe during microwave irradiation. The tips of both probes were set at nearly the same point in the agar phantom made of 0.5% NaCl and 2% agar gel (Ishida and Kato, 1980). Values indicated by the metallic needle probe (A) always exceeded those by the flexible type 1 probe (B), and the difference tended to increase according to the increase of microwave power. The same trends were observed with flexible types 2 and 3. When probes were immersed into liquid egg white, coagulation occurred occasionally around the metallic needle during microwave irradiation; this was never observed around the flexible probes, indicating that an abnormal hot spot sometimes occurring around metallic probes may cause discomfort or even burn patients.

In order to ascertain whether or not there was an abnormal hot spot around the flexible-type probes, the temperature of the phantom adjacent to the probe was measured. Tips of the probe (A) and Teflon tube (B) were placed in close proximity in the phantom during microwave irradiation, and the second probe was introduced through the Teflon tube (B) immediately after cutting the power, in order to assess the temperature without the influence of microwave (Fig. 4). Curve A shows the temperature

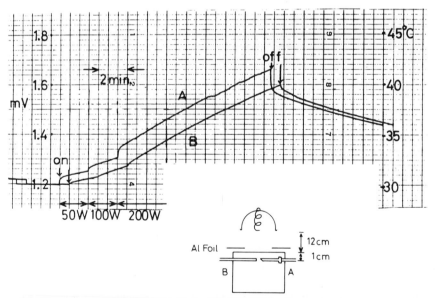

Fig. 3. Temperature records under 2450-MHz microwave irradiation. (A) Metallic needle probe. (B) Flexible type 1 probe. Time lag of curves in abscissa is related to characteristics of the recorder.

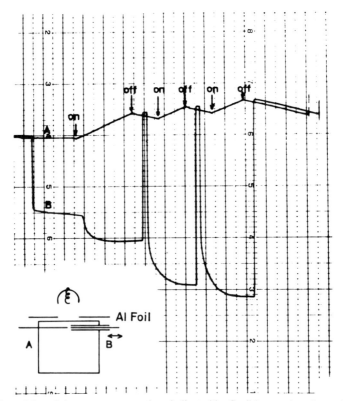

Fig. 4. Validity of the temperature values indicated by flexible type 1 probe under 2450-MHz microwave irradiation. (A) Retained probe; (B) inserted probe after turning off microwave.

record of the retained probe (A), and curve B that of the second probe introduced after the cessation of the microwave. The values indicated by both probes were practically equal, indicating that abnormal hot spots did not develop around the flexible-type probes. Our flexible-type probes show the correct temperature, even during 2450-MHz microwave irradiation.

Figure 5 shows the temperature record during 2450-MHz microwave heating in a patient with neck node metastasis from laryngeal cancer. Probe A was placed at 1 cm depth in the tumor, B on the skin surface, and C in the axillary region. The power can be regulated easily to maintain the desired temperature in the tumor, above 43°C in this case, under continuous monitoring by flexible-type thermocouple probes.

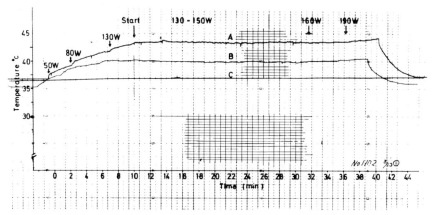

Fig. 5. Temperature record in a patient with neck node metastasis, under conditions of 2450-MHz microwave exposure. Probe A placed at 1-cm depth in tumor (43.2°C), B on skin surface (40.0°C), and C in axillary region (37.1°C).

2. *Radiofrequency (RF), 6 MHz*

Because a hot spot develops around the metallic probe in microwave heating, response in the radiofrequency field was tested only in case of the flexible-type probes. Tips of the three types of probes were set at the nearly the same point in the phantom irradiated with 6-MHz RF (Fig. 6). Temperature curves A and B (probes of types 1 and 2) exceeded curve C (type 3 probe) and showed an abrupt temperature elevation after turning on the RF. This phenomenon closely resembles behavior of the metallic probe in the microwave field and suggests the development of a hot spot around types 1 and 2 probes in the RF field.

To examine further the validity of the temperature reading, a type 3 probe was retained in the phantom during RF irradiation, and the other was inserted immediately after the cessation, as in the case of microwave. Comparison of the values indicated by both probes verified the validity of the temperature measurement by the flexible type 3 probe, even during 6-MHz RF irradiation (Fig. 7). We use this type of probe clinically for continuous temperature monitoring in hyperthermic treatment by 6-MHz RF. Figure 8 shows the temperature record in case of the type 3 probe, in a patient with advanced left breast cancer and treated with 6-MHz RF hyperthermia combined with radiotherapy. Probes A and B were inserted at 2 cm and 4.5 cm depths in the tumor, and probe C on the skin surface, respectively. The surface was cooled by circulating water through the electrodes.

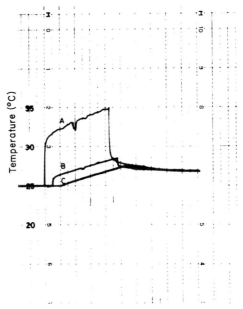

Fig. 6. Responses of three kinds of probes inserted into an agar phantom, under conditions of 6-MHz RF irradiation, 7.5 mm/min.

3. Radiofrequency, 13.56 MHz

Validity of the temperature indicated by the type 3 probe under 13.56-MHz RF was examined by comparing the indicated values of the retained probe (A) and those of the probe inserted immediately after the cessation (B) (Fig. 9). Our thermometer system did not function well, as there was contamination of electromagnetic noise. Nevertheless, a valid temperature was recorded within a few seconds after turning off the RF. Figure 10 shows a representative record taken by the type 3 probe every 10 min in a patient with hemangiopericytoma in the right arm. Probe A was inserted at 1.5 cm in the tumor, and B was placed on the skin surface.

C. Applicability of Thermocouple to Clinical Thermometry in Electromagnetically Induced Hyperthermia

Erroneous behavior of a thermometer equipped with a metallic probe such as a thermocouple has been reported by several authors, and this is regarded as one of the most troublesome problems in hyperthermic treat-

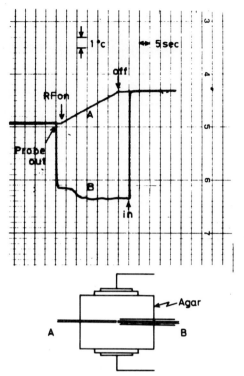

Fig. 7. Validity of the temperature measurement indicated by flexible type 3 probe, under conditions of 6-MHz RF irradiation. (A) Retained probe; (B) inserted probe after turning off RF irradiation.

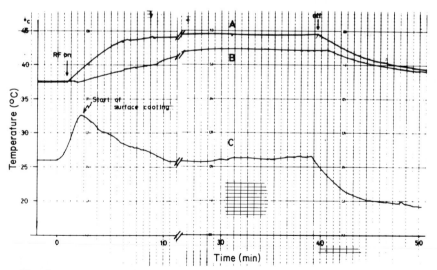

Fig. 8. Temperature record in a patient with breast cancer, under conditions of 6-MHz RF irradiation.

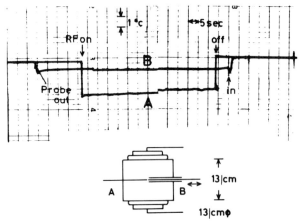

Fig. 9. Validity of the temperature indicated by a flexible type 3 probe under conditions of 13.56-MHz RF irradiation. (A) Retained probe; (B) inserted probe after turning off RF irradiation. Values by the retained probe did not indicate true temperature during 13.56-MHz RF irradiation.

ment by electromagnetic waves. Although various components of the thermometer can be influenced by the electromagnetic field, an electric current that flows from a metallic probe to the ground through the thermometer is probably responsible for the abnormal response of the thermometer and development of a hot spot around the tip of the probe (Eno et al., 1981). This phenomenon was observed in our experiment using the

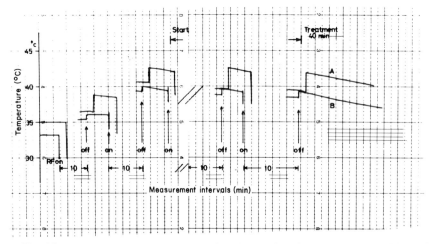

Fig. 10. Temperature record in a patient with a hemangiopericytoma, under conditions of 13.56-MHz RF irradiation. Temperature measurement was made every 10 min.

TABLE I

Applicability of Each Type of Probe under Three
Different Frequencies of Electromagnetic Waves[a]

	Frequency (MHz)		
Type of probe	2450	13.56	6
Metallic needle	X	X	X
Polyethylene (epoxy resins insulation)	O	△*	O*
Teflon (epoxy resins insulation)	O	△*	O*
Teflon (Teflon insulation)	O	△	O

[a] Symbols are as follows: O, Continuous temperature measurement possible; △, temperature measurement possible within 5 sec after cessation; X, temperature measurement practically impossible; *, reliability questionable.

metallic needle probe, under 2450-MHz microwave (Fig. 3), and types 1 and 2 flexible probes under 6-MHz RF (Fig. 6). We attempted to insulate the probe with various materials such as polyethylene, Teflon, and epoxy resins. Behavior of the insulated flexible probes differs according to the frequency of the electromagnetic waves (cf. Figs. 4, 6, 7, and 9, and Table I). Continuous temperature measurement is feasible in the field of 2450-MHz microwave, with all types of probes except the metallic needle type. A Teflon-insulated type 3 probe allowed for continuous assessment of the temperature in the field of 6-MHz RF but not that of 13.56-MHz RF. A valid temperature could be obtained within 5 sec after the cessation in the latter case. Thus the influence of the electromagnetic field on the thermocouple can be reduced markedly by electrical insulation of the probe, and the insulation required to prevent the electric current varies with the frequency of the electromagnetic waves. We consider that a valid temperature reading can be obtained by the thermocouple probe providing there is proper insulation for frequencies of electromagnetic waves.

III. Temperature Distribution

Temperature distribution in the tumor and its surrounding normal tissues has to be determined for localized hyperthermia, just as dose distribution must be determined for radiation therapy. Noninvasive thermometry (Johnson et al., 1975; Sachs and Tanney, 1977) is ideal for this purpose; however, at this writing it is not available. Temperature distributions, obtained by invasive methods in vivo or measured in the tissue-equivalent phantom, are usually used in the planning of heat treatment. It is neither desirable nor possible to implant a large number of probes to assess the total temperature profile, *in vivo*. However, if an accurate temperature distribution could be determined in a phantom study, the measurements obtained at several representative points would aid in temperature monitoring. Development of a thermometric instrument to acquire additional temperature information less invasively has to be considered. Phantom studies, which are the most useful way to determine dose distribution in radiation therapy, are useful in hyperthermia to a certain degree (e.g., power deposition study) (Connor *et al.*, 1977; Cetas and Connor, 1978); however, the applicability of the results for prediction of the temperature profile *in vivo* is limited because of the heterogeneous tissue composition and blood circulation (Cetas, 1981). The bio-heat transfer function,

$$\rho c \frac{\partial T}{\partial t} = V(k\Delta T) + \dot{q}_m + \dot{q}_b + \dot{q}_p$$

is widely used to describe the heat balance in a tissue region, where ρ is tissue density, c is heat capacity, k is thermal conductivity, T is temperature, t is time, q is energy/unit time/unit volume, and the subscripts m, b, and p refer to metabolism, perfusion (blood flow), and external power deposition, respectively. The term on the left represents thermal energy storage, and the four terms on the right represent thermal energy diffusion, metabolic heat generation, perfusion of solids by liquids (primarily by blood), and external thermal deposition, in that order. The fourth term on the right is added to the classical bio-heat transfer equation for application of the equation to hyperthermic treatment. Taking these factors into consideration, two types of phantom—static and dynamic—were prepared. A static (not perfused) phantom, which was made of 0.5% NaCl and 2% agar gel, was used to represent mainly the fourth term of the equation (i.e., power deposition); a dynamic (perfused) phantom, in which the sponge was perfused with saline solution (Cetas and Connor, 1978; Sandhu *et al.*, 1981), represented mainly the third (i.e., blood flow) and fourth terms. Temperature profile and heating pattern in both types during electromagnetic heating were compared to determine the effect of blood flow and to examine the applicability of these results for estimation of the temperature distribution *in vivo*.

A. Invasive Measurement of Temperature Distribution

Figure 11 shows an example of a temperature profile along the central axis in a patient treated using the 6-MHz RF machine with a pair of water-

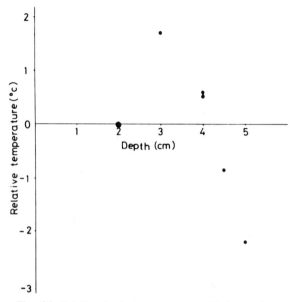

Fig. 11. Relative depth–temperature profile in a patient.

cooled electrodes, 13 and 18 cm in diameter. We use three thermocouple probes in most cases, one placed on the skin surface and the other two inserted into the tumor at different depths. The relative depth–temperature curve (temperature at 2 cm depth as the reference) was drawn on the basis of the collected data from five sessions of hyperthermia. Temperature reached the peak at 3 cm depth and fell rapidly with the effective depth ranging from 4 to 5 cm, in this particular case. Collection of such temperature data in patients is relevant to the clinical practice of hyperthermia and to the development of new machines. The number of probes feasible for application *in vivo* limits the precision of the resulting temperature distribution. Thermometric instruments that yield more temperature-related information without increasing the burden on the patients have to be developed. We designed two methods for this purpose: One is the use of a thermocouple with multiple hot junctions (multiple sensor spots) on one probe, and the other is an instrument that can move the probe intermittently during heating.

The multisensor probe has several hot junctions on the same probe (Fig. 12). Spacing between the hot junctions can be arbitrarily selected and is prepared according to our design. Although temperatures at multiple points that are equivalent to the number of hot junctions can be taken continuously and concomitantly, our chart recorder simultaneously records only three temperatures. However, we can obtain temperature data

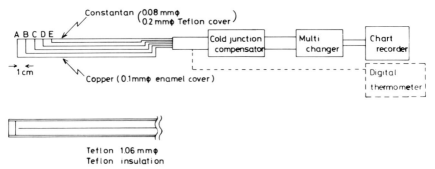

Fig. 12. Structure of the multisensor probe and a block diagram.

intermittently at nine points by using a multichanger for the recording system. Figure 13 shows the temperature record in a patient with neck node metastasis from soft palate carcinoma. Temperatures of A, B, and C were taken by the multisensor probe, and those of C, D, and E were recorded on the chart recorder by selecting the point, using a multi-changer.

The second method of obtaining a multiple temperature reading is the use of a thermometric probe that can move intermittently. A step motor system was developed to move the probe through a Teflon tube inserted into the tissue, according to the prescribed time program. Figure 14 shows the temperature profile in a phantom, in which the probe sweeps over at a speed of 1 cm/sec with 2 sec standstill time every 1 cm. Ripples on the curve result from the time constant of the probe. Technical problems, in particular the simultaneously recorded temperatures, are inevitably associated with this kind of measurement; however, this method does yield information on temperature distribution in the steady state.

B. Temperature Distribution in the Static Phantom

Thermography (Fujitsu Infra Eye 150) was mainly used in the study of temperature distribution in the static phantom. A thermogram of the plane indicated in Fig. 15 was taken immediately after the temperature at the reference point had reached the prescribed value. Figure 16A shows the temperature distribution on the central internal plane of the homogeneous phantom irradiated from above with 2450-MHz microwave. Size of the heated area was controlled by shielding the microwave with aluminum foil placed on the incident surface. The temperature pattern suggests that 2450-MHz microwave can be applicable only to the superficial lesions.

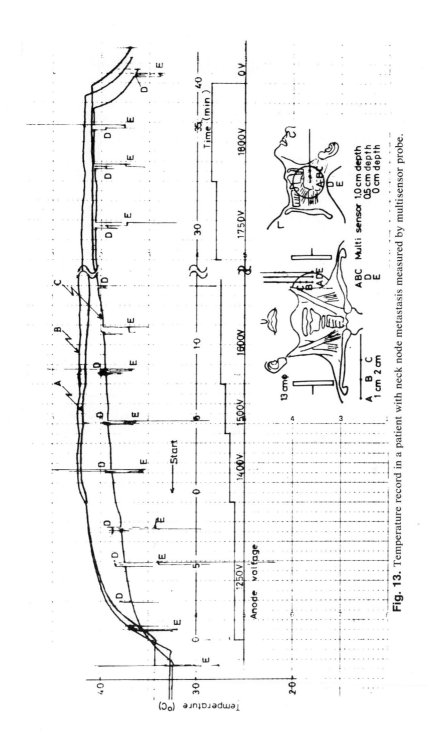

Fig. 13. Temperature record in a patient with neck node metastasis measured by multisensor probe.

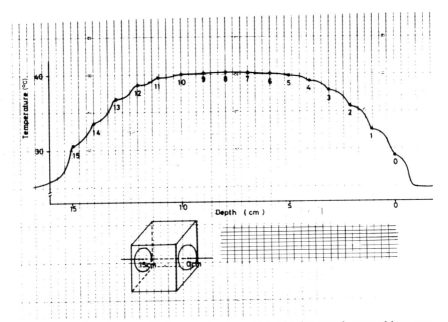

Fig. 14. Temperature profile in agar phantom obtained using a probe moved by a step motor.

Figure 16B shows the temperature distribution by 6 MHz capacitive heating. A pair of water-cooled electrodes was placed at the top and bottom of the phantom. In capacitive heating, treatment volume can be altered by changing the combination of electrodes of various diameters (Fig. 16C).

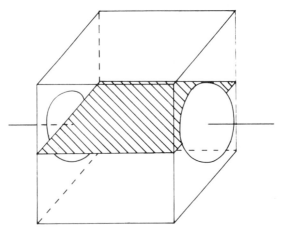

Fig. 15. The plane on which thermography was taken.

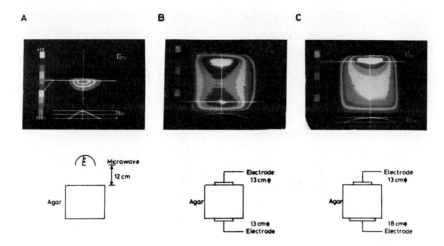

Fig. 16. Temperature distribution in the agar phantom. (A) 2450-MHz microwave irradiation; (B and C) 6-MHz RF irradiation.

Temperature distributions indicated by thermography do not agree strictly with the pattern of power deposition, because the first term of the bio-heat transfer equation (thermal energy diffusion) cannot be neglected in this type of experiment; however, a qualitative study on the tendency of the deposit pattern is feasible.

Figure 17 is a thermogram that illustrates the problem of tissue heterogeneity. Phantoms containing fresh bovine femur (A) and fat layer (B), both of which have low electrical conductivity as compared with muscle, were heated by 6-MHz RF. The fat layer is heated to a greater extent than the surrounding agar gel, because the high-resistive fat acts as a series resistor. The bone acts as a parallel resistor in this case, the current flowing around the bone, leaving it cold, and producing bilateral hot regions.

Study of the static phantom, especially with the use of thermography, is very convenient and time-saving when attempting to assess the temperature pattern in a qualitative or semiquantitative manner. Thus it is helpful to select the heating machine and the combination of electrodes and/or to estimate the effect of tissue heterogeneity (Guy, 1971; Guy *et al.,* 1974; Manning *et al.,* 1982). However, the results in the static phantom cannot be directly applied to predict the temperature distribution *in vivo,* as the physiological system is absent, particularly the blood flow. Temperature records obtained in a rabbit irradiated with 6-MHz RF revealed an interesting curve that showed the influence of blood flow in local hyperthermia (Fig. 18). Thermocouple probes were inserted into the dorsum; the tem-

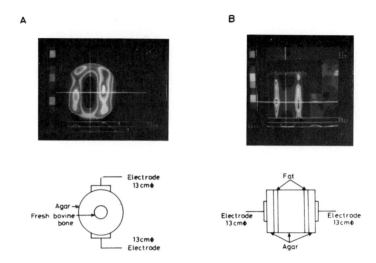

Fig. 17. Temperature distribution in the heterogeneous agar phantom. (A) Fresh bovine bone was incorporated in the center. (B) Fat layers were placed on each side of the phantom.

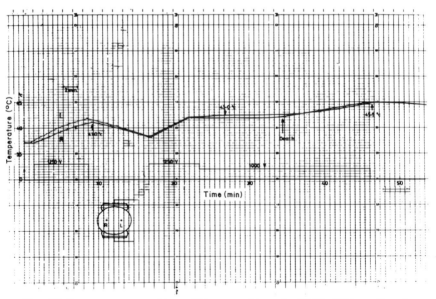

Fig. 18. Temperature record in a rabbit exposed to under 6 MHz RF hyperthermia.

perature increased with time, then fell rapidly when the heat was turned off. After resumption of RF heating, the temperature was maintained at a constant level by adjusting the power. The rabbit was then given an over-dose of pentobarbital sodium; with this, the temperature began to rise again despite equal application of power, and it did not fall so rapidly after the cessation of power as in the live rabbit. The finding that more power was needed to heat the living rabbit may be attributed to the cooling effect of the blood flow. These results suggest the limitation of applicability of the static phantom for studies on clinical hyperthermia and also the neces-sity for studies using an appropriate dynamic (perfused) phantom.

C.   Dynamic Phantom for Hyperthermia

Because of the complexity of hemodynamics *in vivo,* it is impossible to simulate entirely the blood circulation using a phantom model (Cetas and Connor, 1978; Bowman, 1980; Chen and Holmes, 1980). A sponge block perfused with saline solution was used as a simple model (Fig. 19). A block of polyurethane sponge (polyurethane foam 20 12 INOAC) was packed in an acrylic box (15 × 28 × 20 cm) and perfused with saline solution driven by gravity with flow rates ranging from 0 to 4.5 ml/cm^2/min. At the point where electrodes are attached, thickness of the wall is

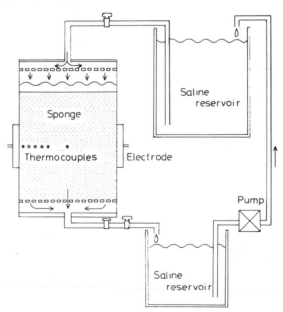

Fig. 19. Structure of the dynamic phantom.

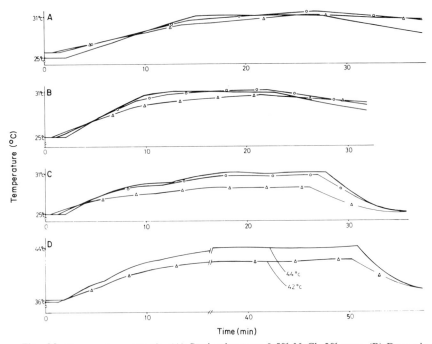

Fig. 20. Temperature records. (A) Static phantom: 0.5% NaCl, 2% agar. (B) Dynamic phantom, 0.1% NaCl, perfusion 0. (C) Same as (B) but perfusion 1.5 ml/cm²/min. (D) Patient data. Probe depth: (——) 1 cm, (○) 2 cm, (△) 3 cm.

reduced to 1 mm to minimize influence of the wall material. Figure 20 shows temperature–time curves at 1, 2, and 3 cm depth from the surface of the phantoms heated by 6-MHz RF. A marked resemblance of temperature variations at each depth is noted between the static agar phantom (Fig. 20A) and the dynamic phantom without perfusion (Fig. 20B; flow rate = 0). If the temperature at a given depth (1 cm in the figure) is maintained constant by adjusting the RF power, temperatures at different depths vary with time in the nonperfused phantom.

A steady state of temperature, which is usually observed *in vivo* as shown in Fig. 20D, is not evident in the static phantom. Steady state refers to the equivalence of heat production and heat loss due to conduction and circulation. Such a state of temperature–time curves occurs in the perfused phantom (Fig. 20C), as it does clinically. Furthermore, patterns of temperature decrease after turning off the power in the dynamic phantom are approximately similar to those seen in patients. Figure 21 shows curves of temperature decrease after cessation of RF at 1 cm depth in the dynamic phantom perfused with saline solution of various flow

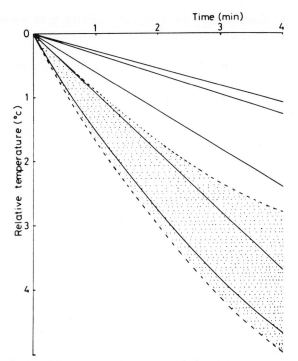

Fig. 21. Cooling curves in the dynamic phantom after cessation of RF at 1 cm depth at various flow rates (ml/cm²/min), from top to   bottom: 0, 0.5, 1.0, 1.5, and 2.0. Shaded portion: patient data.

rates. Collected data of cooling curves in patients, indicated by the shaded portion in the figure, correspond to the flow rate of about 1.5 ml/cm²/min in the dynamic phantom. These results suggest that temperature variations *in vivo* can be simulated by this type of simple model, with regard to the cooling effect by perfusion.

Our study of the dynamic phantom is still in a preliminary state. For example, factors such as the properties of the sponge and the concentration and flow rate of saline solution have yet to be determined according to each term of the bio-heat transfer equation (Balasubramanian and Bowman, 1974, 1977; Jain, 1980).

IV. Evaluation of Clinical Temperature Data

In Osaka City University Medical School, a clinical trial of localized hyperthermia combined with radiotherapy is in progress, and 36 patients with advanced malignancies are included in the trial as of April 1982. Two sources for local heat are used; 2450-MHz microwave, and 6- or 13.56-MHz radiofrequency of the capacitive type. Temperatures in the tumor or normal tissue were measured invasively with our handmade thermocouple probe.

Although some encouraging results on the beneficial effect were observed, temperatures achieved by these heat sources were affected by various factors, such as slight inadequacy in the arrangement of electrodes, unevenness of the skin surface, site of the lesion, and heat sensitivity of the patient; thus the prescribed tumor temperature could always be reached. Peak value and pattern of the temperature–time curve may vary remarkably in each session of the heat treatment, even in the same patient. In addition, it is impossible using equipment presently available to heat the entire large tumor uniformly and to the prescribed temperature. Considering variation of the temperature in time and place, it is important to develop a system of evaluating heat dose that includes the relative biological effectiveness of different temperatures, in order to evaluate quantitatively the effect of hyperthermia. Because of the complexity of factors involved, computerized data processing is in progress in our department.

A. Clinical Results of Radiothermotherapy

Of the 36 patients treated with hyperthermia, 17 were exposed 105 times to microwaves and 23 were exposed 143 times to RF. Four patients received both microwave and RF. There were 18 with neck node metastases mainly from head and neck tumors, 7 with chest wall tumors, and 11 with tumors of different sites and kinds (Table II). Heating with 2450-MHz microwaves with a helical antenna was mainly applied to superficial lesions because of its penetration to about 2 cm from the skin surface, whereas the relatively deep or large tumors were treated with RF capacitive heating (Johnson and Guy, 1972; LeVeen et al., 1976; Kim et al., 1978; Sugaar and LeVeen, 1979; U et al., 1980; Hand and Haar, 1981). Heat treatments at 42.5°C for 30 to 40 min were repeated biweekly after the irradiation of 4 Gy. The following examples demonstrate the effect of combined treatment of hyperthermia and irradiation.

Figure 22 shows an inoperable huge breast cancer (16 × 16 × 6 cm) with an allied tumor (4 × 4 × 4 cm) in its left upper quadrant before and after treatment. Seven sessions of tangential irradiation of 2 Gy each with 10-MV X ray (total dose: 7 × 2 = 14 Gy) resulted in no tumor regression; therefore, RF hyperthermia, using a circular 13-cm electrode on the front

TABLE IIA

Distribution of Histology and Tumor Response to Microwave Hyperthermia

Site	Histology	No. of cases	CR	PR	NR	NM
			Response[a]			
Neck	Epidermoid carcinoma	5 + (1)[b]	2	2	1	0
	Medullary tubular carcinoma	2	0	0	1	1
	Papillary carcinoma	1	1	0	0	0
	Adenocarcinoma	1	0	1	0	0
Chest wall	Medullary tubular carcinoma	2	2	0	0	0
	Scirrhous carcinoma	1	1	0	0	0
	Intraductal adenocarcinoma	1	0	1	0	0
Abdomen	Adenocarcinoma	1	0	1	0	0
Face	Epidermoid carcinoma	1	0	1	0	0
Groin	Malignant melanoma	1[b]				
		15 + (2)[b]	6	6	2	1

[a] Abbreviations: CR, complete regression; PR, partial regression; NR, no response; NM, not measurable.

[b] Evaluated in the RF hyperthermia group.

TABLE IIB

Distribution of Histology and Tumor Response to RF Hyperthermia

Site	Histology	No. of cases	CR	PR	NR	NM
			Response[a]			
Neck	Epidermoid carcinoma	7	2	3	2	0
	Adenocarcinoma	1 + (1)[b]	0	1	0	0
	Renal cell carcinoma	1	0	0	1	0
Chest wall	Medullary tubular carcinoma	1	0	1	0	0
	Papillotubular carcinoma	1	0	1	0	0
	Large cell carcinoma	1	0	1	0	0
Back	Malignant melanoma	1	0	0	0	1
Abdomen	Epidermoid carcinoma	2	1	0	1	0
	Malignant hystiocytoma	1	0	0	1	0
	Transitional cell carcinoma	1	0	0	0	1
	Hepatoma	1	0	1	0	0
	Adenocarcinoma	1[b]				
Arm	Hemangiopericytoma	1	0	0	1	0
Groin	Epidermoid carcinoma	1	0	0	0	1
	Malignant melanoma	1	0	0	1	0
		21 + (2)[b]	3	8	7	3

[a] Abbreviations as in Table IIA.

[b] Evaluated in the microwave hyperthermia group.

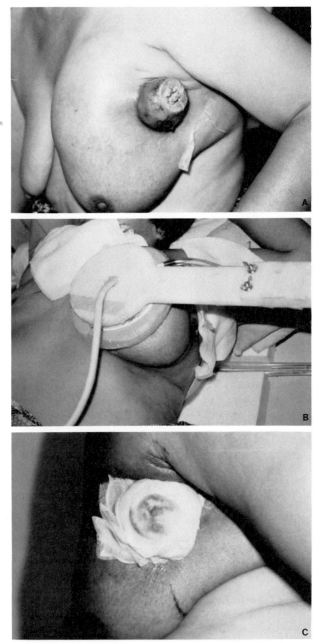

Fig. 22. Hyperthermic treatment of breast carcinoma. (A) Pretreatment, (B) RF hyperthermic treatment, (C) Posttreatment.

and an 18-cm one on the back of the patient, was administered biweekly after irradiation with a dose of 4 Gy. Temperature–time curves in this case are shown in Section II,B,2 (Fig. 8). After six sessions of combined treatment, the main tumor had shrunk to 8 × 6 × 3 cm in size and was successfully resected.

Figure 23 demonstrates a chest wall mass (8 × 8 × 4 cm), metastasized from a large cell carcinoma of the left lung. After 10 sessions of irradiation with 13-MeV electron beam followed by RF hyperthermia, the tumor disappeared on palpation. The effect in this case was evaluated as one of partial regression because of a small residual mass demonstrated by computed tomography.

Exact evaluation of the beneficial effect of hyperthermia in the present series is difficult, because the prescribed temperature could not be achieved in some patients and most were given heat treatment after conventional radiotherapy, with the dose ranging from 10 to 45 Gy. However, as shown in Table II, remarkable tumor regression was observed in 23; complete regression in 9 and partial regression of over 50% in 14 of the evaluable 35 patients with radioresistant tumors. Although further study and longer follow-up data are required, these results do provide evidence for the effectiveness of thermotherapy combined with radiation.

B. Tumor Temperature in Patients

In each session of hyperthermia, temperatures at the skin surface, subcutaneous tissue, and whenever possible in the tumor were monitored using our handmade thermocouple probe. The 18-gauge Teflon catheter containing a metallic needle was inserted into the tumor (under local anesthesia), and location of the tip was determined by bidirectional radiography taken with an X-ray simulator for radiotherapy planning. The thermocouple probe was threaded through the catheter and left in place throughout the heat treatment. Temperature variation was recorded continuously on a chart recorder in the case of 2450-MHz microwave and 6-MHz RF, and intermittently in 13.56-MHz RF. A 24-channel digital temperature recorder (Yokogawa Electronics Works Ltd., Yew type 3874) was also used to measure the temperature at multiple points, every 5 min.

Temperature in the tumor was measured 182 times in 248 hyperthermic sessions. A median value of temperatures, obtained every 10 min after reaching the constant level, was defined arbitrarily as the representative of treatment temperature in the session, because variation in temperature was occasionally observed, even during the "plateau" period. Hyperthermic sessions in which treatment temperature was over 42°C, between 40

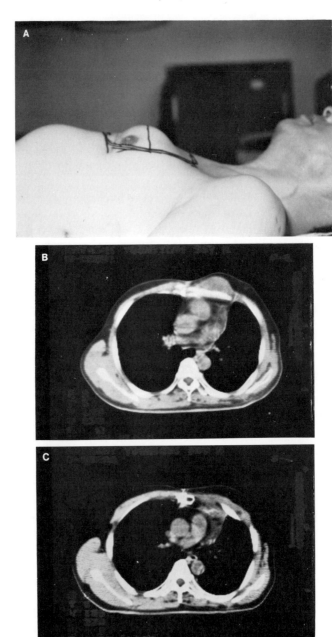

Fig. 23. Hyperthermic treatment of chest wall metastasis from lung carcinoma. (A) Pretreatment, (B) pretreatment CT, (C) Posttreatment CT.

and 42°C, and under 40°C, were designated as groups A, B, and C, respectively (Table III). Treatment temperature over 42°C (A) was achieved in 31.5% of the patients treated by RF and in 53.5% of those exposed to microwaves, and treatment temperature (B) in 40.3 and 31.0%, respectively. This result does not indicate the superiority of microwave heating, however, because tumors exposed to RF were generally deep seated. For example, there were two patients with uterine cancer in the RF series. Treatment temperature achieved by electromagnetic heating tends to vary according to site of the lesion. Heating over 42°C (A) can be achieved more frequently in case of lesions of the chest wall, back, and thigh; however, this is not the case with neck tumors. The difference may be attributed in part to the technical difficulty of achieving close contact between the electrode and the skin surface and the abundant blood flow in the neck region. In addition, treatment temperature may vary in each session and even in the same patient; therefore the temperature has to be measured at each session of heat treatment.

In view of the temperature dependence of thermal radiosensitizing effect (Henle and Dethlefsen, 1980; Storm *et al.,* 1980; Luk *et al.,* 1981), development of a method that can express the equivalent effect of heat given under conditions of various treatments will enable a quantitative evaluation of the efficacy of hyperthermia in cancer therapy.

C. Computerized Processing of Temperature Data

In clinical hyperthermia induced by the available electromagnetic instruments, unlike experiments involving *in vitro* cells or animal tumors, the prescribed temperature cannot always be achieved and maintained during every session of heat treatment. The gradient of the temperature increase curve may also vary with each session. Because these factors affect the degree of the sensitizing effect of hyperthermia, a more detailed analysis of the temperature data is required for a quantitative evaluation of the effects of heat. We developed a computerized data processing system, in which temperature data are automatically stored in a floppy disk by tracing the temperature curves obtained by the chart recorder on the curve digitalyzer (Siemens Evados). Various parameters of the treatment, such as maximum, minimum, median, and mean temperatures, with standard deviation, etc., are rapidly printed out by data processing. We are now developing a new real-time system that will allow for a direct input of the temperature from the thermometer.

Figure 24 shows temperature–time curves redrawn from the data of the

TABLE IIIA

Tumor Temperatures Achieved in Each Microwave Hyperthermia Session

Site	No. of cases	No. of measurements	Median temperature[a]		
			A	B	C
Neck	8	31	14	11	6
			(45.2%)	(35.5%)	(19.4%)
Chest wall	2	12	8	3	1
			(66.7%)	(25.0%)	(8.3%)
Abdomen	1	7	4	2	1
			(57.1%)	(28.6%)	(14.3%)
Face	1	6	3	2	1
			(50.0%)	(33.3%)	(16.7%)
Groin	1	2	2	0	0
	13	58	31	18	9
			(53.5%)	(31.0%)	(15.5%)

[a] Median temperatures: group A, >42°C; B, 40–42°C; C, <40°C.

TABLE IIIB

Tumor Temperatures Achieved in Each RF Hyperthermia Session

Site	No. of cases	No. of measurements	Median temperature[a]		
			A	B	C
Neck	9	53	8	31	14
			(15.1%)	(58.5%)	(26.4%)
Chest wall and back	4	34	22	9	3
			(64.7%)	(26.5%)	(8.8%)
Abdomen	5	20	1	7	12
			(5.0%)	(35.0%)	(60.0%)
Arm	1	9	2	1	6
			(22.2%)	(11.1%)	(66.7%)
Groin	1	8	6	2	0
			(75.0%)	(25.0%)	
	20	124	39	50	35
			(31.5%)	(40.3%)	(28.2%)

[a] Median temperatures same as in Table IIIA.

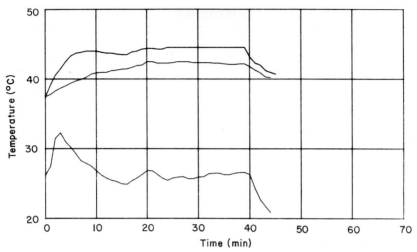

Fig. 24. Temperature record reconstructed by the computer from stored data, for the patient described in Fig. 8.

patient illustrated in Fig. 8. Figure 25 demonstrates a printout of all temperature data every 1 min at 2 cm depth in the tumor, from the start to the end of heat treatment. Maximum, median, mean, and minimum temperatures during the session were 44.5, 44.0, 43.4, and 37.5°C, respectively. Length of the period over which parameters are calculated can be selected. Temperature parameters between 13 and 45 min after the initiation of hyperthermia, during which time the temperature was maintained fairly constant, were 44.5, 44.4, 43.7, and 40.5°C, respectively. In general, maximum and median temperatures were less influenced according to different selections of the calculation range.

An attempt to evaluate accumulated heat dose given under different conditions was made by adopting the concept of equivalent time calculated by computer (Sapareto and Dewey, 1982). Equivalent time means summation of the products of the time duration and the relative effectiveness of heat, at that temperature. All heat exposure to different temperatures is converted to the length of time at the reference temperature, 43°C in this case. Conversion factors for relative effectiveness, 2 per 1°C for temperature above 43°C and $\frac{1}{4}$ per 1°C below 43°C, were used temporarily on the basis of reported results (Fig. 26) (Crile, 1963; Dewey *et al.*, 1977; Dickson and Shah, 1977; Henle and Dethlefsen, 1980). Equivalent time at 43°C in the case shown in Figs. 8 and 24 was 84.2 min at 2 cm depth, 9.8 min at 4.5 cm, and 5.7×10^{-7} min on the skin surface.

Equivalent time in every session can be added theoretically, and the total length of equivalent time represents the total heat dose administered

HISTOGRAM

Number	Lower limit		Upper limit	Frequency
1	37.00	----	37.50	0
2	37.50	----	38.00	1
3	38.00	----	38.50	0
4	38.50	----	39.00	0
5	39.00	----	39.50	1
6	39.50	----	40.00	0
7	40.00	----	40.50	0
8	40.50	----	41.00	2
9	41.00	----	41.50	2
10	41.50	----	42.00	1
11	42.00	----	42.50	2
12	42.50	----	43.00	1
13	43.00	----	43.50	2
14	43.50	----	44.00	9
15	44.00	----	44.50	9
16	44.50	----	45.00	16

Class Interval = 0.50
Number of Class = 16
Number of Data = 46
Maximum : 44.500
Minimum : 37.500
Average : 43.428
Standard deviation : 1.5641
Coefficient of variation : 0.0360
Median : 44.000

Fig. 25. Example of data processing.

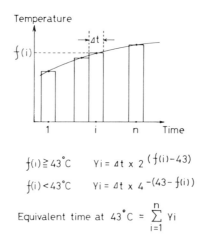

$$f(1) \geqq 43°C \quad Y_i = \Delta t \times 2^{(f(i)-43)}$$

$$f(i) < 43°C \quad Y_i = \Delta t \times 4^{-(43-f(i))}$$

$$\text{Equivalent time at } 43°C = \sum_{i=1}^{n} Y_i$$

Fig. 26. Expression of the equivalent time at 43°C.

to the patients. The patient in Fig. 8 received six sessions of heat treatment. Although points of temperature measurement were not at the same depth in each of the six sessions, when the highest temperature curve in each treatment was selected as a representative value, the cumulative length of equivalent time at 43°C in this case was 192.3 min, occupying about 70% of the actual treatment time of 276 min. Introduction of the concept of equivalent time into hyperthermia facilitates evaluation of the effect of heat treatment given under different conditions and provides a clue for a quantitative analysis of the dose. Additional biological and clinical data on the temperature–effect relationship of thermal radiosensitization are required to assess the validity of hyperthermia treatment.

V. Conclusions

Clinical trials and experimental studies of localized hyperthermia were carried out to assess its effectiveness in cancer radiotherapy and to elucidate the technical problems. Special reference was made to the measurement and control of temperatures *in vivo,* during the heat treatment. The results of our studies can be summarized as follows:

1. Thermocouple probes with appropriate electrical insulation can be used for temperature measurement during exposure to microwaves or radiofrequency, with a clinically sufficient accuracy. Multisensor thermocouple probes will facilitate acquisition of temperature data *in vivo,* and the extent of invasion will be diminished.

2. The value of phantom study for estimating the temperature distribution *in vivo* (unlike the case of radiation) is limited because of a lack of blood circulation in the usual static phantom. A prototype of a dynamic (perfused) phantom was developed, and interesting results on the effect of perfusion were obtained in comparative studies using data obtained with the phantom and from patients. This approach should be useful in developing a theoretical method for estimation of temperature distribution *in vivo.*

3. The prescribed temperature cannot always be achieved and maintained during each session of heat treatment. To evaluate the heat dose (administered under different temperature conditions), a concept of "equivalent time" at 43°C was introduced, and a computer system was used for calculation. Further biological and clinical studies on the temperature–time relationship have to be done to assess its validity in clinical hyperthermia; however, the concept of equivalent time does provide a clue with regard to quantitative evaluation of the heat dose.

4. The combined modality is a feasible and promising method for treating radioresistant tumors, and with improvement of heating and thermometric equipment, even better results can be expected.

Acknowledgments

We thank K. Ito, A. Izumi, M. Ono, N. Shiizaki, and M. Tsuji for technical assistance. This work was supported by Grants No. 501063 and 56010065 from the Japanese Ministry of Education, and Grant No. 55-5 from the Japanese Ministry of Health and Welfare.

References

Arcangelli, G., Barni, E., Cividallou, A., Mauro, F., Spano, M., and Tabocchini, A. (1980). Effectiveness of microwave hyperthermia combined with ionizing irradiation: clinical results on neck node metastases. *Int. J. Radiat. Oncol. Biol. Phys.* **6,** 143–148.

Balasubramanian, T. A., and Bowman, H. F. (1974). Temperature field due to a time dependent heat source of spherical geometry in an infinite medium. *J. Heat Transfer, Trans ASME* **96,** 296–299.

Balasubramanian, T. A., and Bowman, H. F. (1977). Thermal conductivity and thermal diffusivity of biomaterials: a simultaneous measurement technique. *J. Biomech. Eng., Trans ASME* **99** (Series K, No. 3), 148–154.

Bicher, H. I., Sandhu, T. S., and Hetzel, F. W. (1980). Hyperthermia and radiation in combination. *Int. J. Radiat. Oncol. Biol. Phys.* **6,** 867–870.

Bowman, H. F. (1980). The bioheat transfer equation and discrimination of thermally significant vessels. *Ann. N.Y. Acad. Sci.* **335,** 155–160.

Bowman, R. R. (1976). A probe for measuring temperature in radio-frequency-heated material. *IEEE Trans. Microwave Theory Tech.* **24,** 43–45.

Cetas, T. C. (1981). The philosophy and use of tissue-equivalent electromagnetic phantom. *In* Textbook of AAPM Summer School on "Physical Aspects of Hyperthermia" (C. Streffer *et al.,* eds), pp. 1–14. Urban & Schwarzenberg, Balitmore and Munich.

Cetas, T. C., and Connor, W. G. (1978). Thermometry considerations in localized hyperthermia. *Med. Phys.* **5,** 79–91.

Cetas, T. C., Connor, W. G., and Boone, M. L. M. (1978). Thermal dosimetry: some biological consideration. *In* "Cancer Therapy by Hyperthermia and Radiation" (D. von Beuninger, F. Dretzel, E. Röttinger, J. E. Robinson, E. Scherer, S. Seeber, and K.-R. Trott, eds.), pp. 3–12. Urban & Schwarzenberg, Baltimore and Munich.

Chen, M. M., and Holmes, K. R. (1980). Microvascular contributions in tissue heat transfer. *Ann. N.Y. Acad. Sci.* **335,** 137–150.

Christensen, D. A. (1977). A probe for measuring temperature in radiofrequency-heated material. *IEEE Trans. Microwave Theory Tech.* **24,** 43–45.

Christensen, D. A. (1979). Thermal dosimetry and temperature measurement. *Cancer Res.* **39,** 2325–2327.

Connor, W. G., Gerner, E. W., Miller, R. C., and Boone, M. L. M. (1977). Prospects for hyperthermia in human cancer therapy. *Radiology (Easton, Pa.)* **123,** 497–503.

Crile, G., Jr. (1963). The effects of heat and radiation on cancers implanted on the feet of mice. *Cancer Res.* **23**, 372–380.

Dewey, W. C., Hopwood, L. E., Sapareto, S. A., and Gerweck, L. E. (1977). Cellular responses to combinations of hyperthermia and radiation. *Radiology* (*Easton, Pa.*) **123**, 463–474.

Dickson, J. A., and Shah, S. A. (1977). Technology for the hyperthermic treatment of large solid tumors at 50°C. *Clin. Oncol.* **3**, 301–318.

Dickson, J. A., Shah, S. A., Waggot, D., and Whalley, W. B. (1977). Tumor eradication in the rabbit by radiofrequency heating. *Cancer Res.* **37**, 2162–2169.

Eno, K., Kato, H., Nishida, T., Kano, E., Sugahara, T., Tanaka, H., and Ishida, T. (1981). Physical basis of RF hyperthermia for cancer therapy III. A nonperturbed and nonperturbing thermometer at RF heating. *J. Radiat. Res.* **22**, 265–273.

Gerweck, L. E., Gillette, E. L., and Dewey, W. C. (1975). Effect of heat and radiation on synchronous Chinese Hamster cells: killing and repair. *Radiat. Res.* **64**, 611–623.

Guy, A. W. (1971). Analyses of electromagnetic fields induced in biological tissues by thermographic studies on equivalent phantom models. *IEEE Trans. Microwave Theory Tech.* **19**, 205–214.

Guy, A. W., Lehmann, J. F., and Stonebridge, J. B. (1974). Therapeutic applications of electromagnetic power. *Proc. IEEE.* **62**, 55–75.

Hahn, E. W., and Kim, J. H. (1980). Clinical observations on the selective heating of cutaneous tumors with the radio-frequency inductive method. *Ann. N.Y. Acad. Sci.* **335**, 347–351.

Hand, J. W., and Haar, G. (1981). Heating techniques in hyperthermia. *Br. J. Radiol.* **54**, 443–466.

Henle, K. J., and Dethlefsen, L. A. (1980). Time-temperature relationships for heat induced killing of mammalian cells. *Ann. N.Y. Acad. Sci.* **335**, 234–252.

Ishida, T., and Kato, H. (1980). Muscle equivalent agar phantom for 13.56 MHz RF-induced hyperthermia. *Shimane J. Med. Sci.* **4**, 134–140.

Jain, R. K. (1980). Temperature distributions in normal and neoplastic tissues during normothermia and hyperthermia. *Ann. N.Y. Acad. Sci.* **335**, 48–64.

Johnson, C. C., and Guy, A. W. (1972). Nonionizing electromagnetic wave effect in the biological materials and systems. *Proc. IEEE.* **60**, 692–718.

Johnson, S. A., Greenleaf, J. F., Samayoa, W. A., Duck, F. A., and Sjostand, J. (1975). Reconstruction of three-dimensional velocity fields and other parameters by acoustic ray tracing. *Ultrasonic Symp. Proc. 1975,* CHO 994–945 (IEEE Catalog No. 75).

Kim, J. H., Hahn, E. W., and Tokita, N. (1978). Combination hyperthermia and radiation therapy for cutaneous malignant melanoma. *Cancer* (*Philadelphia*) **41**, 2143–2148.

Kim, S. H., Kim, J. H., and Hahn, E. W. (1975). The radiosensitization of hypoxic tumor cells by hyperthermia. *Radiology* (*Easton, Pa.*) **114**, 727–728.

Kim, S. H., Kim, J. H., and Hahn, E. W. (1976). The enhanced killing of irradiated Hela cells in synchronous culture by hyperthermia. *Radiat. Res.* **66**, 337–345.

Larsen, L. E., Moore, R. A., and Acevedo, J. (1974). A microwave decoupled brain temperature transducer. *IEEE Trans. Microwave Theory Tech.* **22**, 438–444.

LeVeen, H. H., Wapnick, S., Piccone, V., Falk, G., and Ahmed, N. (1976). Tumor eradication by radiofrequency therapy, response in 21 patients. *JAMA J. Am. Med. Assoc.* **235**, 2198–2200.

LeVeen, H. H., Ahmed, N., Piccone, V. A., Sugaar, S., and Falk, G. (1980). Radiofrequency therapy: clinical experience. *Ann. N.Y. Acad. Sci.* **335**, 362–371.

Luk, K. H., Purser, P. R., Castro, J. R., Meyler, T. S., and Phillips, T. L. (1981). Clinical experiences with local microwave hyperthermia. *Int. J. Radiat. Oncol. Biol. Phys.* **7,** 615–619.

Manning, M. R., Cetas, T. C., Miller, R. C., Oleson, J. R., Connor, W. G., and Gerner, E. W. (1982). Clinical hyperthermia: results of a phase 1 trial employing hyperthermia alone or in combination with external beam or interstitial radiotherapy. *Cancer (Philadelphia)* **49,** 205–216.

Overgaard, J. (1981). Effect of hyperthermia on the hypoxic fraction in an experimental mammary carcinoma *in vivo. Br. J. Radiol.* **54,** 245–249.

Overgaard, J., and Bichel, P. (1977). The influence of hypoxia and acidity on the hyperthermic response of malignant cells in vitro. *Radiology (Easton, Pa.)* **123,** 511–514.

Sachs, T. D., and Tanney, C. S. (1977). A two-beam acoustic system for tissue analysis. *Phys. Med. Biol.* **22,** 327–340.

Sandhu, T. S. (1982). Thermal dosimetry system with blood flow simulation. *Natl. Cancer Inst. Monogr.* **61,** 513–515.

Sapareto, S. A., and Dewey, W. C. (1982). Thermal dose determination in cancer therapy. *Annu. Meet. Hyperthermia Group 2nd,* p. 27.

Song, C. W., Kang, M. S., Rhee, J. G., and Levitt, S. H. (1980). Effect of hyperthermia on vascular function in normal and neoplastic tissues. *Ann. N.Y. Acad. Sci.* **335,** 35–43.

Storm, F. K., Harrison, W. H., Elliott, R. S., Hazitheofilou, C., and Morton, D. L. (1979a). Human hyperthermia therapy: relation between tumor type and capacity to induce hyperthermia by radiofrequency. *Am. J. Surg.* **138,** 170–174.

Storm, F. K., Harrison, W. H., Elliott, R. S., and Morton, D. L. (1979b). Normal tissue and solid tumor effects of hyperthermia in animal models and clinical trials. *Cancer Res.* **39,** 2245–2251.

Storm, F. K., Harrison, W. H., Elliot, R. S., and Morton, D. L. (1980). Hyperthermic therapy for human neoplasms: thermal death time. *Cancer (Philadelphia)* **46,** 1849–1854.

Sugaar, S., and LeVeen, H. H. (1979). A histopathological study on the effect of radiofrequency. *Cancer (Philadephia)* **43,** 767–783.

Suit, H. D. (1977). Hyperthermic effects on animal tissues. *Radiology (Easton, Pa.)* **123,** 483–487.

U, R., Noell, K. T., Woodward, K. T., Worde, B. T., Fishburn, R. T., and Miller, L. S. (1980). Microwave-induced local hyperthermia in combination with radiotherapy of human malignant tumors. *Cancer (Philadelphia)* **45,** 638–646.

22 Radiothermotherapy in the Management of Refractory Malignant Neoplasms: Radiobiological Rationale, Technique, and Results

Raymond U
Boyd T. Worde

Department of Radiology
Duke University and
V.A. Medical Centers
Durham, North Carolina

I. Introduction

The current experimental strategy for improved management of refractory cancer includes developing effective treatment against relatively ra-

Modification of Radiosensitivity in Cancer Treatment

415

dioresistant hypoxic tumor cells having poor accessibility to chemotherapeutic agents, reducing variation of cell cycle-specific drug susceptibility or radiosensitivity, inhibiting repair of sublethal damage (SLD) and potentially lethal damage (PLD) of tumor cells after treatment with radiation or chemotherapeutic agents, and diverse fractionation techniques, along with increasing normal tissue tolerance to radiation therapy or chemotherapy.

Another development is the interest in hyperthermia for cancer therapy, either by itself or in combination with radiation or other therapeutic modalities. This prospect is based on considerable biological and increasing clinical evidence.

Rationale for hyperthermia in cancer therapy is as follows:

1. The log of cell survival, as a function of exposure time to moderate levels of heat, resembles X-ray dose–response cell survival curves, and at temperatures above 43°C, there is a 50% reduction factor in the heating time, to a given cell survival level for each degree of increased temperature, although heat sensitivity of different mammalian cell lines varies to a greater extent than expected with X irradiation (Westra and Dewey, 1971; Dewey *et al.*, 1977). Thus quantitative relationships of heat exposure to cellular response are predictable.

2. Malignant tumors are more vulnerable to destruction by heat than are the surrounding normal tissues (Crile, 1961; Cavaliere *et al.*, 1967; Chen and Heidelberger, 1969; Turans *et al.*, 1970; Kase and Hahn, 1975; Hoffer *et al.*, 1976; Rossi-Fanelli *et al.*, 1977). This selective difference in heat sensitivity has been attributed to tumor microenvironmental conditions such as hypoxia (Gerweck *et al.*, 1974, 1979; Kim *et al.*, 1975; Bass *et al.*, 1978; Dewhirst *et al.*, 1980), low pH (Ashby, 1966; Overgaard, 1976a; Bichel and Overgaard, 1977; Gerweck, 1977; Overgaard and Bichel, 1977; Meyer *et al.*, 1979; von Ardenne and Reitnauer, 1980; Li *et al.*, 1980; Freeman *et al.*, 1981), and nutritional deficiencies (Hahn, 1974; Li *et al.*, 1980). Also the tumor vascular beds appear to be far more sensitive to a heat-induced destructive effect than are the vascular beds in surrounding normal tissues (von Ardenne, 1978; Song, 1978; Endrich *et al.*, 1979; Vaupel, 1979; Eddy, 1980; Emami *et al.*, 1980; Dickson and Calderwood, 1980; Song *et al.*, 1980). In addition, many tumors selectively absorb more heat than normal tissues because their neovascularity is physiologically inefficient to handle thermal stress and is incapable of regulating and augmenting blood perfusion (LeVeen *et al.*, 1976; Storm *et al.*, 1979; Emami *et al.*, 1980; Dickson and Calderwood, 1980; Bicher *et al.*, 1980b).

3. Cells in mid- to late S phase, which are usually radiation resistant, are most sensitive to heat, and the differences in radiosensitivity among

cells at various stages in the cell cycle are minimized by heat (Westra and Dewey, 1971; Palzer and Heidelberger, 1973, 1974; Schulman and Hall, 1974; Gerweck et al., 1975; Kim et al., 1976; Dewey et al., 1977; Bhuyan et al., 1977; Gerner et al., 1979).

4. Hyperthermia enhances ionizing radiation damage (Selawry et al., 1958; Belli and Bonte, 1963; Crile, 1963; Ben-Hur and Elkind, 1974; Ben-Hur et al., 1974, 1978; Robinson et al., 1974; Gerweck et al., 1975; Braun and Hahn, 1975; Thrall et al., 1975; Yerushalmi, 1975; Harris et al., 1976, 1977; Li et al., 1976; Dewey et al., 1977, 1979; Harisiadis et al., 1977; Stewart and Denekamp, 1978; Witcofski and Kremkau, 1978; Bichel et al., 1979; Field et al., 1979; Gillette, 1979; Suit and Gerweck, 1979), and inhibits the repair of SLD and PLD. Heat also accentuates the effects of selected antitumor drugs (Shingleton et al., 1962; Suzuki, 1967; Hahn et al., 1975, 1977; Hahn and Strande, 1976; Bhuyan et al., 1976; Overgaard, 1976b; Giovanella et al., 1977; Goss and Parsons, 1977; Bleecheu et al., 1977, 1978; Hahn, 1978, 1979; Twentyman et al., 1978; Yatvin et al., 1978; Herman et al., 1979; Marmor, 1979; Bhuyan, 1979; Kowal and Bertino, 1979; Goldfeder et al., 1979; Arcangeli et al., 1979; Magin et al., 1979; Weinstein et al., 1979; Meyn et al., 1980; Hones et al., 1980; Nakamura and Nakayama-Sato, 1981).

5. Early clinical investigations on malignant tumors using moderate doses of repeated hyperthermia, either alone or with radiation therapy or other therapeutic modalities, have shown encouraging results, and complications involving normal tissue are not enhanced (Pettigrew et al., 1974; Stehlin et al., 1975; Hornback et al., 1977, 1979; Kim et al., 1977, 1978, 1982; Mendecki et al., 1978; Steinhagen et al., 1978; Arcangeli et al., 1979; Caldwell, 1979; Larkin, 1979; Bull et al., 1979; Marmor et al., 1979; Parks et al., 1979; Abe et al., 1980; Bicher et al., 1980a; Holt, 1980; LeVeen et al., 1980; Luk et al., 1980; Marmor and Hahn, 1980; Stehlin, 1980; Storm et al., 1980; U et al., 1980; Bicher, 1981; Hiraoka and Abe, 1981; Joseph et al., 1981; Overgaard, 1981; Perez et al., 1981; Baker et al., 1982; Manning et al., 1982). With regional or localized hyperthermia and a cautious approach, side effects can be diminished. Untoward events are seldom serious despite the early stages of development of thermotherapy techniques and equipment.

In 1976 we began clinical investigations using microwave-induced localized hyperthermia and ionizing radiation to evaluate the safety and biological response of normal tissue as well as the regression of refractory malignant tumors. Of further interest are the obvious needs for identifying directions for improved thermotherapy equipment and techniques. Summarized in this chapter are the results of 63 individual treatment sites in 50 patients.

II. Materials and Methods

A. Patient Selection and Tumor Histologies

In patients with biopsy-confirmed and locally accessible refractory malignant tumors, external beam radiation therapy followed by 915-MHz (two cases) and 2450-MHz (all other cases) microwave-induced localized hyperthermia was prescribed for selected patients, with a life expectancy of at least 2 months, meeting some or all of the following criteria:

1. Tumors were medically or technically inoperable, or recommended surgery was refused by patient.
2. Disease was known to be resistant to radiation.
3. Applicability of conventional radiation therapy was limited because of tumor recurrence in a previously irradiated volume.
4. Chemotherapeutic and/or immunotherapeutic options were exhausted.

Patients in this trial have had malignant melanoma, adenocarcinoma of the breast, squamous cell carcinoma, plasmacytoma, epithelioid sarcoma, undifferentiated carcinoma, and other types of malignancy.

B. Informed Consent

This investigation was conducted with the approval of the Duke University Medical Center Committee for Clinical Investigations or the U.S. Veterans Administration Medical Center Research and Development Committee and Human Studies Subcommittee. Informed consent meeting the criteria of this governing body was obtained from each patient.

C. Ionizing Radiation Sources and Techniques

Ionizing radiation sources were ^{60}Co, 280 kVp, 4- to 20-MeV linear accelerators. Calibration, collimation, and beam-blocking techniques were those used routinely in conventional radiation therapy.

D. Heating Methods

Air-filled microwave guides of 12 × 12 × 12 cm or 16 × 14 × 12 cm size were used with further shaping and reduction of the hyperthermia field size, according to need, by applying lightly padded aluminum tape, an effective microwave insulator. Both of the microwave applicators used had an input capacity of 100 W. A RAHAM radiation hazard meter (General Microwave Corporation, Model 2) was utilized to detect excessive microwave leakage beyond the immediate heating area.

E. Thermometry

Temperature measurements were performed using 22-gauge YSI needle-type thermistors via digital thermometers in our initial trials, and for all later cases, we used a very fine-gauge Teflon-coated copper constantan thermocouple probe via Clinical Thermometer TM-10 (Bailey Co.) digital monitoring system. Thermocouple sensors were placed through 18- to 21-gauge catheters and the metallic needle withdrawn with the tip of the sensor remaining in the desired spot throughout heat measurements. These temperature sensors were frequently calibrated both before and after a hyperthermia session against a mercury thermometer traceable to the National Bureau of Standards, accurate to 0.1°C. The mains leading to the thermometer digital system included low-pass filters to minimize RF interference. Temperatures were recorded every 15–30 sec from the start of heating until steady-state hyperthermic temperatures were attained, then every 1–5 min throughout each hyperthermia session. Precautions to minimize microwave interference included implanting the temperature-sensing probes perpendicular to the microwave field and interrupting the microwave power for a few seconds to sample temperatures; during this interval, recorded digital temperatures declined only 0.1–0.2°C. Temperature within the heating field of both tumors and adjoining tissues was monitored by multiple sensors.

Lidocaine (1%) anesthesia was used at the catheter insertion puncture sites only. No other anesthesia or analgesia was required. With invasive thermometry, more than three or four sites within the heating field were not practical.

F. Radiothermotherapy Techniques

Fractionated doses of hyperthermia combined with ionizing radiation treatment were administered according to the following schedule: Usually 3 Gy photon or electron beam irradiation was immediately followed by 45 min of hyperthermia at 42 to 43.5°C for a total of 6 to 10 combined treatments, consisting of 2 to 3 treatments/week (Monday, Wednesday, and Friday or Monday and Thursday) over a maximum of 21 days.

G. Pretreatment Evaluation and Criteria of Response

Each tumor selected for inclusion in this trial was measured in millimeters in two diameters—where possible, three—using Vernier calipers, and depth of the tumor was estimated. Photographic and written evaluations were instituted to document initial clinical examinations and the subsequent treatment responses and side effects. Tumor response was graded as complete (CR) or partial (PR). Complete regression was defined as clinical disappearance of palpable tumor; partial regression signifies 50% or more decrease in tumor volume, and no response (NR) signifies less than a 50% decrease in tumor volume.

III. Results

A. Summary of the Treatment Parameters and Anatomical Sites

Table I summarizes the treatment parameters for our clinical study involving radiation therapy in combination with hyperthermia. Although the total radiation dose used and the number of fractions employed among other factors were in a wide range, the majority of treatment was based on the following modes: Ionizing radiation doses were 30 Gy delivered in 10 fractions over 21 elapsed days, and the TDF factors were 57. Each hyperthermia session consisted of 42.0 to 43.5°C (± 0.5) for 45 min immediately

TABLE I

Summary of Treatment Parameters:
Radiation Therapy and Hyperthermia

Treatment parameter	Range	Mode
Radiation dose (Gy)	18–48	30
Fractions	5–20	10
No. of days of treatment	2–28	21
TDF[a]	30–124	57
Hyperthermia sessions[b]	2–10	10
Follow-up duration (months)	1–34	3

[a] Time dose fractionation (TDF): Taken from tables of Orton (1972).

[b] Hyperthermia session: 42.0–43.5°C for 45 min each session.

following radiation therapy, and the duration of follow-up was from 1 month to 32 months, with an average of 3 months.

Anatomical sites of the treatment included chest wall, abdomen, shoulder, flank, leg, thigh (calf, popliteal fossa), arm, palm, foot, external genitalia, and in the head and neck region.

B. Thermometry—Tumor and Normal Tissues

Five to ten minutes of microwave irradiation, while adjusting the energy requirement and fine alignment of waveguide angles to reduce temperature variations within the tumor target, were needed to achieve the desired tumor temperature levels. Another technique was scanning of the catheter tube in the target tissues by moving only thermocouple positions. In addition, patients were often able to describe a feeling of unevenness of the heating pattern and the presence of hot spots, thus enabling adjustment of waveguide angles or position to achieve improved heating while using a minimum of only two or three temperature-sensing probes (i.e., tumor and normal tissues).

Steady-state tumor–normal tissue temperature differences were noted with tumor temperature 1–5°C above that of normal tissue without cooling. This selective tumor heating has been attributed to inefficient heat dissipation capacity in many tumors because of the neovascularity relative to surrounding normal tissues (LeVeen *et al.*, 1976; Storm *et al.*, 1979; Bicher *et al.*, 1980b; Emami *et al.*, 1980; Dickson and Calderwood, 1980).

In general, the first several heating sessions were most difficult to conduct with each new patient. This is because incident energy requirement to achieve desired levels of hyperthermia has to be determined in each case, according to tumor size, density, bio-heat transfer factor, and the possible influence of anatomical location.

C. Tumor Response

Table II summarizes the response of refractory tumors to radiation therapy in combination with hyperthermia. Of the 63 evaluated lesions in 50 patients, the histological types consisted of 32 malignant melanoma (51%), 10 adenocarcinoma of the breast (16%), 6 squamous cell carcinoma (9%), and 15 other types of neoplasms (24%), which comprised plasmacytoma, liposarcoma, epithelioid sarcoma, undifferentiated carcinoma, basal cell carcinoma, and chondrosarcoma. Tumor sizes varied from less than 5-mm pellets under the skin to larger than $100 \times 100 \times 100$ mm

TABLE II

Response of Refractory Malignant Tumors to Radiation Therapy and Hyperthermia

Tumor types	No. of points	No. of sites	Response			
			CR	PR	NR	CR + PR
Melanoma	28	32	20 (62.5%)	2 (6.2%)	10 (31.2%)	22 (68.7%)
Adenocarcinoma of breast	9	10	7 (70.0%)	3 (30.0%)	—	10 (100.0%)
Squamous cell carcinoma	4	6	5 (83.3%)	—	1 (16.7%)	5 (83.3%)
Other types	9	15	11 (73.3%)	2 (13.3%)	2 (13.3%)	13 (86.7%)
	50	63	43 (68.2%)	7 (11.1%)	13 (20.6%)	50 (79.4%)

masses with an average of 20- to 60-mm^2 sizes. All tumors were either cutaneous or subcutaneous, involving various anatomical locations; however, the majority were in the head and neck regions. The current overall complete response rate was over 68% without concomitant increase in normal tissue complications.

D. Radiosensitization by Hyperthermia

The present updated analysis includes in part our early pilot study data reported in 1980 (U et al., 1980). Nine patients were selected to study the effectiveness of low-dose radiation combined with hyperthermia. Multiple metastatic superficial tumors (20–40 mm in diameter and less than 30 mm deep) involving the patient's own tumors served as the controls. The results showed that seven of nine achieved CR (77.7%) with the two combined treatments, and there was no evidence of toxicity to the normal tissue. However, the response of similarly sized lesions treated with hyperthermia alone was limited, without a single CR and only three PR of seven lesions (43%), whereas the low-dose radiation treatment alone produced one CR and four PR of nine (CR 11%; PR 44%). The follow-up at this writing is 1–7 months. A much longer follow-up is obviously required.

E. Tolerance and Normal Tissue Reaction

The treatment did not have to be discontinued in any patient as a result of hyperthermia-related discomfort. In general, locally induced hyperthermia at moderate levels of elevated temperatures up to 44°C was tolerated well. Some patients complained of localized but bearable discomfort, slight aching sometimes associated with tingling sensations, or some pressure in the treated area—all of which usually disappeared immediately on cessation of microwave application. Once routine procedures were established, patients often fell asleep during subsequent hyperthermia sessions.

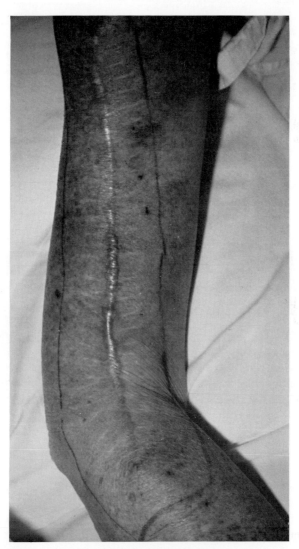

Fig. 1. Appearance of skin reaction immediately following 43.5°C thermotherapy for 45 min on the surface of the arm.

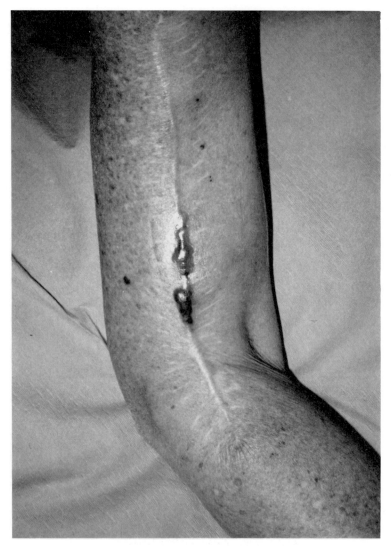

Fig. 2. Example showing the presence of blisters along the ridges of surgical wound scar. Photo taken 48 h following the first thermotherapy session (Fig. 1).

Blisters formed in 12 of 63 sites over 600 hyperthermia sessions (2%), with rapid healing vesicles in 8 and full-thickness skin loss in 4. These blisters seemed to be caused by hot spots and did not correspond to the shape of the field of treatment.

In patients who completed treatment, we assessed the normal tissue (skin) reaction in both hyperthermia alone or combined with radiation

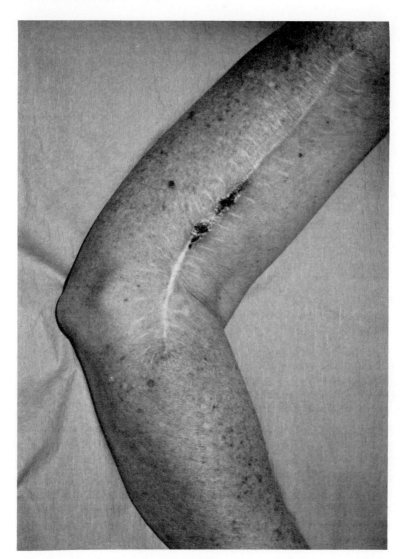

Fig. 3. Example of the prompt healing without special care. Photo taken 1 week following the first thermotherapy session (Figs. 1 and 2).

therapy. The responses were virtually the same in case of a short transient period of erythema. On rare occasions, the radiothermotherapy response of the skin took the form of modest desquamation and residual erythema that lasted 2–3 weeks.

Figure 1 illustrates appearance of the skin reaction immediately following 43.5°C thermotherapy for 45 min, on the surface of the arm with a long surgical scar. The relatively similar erythematous skin reaction of the entire treatment field shows the uniformity of heating. Figure 2 shows a good example of selective heat absorption in the neovascular scar. This could be due to a poor dissipation of heat in such tissues relative to the well-vascularized surrounding tissue (photo taken 48 h following the first thermotherapy session). Figure 3 shows the healing of blisters, within 1 week.

Therefore, caution is advised when including scar tissue in the field exposed to hyperthermia.

IV. Case Report

A 73-year-old white male presented on January 19, 1981 with a firm, nontender mass measuring 50 × 50 × 20 mm in the left parotid region. This was diagnosed as recurrent metastatic malignant melanoma. He was sent to us for consideration for radiothermotherapy, according to protocol. He had undergone a left superficial parotidectomy in March 1980. Surgical incisional biopsy on January 12, 1981 revealed a metastatic undifferentiated tumor consistent with malignant melanoma. He had already received immunotherapy and later chemotherapy but with limited improvement.

Figure 4 is a photo taken before the initiation of 10 sessions of radiothermotherapy (January 21, 1981). His eyes, ear, and normal tissue outside the intended heating field were protected by insulated aluminum tape covered with thin cheesecloth. Thermocouple temperature-sensing wires were inserted into the tumor and adjacent tissue before placing the microwave heating applicator on top of the field. As with all other cases in this investigation, measurement of temperature both in the tumor and adjacent tissue was repeated in each of the 10 thermotherapy sessions.

Tumor and normal tissue temperature data depicting the average basal temperature, maximum temperature, and average treatment temperature range of the 10 thermotherapy sessions are as follows:

Tissue	Basal temperature range (°C)	Maximum temperature (°C)	Treatment temperature[a] range (°C)
Tumor	36.2–36.8	43.6	42.9–43.6
Normal	35.0–36.6	42.2	38.6–42.2

[a] Temperature maintained for 45 min/session, repeated 10 times over 19 days.

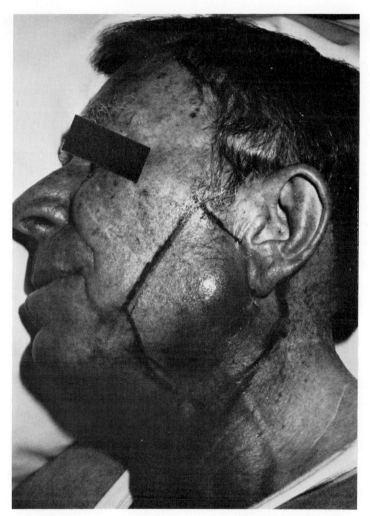

Fig. 4. Recurrent malignant melanoma to the left parotid region, before treatment (Section IV, Case Report).

A single left lateral 7.5 × 9.0 cm field was used under the 10-MeV electron beam at 95 cm source-to-skin distance. A total dose of 30 Gy was given in 10 sessions over 19 days. Each electron beam radiation therapy session was promptly followed by thermotherapy at a temperature of 42.9 to 43.6°C, which was maintained for 45 min/session.

On the fifth day of the treatment, the tumor mass measured 45 × 35 × 15 mm, and at the completion it measured 45 × 25 × 15 mm. The patient

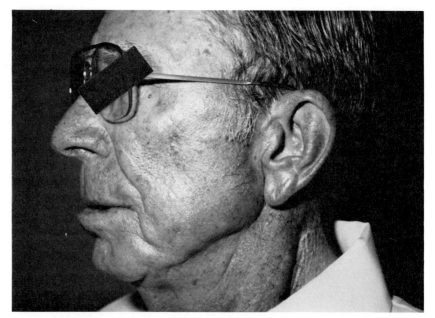

Fig. 5. Same patient as in Fig. 4, photograph taken at 7-month posttreatment follow-up.

tolerated the scheduled treatment well, and only a modest degree of desquamation and erythema occurred. At 2 weeks posttreatment follow-up, the size of the mass was unchanged. However, at the 2-month interval follow-up, the mass was reduced to about 3 × 13 × 10 mm in maximum perpendicular diameters in the sagittal plane. The 4-month follow-up examination showed complete resolution of the residual tumor. Thus, complete response to thermoradiotherapy was noted with no adverse normal tissue complication. The photo in Figure 5 was taken September 30, 1981 (at the 7-month posttreatment follow-up). Recurrence in the site of treatment and adverse tissue effects in the treated area were nil. The patient has a follow-up record of over 15 months postthermoradiotherapy with no sign of recurrence, and the irradiated skin is in excellent condition.

In most instances, complete regression of the tumor mass following thermoradiotherapy was noted at the time of treatment completion, or at most, within a 3- to 4-week period. The slow resolution of the residual tumor mass seen in this patient was an exception. This signifies that the tumor response criteria in terms of size reduction alone within a couple of months may lead to an inaccurate assessment.

V. Discussion

The results of this clinical investigation demonstrate that localized thermotherapy alone or thermoradiotherapy is generally safe, and normal tissue tolerance is excellent provided that the tissue temperatures are carefully monitored and controlled. It also shows that results of heat combined with low doses of radiation for the treatment of malignant tumors are superior to separate applications. Instances of blisters in normal tissues are likely due to technical difficulties in temperature measurements of multiple points in a larger heating field, when local temperatures are at moderate levels. The few and seldom serious complications in normal tissue are gratifying when considering the prototype heating and temperature-measuring system used. These observations reinforce the idea of a potential therapeutic benefit and radiation-sensitizing effects of radiothermotherapy against refractory tumors, without concomitant increase in normal tissue complications.

Further investigation and a longer follow-up of diverse anatomical sites are required to establish optimal forms of thermotherapy and/or radiothermotherapy in the management of refractory neoplasms. Accumulating evidence from an ever-increasing number of clinical hyperthermia trials confirms the prospect of such a therapeutic approach, either alone or combined with other tumor therapeutic methods.

Many of the reported tumor–normal tissue responses to hyperthermia are difficult to compare because the heating–thermometry systems and/or techniques are different. Also a uniform quality assurance system is only now being developed. Other technical problems are accuracy and reliability of reproducing temperature distribution, temperature energy requirements versus time and relationships per given quantity of target tissues at different locations.

As practiced in radiation oncology and chemotherapy, the optimal forms of applying hyperthermia may also be utilized in multifractionation regimens. Thus the question of biological and physiological factors arises, as related to thermotolerance (thermal resistance phenomena) in the target tissues. Are the levels of thermotolerance different in tumor and normal tissues? Is it possible to observe such thermotolerance phenomena in relatively large tumors, in that microenvironmental conditions and the intrinsic anatomical and functional differences in tumors and normal tissues *in vivo* may significantly alter heat response patterns? Can the fractionation schedules that may selectively protect the normal tissue with differential thermotolerance factors be manipulated between target tissues?

With such a potential of therapeutic gain with the proper use of heat, much additional research remains to be conducted.

An improved hyperthermia delivery system for advanced clinical trials is being prepared.

Meanwhile, some of the available heating systems are acceptable, but there is room for improvement. Instituting further research with superficial tumor target tissues should facilitate determination of the requirements and practical feasibility of time–temperature relationships for optimal treatment.

Radiothermotherapy may well become the treatment of choice for neoplastic disease. Heat alone or in combination with radiation or chemotherapy should be effective for selective tumors that are either radioresistant or that respond poorly to other modalities. For selected cases a localized radiation field boost may be utilized. This alternative may increase the effect of the boost dose and decrease the morbidity.

VI. Summary

Resurging interest in hyperthermia for cancer therapy is based on considerable thermobiological and increasing clinical evidence that tumors are more vulnerable than normal tissue to heat. Since 1976, 63 assessable lesions in 50 patients with advanced, locally accessible refractory superficial tumors were treated with radiation and hyperthermia to assess the safety and biological response of normal tissue as well as the regression of refractory malignant tumors. Of further interest in this investigation is the obvious need for identifying directions for an improved thermotherapy delivery system and optimal techniques.

Although the total radiation dose used and the number of fractions utilized, among other factors, were in a wide range, most treatments involved a 3-Gy tumor dose three times weekly for 10 treatments. Each hyperthermia session consisted of 42 to 44°C for 45 min immediately after each radiation treatment. The duration of follow-up averaged 3 months. Temperature measurements both in the tumor and in adjacent normal tissue were repeated in each of 10 hyperthermia sessions. Each thermotherapy summary record included the basal temperature prior to the hyperthermia sessions, maximum temperature during treatment, treatment temperature range, and duration. Temperature within the heating field was monitored by multiple sensors (26-gauge Teflon-coated copper constantan thermocouples) inserted into the 18-gauge catheter tube, which had already been inserted into target tissues. Temperature distribution profiles were checked by scanning 1- to 2-cm track lengths from the tip inside of the catheter tube by moving only the thermocouple. The tumor histologies consisted of malignant melanoma, adenocarcinoma of the breast, squamous cell carcinoma, and other types. The total response rate for thermoradiotherapy was 43 complete regressions (CR) and 7 partial regressions (PR) of 63 (CR 68%; PR 11%). Normal tissue toxicity has been minimal. Twelve instances of blisters over 600 hyperthermia sessions (2%) were noted.

Another type of study was done to determine whether the effectiveness of irradiating tumors was enhanced by the use of hyperthermia, as compared with the similarly matched nodules exposed to the same doses with either heat or radiation alone. There were 17 additional assessable lesions in this study that involved 9 of the previously mentioned 50 patients studied. Multiple metastatic superficial tumors involving the patient's own tumor served as the control. Response from the two combined treatments showed 7 CR of 9 (77.7%). However, response of similarly sized lesions in the same patients with heat alone showed no CR and 3 PR of 7 (42%), whereas the radiation treatment-alone group responses were 1 CR and 4 PR of 9 (CR 11%; PR 44%).

The potentially significant impact on clinical cancer therapy, whether of curative or palliative intent, by moderate thermotherapy or thermoradiotherapy is evident. Technical advances to optimize such therapeutic approaches including delivery of a known localized quantity of heat to tumors in various locations in the body are expected to be rapid.

References

Abe, M., Hiraoka, M., Takahashi, M., Ono, K., and Nohara, H. (1980). Clinical experience with microwave and radio frequency thermotherapy in the treatment of advanced cancer. *Proc. Int. Symp. Cancer Ther. Hyperthermia Drugs Radiat. 3rd,* Abstr. No. tT–III–1, p. 116.

Arcangeli, G., Cividalli, A., Mauro, F., Nervi, C., and Pavin, G. (1979). Enhanced effectiveness of adriamycin and bleomycin combined with local hyperthermia in neck node metastases from head and neck cancers. *Tumori* **65,** 481–486.

Ashby, B. S. (1966). pH studies in human malignant tumors. *Lancet* **2,** 312–315.

Baker, H. W., Snedecor, P. A., Goss, J. C., Galen, W. P., Gallucci, J. J., Horowitz, I. J., and Dugan, K. (1982). Regional hyperthermia for cancer. *Am. J. Surg.* **143,** 586–590.

Bass, H., Moore, J. L., and Coakley, W. T. (1978). Lethality in mammalian cells due to hyperthermia under oxic and hypoxic conditions. *Int. J. Radiat. Biol.* **33,** 57–67.

Belli, J. A., and Bonte, F. J. (1963). Influence of temperature on the radiation response of mammalian cells in tissue culture. *Radiat. Res.* **18,** 272–276.

Ben-Hur, E., and Elkind, M. M. (1974). Thermally enhanced radioresponse of cultured Chinese hamster cells. Damage and repair of single stranded DNA and a DNA complex. *Radiat. Res.* **59,** 484–495.

Ben-Hur, E., Elkind, M. M., and Bronk, B. V. (1974). Thermally enhanced radioresponse of cultured Chinese hamster cells. Inhibition of sublethal damage and enhancement of lethal damage. *Radiat. Res.* **58**, 38–51.

Ben-Hur, E., Elkind, M. M., and Riklis, E. (1978). The combined effects of hyperthermia and radiation in cultured mammalian cells. *In* "Cancer Therapy by Hyperthermia and Radiation" (C. Streffer, D. von Beuningen, F. Dretzel, E. Röttinger, J. E. Robinson, E. Scherer, S. Seeber, and K.-R. Trott, eds.), pp. 29–36. Urban & Schwarzenberg, Baltimore, Maryland.

Bhuyan, B. K. (1979). Kinetics of cell kill by hyperthermia. *Cancer Res.* **39**, 2277–2284.

Bhuyan, B. K., Loughman, B. E., Fraser, T. J., and Day, K. J. (1976). Comparison of different methods of determining cell viability after exposure to cytotoxic compounds. *Exp. Cell Res.* **97**, 275–280.

Bhuyan, B. K., Day, K. J., Edgerton, C. E., and Ogunbase, O. (1977). Sensitivity of different cell lines and of different phases in the cell cycle to hyperthermia. *Cancer Res.* **37**, 3780–3784.

Bichel, P., and Overgaard, J. (1977). Hyperthermic effect on exponential and plateau ascites tumor cells *in vitro* dependent on environmental pH. *Radiat. Res.* **70**, 449–454.

Bichel, P., Overgaard, J., and Nielsen, O. S. (1979). Synergistic cell cycle kinetic effect of low doses of hyperthermia and radiation on tumour cells. *Eur. J. Cancer* **15**, 1191–1196.

Bicher, H. I. (1981). Hyperthermia: clinical results and physiological mechanisms of action. "IAEA Seminar, Prospective Methods of Radiation Therapy in Developing Countries." pp. 157–162. IAEA-TECDOC-266.

Bicher, H. I., Sandhu, T. S., and Hetzel, F. W. (1980a). Hyperthermia and radiation in combination: clinical fractionation regime. *Int. J. Radiat. Oncol. Biol. Phys.* **6**, 867–870.

Bicher, H. I., Hetzel, F. W., Sandhu, T. S., Frinak, S., Vaupel, P., O'Hara, M. D., and O'Brien, T. (1980b). Effects of hyperthermia on normal and tumor microenvironment. *Radiology (Easton, Pa.)* **137**, 523–530.

Bleehen, N. M., Hones, D. J., and Morgan, J. E. (1977). Interaction of hyperthermia and hypoxic cell sensitizer Ro-07-0582 on the EMT6 mouse tumour. *Br. J. Cancer.* **35**, 299–306.

Bleehen, N. M., Honess, D. J., and Morgan, J. E. (1978). The combined effects of hyperthermia and hypoxic cell sensitizers. *In* "Cancer Therapy by Hyperthermia and Radiation" (C. Streffer, D. von Beuningen, F. Dretzel, E. Röttinger, J. E. Robinson, E. Scherer, S. Seeber, and K.-R. Trott, eds.), pp. 62–71. Urban & Schwarzenberg, Baltimore, Maryland.

Braun, J., and Hahn, G. M. (1975). Enhanced cell killing by bleomycin and 43° hyperthermia and inhibition of recovery from potentially lethal damage. *Cancer Res.* **35**, 2921–2927.

Bull, J., Lees, D., Schuette, W., Whang-Peng, J., Smith, R., Bynum, G., Atkinson, E. R., Gottiener, J. S., Gralnick, H. R., Shawker, T. H., and De Vita, V. T. Jr. (1979). Whole body hyperthermia: a phase I trial of a potential adjuvant to chemotherapy. *Ann. Intern. Med.* **90**, 317–323.

Caldwell, W. L. (1979). Clinical instrumentation requirements with a review of the Perth hyperthermia experience. *Cancer Res.* **39**, 2332–2335.

Cavalier, R., Ciocatto, E. C., Giovanella, B. C., Heidelberger, C., Johnson, R. O., Margottin, M., Mondovi, B., Moricca, G. and Rossi-Fanelli, A. (1967). Selective heat sensitivity of cancer cells: biochemical and clinical studies. *Cancer (Philadelphia)* **20**, 1351–1381.

Chen, T. T., and Heidelberger, C. (1969). Quantitative studies on the malignant transformation of mouse prostate cells by carcinogenic hydrocarbons *in vitro*. *Int. J. Cancer* **4**, 166–178.

Crile, G., Jr. (1961). Heat as an adjunct to the treatment of cancer. *Cleveland Clin. Q.* **28**, 75–89.

Crile, G., Jr. (1963). The effect of heat and radiation on cancers implanted on the feet of mice. *Cancer Res.* **23,** 372–380.

Dewey, W. C., Hopwood, L. E., Saparato, S. A., and Gerweck, L. E. (1977). Cellular responses to combinations of hyperthermia and radiation. *Radiology (Easton, Pa.)* **123,** 463–474.

Dewey, W. C., Highfield, D. P., Freeman, M. L., Coss, R. A., Wong, R. S. L., and Barrau, M. D. (1979). Cell biology of hyperthermia and radiation. *Proc. Int. Congr. Radiat. Res. 6th,* pp. 832–840.

Dewhirst, M. W., Ozimek, E. J., Gross, J., and Cetas, T. C. (1980). Will hyperthermia conquer the elusive hypoxic cell? *Radiology (Easton, Pa.)* **137,** 811–817.

Dickson, J. A., and Calderwood, S. K. (1980). Temperature range and selective sensitivity of tumors to hyperthermia: a critical review. *Ann. N.Y. Acad. Sci.* **335,** 327–346.

Eddy, H. A. (1980). Alterations in tumor microvasculature during hyperthermia. *Radiology (Easton, Pa.)* **137,** 515–521.

Emami, B., Nussbaum, G. H., TenHaken, R. K., and Hughes, W. L. (1980). Physiological effects of hyperthermia: response of capillary blood flow and structure to local tumor heating. *Radiology (Easton, Pa.)* **137,** 805–809.

Endrich, B., Intaglietta, M., Reinhold, H. S., and Gross, J. F. (1979). Hemodynamic characteristics in microcirculatory blood channels during early tumor growth. *Cancer Res.* **39,** 17–23.

Field, S. B., Hume, S. P., and Law, M. P. (1979). The response of tissues to heat alone or in combination with radiation. *Proc. Int. Congr. Radiat. Res. 6th,* pp. 847–854.

Freeman, M. L., Boone, M. L., Ensley, B. A., and Gillette, E. L. (1981). The influence of environmental pH on the interaction and repair heat and radiation damage. *Int. J. Radiat. Oncol. Biol. Phys.* **7,** 761–764.

Gerner, E. W., Holmes, P. W., and McCullough, J. A. (1979). Influence of growth state on several thermal responses of EMT 6/AZ tumor cells *in vitro. Cancer Res.* **39,** 981–986.

Gerweck, L. E. (1977). Modification of cell lethality at elevated temperatures. The pH effect. *Radiat. Res.* **70,** 224–235.

Gerweck, L. E., Gillette, E. L., and Dewey, W. C. (1974). Killing of Chinese hamster cells *in vitro* by heating under hypoxic or aerobic conditions. *Eur. J. Cancer* **10,** 691–693.

Gerweck, L. E., Gillette, E. L., and Dewey, W. C. (1975). Effect of heat and radiation on synchronous Chinese hamster cells. Killing and repair. *Radiat. Res.* **64,** 611–623.

Gerweck, L. E., Nygaard, T. G., and Burlett, M. (1979). Response of cells to hyperthermia under acute and chronic conditions. *Cancer Res.* **39,** 966–972.

Gillette, E. L. (1979). Large animal studies of hyperthermia and irradiation. *Cancer Res.* **39,** 2242–2244.

Giovanella, B. C., Stehlin, J. S., and Morgan, A. C. (1976). Selective lethal effect of supranormal temperatures on human neoplastic cells. *Cancer Res.* **36,** 3944–3950.

Giovanella, B. C., Lohman, W. A., and Heidelberger, C. (1977). Effects of elevated temperatures and drugs on the viability of L1210 leukemia cells. *Cancer Res.* **30,** 1623–1631.

Goldfeder, A., Brown, D. A., and Berger, A. (1979). Enhancement of radioresponse of a mouse mammary carcinoma to combined treatment with hyperthermia and radiosensitizer misonidazol. *Cancer Res.* **39,** 2966–2970.

Goss, P., and Parsons, P. G. (1977). The effect of hyperthermia and melphalan on survival of human fibroblast strains and melanoma cell lines. *Cancer Res.* **37,** 152–156.

Hahn, G. M. (1974). Metabolic aspects of the role of hyperthermia in mammalian cells inactivation and their relevance to cancer treatment. *Cancer Res.* **34,** 3117–3123.

Hahn, G. M. (1978). Interactions of drugs and hyperthermia *in vitro* and *in vivo. In* "Cancer Therapy by Hyperthermia and Radiation" (C. Streffer, D. von Beuningen, F. Dretzel, E. Röttinger, J. E. Robinson, E. Scherer, S. Seeber, and K.-R. Trott, eds.), pp. 72–79.

Hahn, G. M. (1979). Potential for therapy of drugs and hyperthermia. *Cancer Res.* **39**, 2264–2268.

Hahn, G. M., and Strande, D. P. (1976). Cytotoxic effects of hyperthermia and adriamycin on Chinese hamster cells. *J. Natl. Cancer Inst. (U.S.)* **57**, 1063–1067.

Hahn, G. M., Braun, J., and Har-Kedar, I. (1975). Thermochemotherapy: syngergisms between hyperthermia (42–43°C) and adriamycin (or bleomycin) in mammalian cell interaction. *Proc. Natl. Acad. Sci. USA* **79**, 937–940.

Hahn, G. M., Li, G. C., and Shiu, E. (1977). Interaction of amphotericin B and 43° hyperthermia. *Cancer Res.* **37**, 761–764.

Harisiadis, L., Sung, D. I., and Hall, E. J. (1977). Thermal tolerance and repair of thermal damage by cultured cells. *Radiology (Easton, Pa.)* **123**, 505–509.

Harris, J. R., Murthy, A. K., and Belli, J. A. (1976). The effects of hyperthermia on the repair of radiation damage in plateau phase cells. *Radiology (Easton, Pa.)* **119**, 227–229.

Harris, J. R., Murthy, A. K., and Belli, J. A. (1977). The effects of delay between heat and X-irradiation on the survival response of plateau phase V-79 cells. *Int. J. Radiat. Oncol. Biol. Phys.* **2**, 515–519.

Herman, T. S., Cress, A. E., and Gerner, E. W. (1979). Collateral sensitivity of methotrexate in cells resistant to adriamycin. *Cancer Res.* **39**, 1937–1942.

Hiraoka, M., and Abe, M. (1981). Hyperthermia combined with radiation in the treatment of cancer. "IAEA Seminar, Prospective Methods of Radiation Therapy in Developing Countries," pp. 163–176. IAEA-TECDOC-266.

Hoffer, K. G., Choppin, D. A., and Hoffer, M. G. (1976). Effect of hyperthermia on the radiosensitivity of normal and malignant cells in mice. *Cancer (Philadelphia)* **38**, 279–287.

Holt, J. A. G. (1980). Alternative therapy for recurrent Hodgkins disease. Radiotherapy combined with hyperthermia by electromagnetic radiation to create complete remission in 11 patients without morbidity. *Br. J. Radiol.* **53**, 1061–1067.

Hones, D. J., Workman, P., Morgan, J. E., and Bleehen, N. M. (1980). Effects of local hyperthermia on the pharmacokinetics of misonidazole in the anaesthetized mouse. *Br. J. Cancer* **41**, 529–540.

Hornback, N. B., Shupe, R., Shidnia, H., Joe, B. T., Sayoc, E., and Marshall, C. (1977). Preliminary clinical results of combined 433 megahertz microwave therapy and radiation therapy in patients with advanced cancer. *Cancer (Philadelphia)* **40**, 2854–2863.

Hornback, N. B., Shupe, R., Shidnia, H., Joe, B. T., Sayo, E., and George, R. (1979). Radiation and microwave therapy in the treatment of advanced cancer. *Radiology (Easton, Pa.)* **130**, 459–464.

Joseph, C. D., Astrahan, M., Lipsett, J., Archambeau, J., Forell, B., and George, F. W. (1981). Interstitial hyperthermia and interstitial iridium 192 implantation: a technique and preliminary results. *Int. J. Radiat. Oncol. Biol. Phys.* **7**, 827–833.

Kase, K., and Hahn, G. M. (1975). Differential heat response of normal and transformed human cells in tissue culture. *Nature (London)* **225**, 228–230.

Kim, J. H., Hahn, E. W., Tokita, N., and Nisce, L. Z. (1977). Local tumor hyperthermia in combination with radiation therapy. I. Malignant cutaneous lesions. *Cancer (Philadelphia)* **40**, 161–169.

Kim, J. H., Hahn, E. W., and Tokita, N. (1978). Combined hyperthermia and radiation therapy for cutaneous malignant melanoma. *Cancer (Philadelphia)* **41**, 2143–2148.

Kim, J. H., Hahn, E. W., and Ahmed, S. A. (1982). Combination hyperthermia and radiation therapy for malignant melanoma. *Cancer (Philadelphia)* **50**, 478–482.

Kim, S. H., Kim, J. H., and Hahn, E. W. (1975). The radiosensitization of hypoxic tumor cells by hyperthermia. *Radiology (Easton, Pa.)* **114**, 727–728.

Kim, S. H., Kim, J. H., and Hahn, E. W. (1976). The enhanced killing of irradiated HeLa cells in synchronous culture by hyperthermia. *Radiat. Res.* **66,** 337–345.

Kowal, C. D., and Bertino, J. R. (1979). Possible benefits of hyperthermia to chemotherapy. *Cancer Res.* **39,** 2285–2289.

Larkin, J. M. (1979). A clinical investigation of total body hyperthermia as a cancer therapy. *Cancer Res.* **39,** 2252–2254.

LeVeen, H. H., Wapnik, S., Piccone, V., Falk, G., and Ahmed, N. (1976). Tumor eradiation by radio-frequency therapy. Response in 21 patients. *JAMA J. Am. Med. Assoc.* **235,** 2198–2200.

LeVeen, H. H., Ahmed, N., and Piccone, V. A. (1980). RF therapy: clinical experience. *Ann. N.Y. Acad. Sci.* **335,** 362–371.

Li, G. C., Evans, R. G., and Hahn, G. M. (1976). Modification and inhibition of repair of potentially lethal X-ray damage by hyperthermia. *Radiat. Res.* **67,** 491–501.

Li, G. C., Shiu, E. V., and Hahn, G. M. (1980). Recovery of cells from heat-induced potentially lethal damage: effects of pH and nutrient environment. *Int. J. Radiat. Oncol. Biol. Phys.* **6,** 577–582.

Luk, K. H., Hulse, M., and Phillips, T. L. (1980). Hyperthermia in cancer therapy. *West. J. Med.* **132,** 179–185.

Magin, R. L., Sikic, B. I., and Cysyk, R. L. (1979). Enhancement of bleomycin activity against Lewis lung tumors in mice by local hyperthermia. *Cancer Res.* **39,** 3792–3795.

Manning, M. R., Cetas, T. C., Miller, R. C., Olesom, J. R., Connor, W. G., and Gerner, E. W. (1982). Clinical hyperthermia: results of a phase I trial employing hyperthermia alone or in combination with external beam or interstitial radiotherapy. *Cancer (Philadelphia)* **49,** 205–216.

Marmor, J. B. (1979). Interactions of hyperthermia and chemotherapy in animals. *Cancer Res.* **39,** 2269–2276.

Marmor, J. B., and Hahn, G. M. (1980). Combined radiation and hyperthermia in superficial human tumors. *Cancer (Philadelphia)* **46,** 1986–1991.

Marmor, J. B., Pounds, D., Postic, T. B., and Hahn, G. M. (1979). Treatment of superficial human neoplasms by local hyperthermia induced by ultrasound. *Cancer (Philadelphia)* **43,** 188–197.

Mendecki, J., Friedenthal, E., and Botstein, C. (1978). Microwave-induced hyperthermia in cancer treatment apparatus and preliminary results. *Int. J. Radiat. Oncol. Biol. Phys.* **4,** 1095–1103.

Meyer, K. R., Hopwood, L. E., and Gillette, E. L. (1979). The thermal response of mouse adenocarcinoma cells at low pH. *Eur. J. Cancer* **15,** 1219–1222.

Meyn, R. E., Corry, P. M., Fletcher, S. E., and Demetriades, M. (1980). Thermal enhancement of DNA damage in mammalian cells treated with cis-diamminedichloroplatinum (II). *Cancer Res.* **40,** 1136–1139.

Nakamura, W., and Nakayama-Sato, T. (1981). Present status of the thermo-chemotherapy of cancer. *Gan-to-Kagaku Ryoho* **8,** 1–8.

Orton, C. G. (1972). *AAPM Quart. Bull.* **6,** 173.

Overgaard, J. (1976a). Influence of extracellular pH on the viability and morphology of tumor cells exposed to hyperthermia. *J. Natl. Cancer Inst. (US)* **56,** 1243–1250.

Overgaard, J. (1976b). Combined adriamycin and hyperthermia treatment of a murine mammary carcinoma *in vivo. Cancer Res.* **36,** 3077–3081.

Overgaard, J. (1981). Fractionated radiation and hyperthermia: experimental and clinical studies. *Cancer (Philadelphia)* **48,** 1116–1123.

Overgaard, J., and Bichel, P. (1977). The influence of hypoxia and acidity on the hyperthermia response of malignant cells *in vitro. Radiology (Easton, Pa.)* **123,** 511–514.

Palzer, R. J., and Heidelberger, C. (1973). Studies on quantitative biology of hyperthermic killing of HeLa cells. *Cancer Res.* **33,** 415–421.

Palzer, R. J., and Heidelberger, C. (1974). Influence of drugs and synchrony on the hyperthermic killing of HeLa cells. *Cancer Res.* **33,** 422–427.

Parks, L. C., Minaberry, D., Smith, D. P., Neely, W. A. (1979). Treatment of far-advanced bronchogenic carcinoma by extracorporeally induced systemic hyperthermia. *J. Thorac. Cardiovasc. Surg.* **78,** 883–892.

Perez, C. A., Kopecky, W., Rao, D. V., Baglan, R., and Mann, J. (1981). Local microwave hyperthermia and irradiation in cancer therapy: preliminary observations and directions for future clinical trials. *Int. J. Radiat. Oncol. Biol. Phys.* **7,** 765–772.

Pettigrew, R. T., Galt, J. M., Ludgate, C. M., and Smith, A. N. (1974). Clinical effects of wholebody hyperthermia on advanced malignancy. *Br. Med. J.* **4,** 679–692.

Robinson, J. E., Wizenberg, M. J., and McCready, W. A. (1974). Combined hyperthermia and radiation suggest an alternative to heavy particle therapy for reduced oxygen enhancement ratios. *Nature (London)* **251,** 521–522.

Rossi-Fanelli, A., Cavaliere, R., Mondovi, A., and Moricca, G. (eds.) (1977). Selective heat sensitivity of cancer cells. *Recent Results Cancer Res.* **59,** 1–185.

Schulman, N., and Hall, E. J. (1974). Hyperthermia: its effect on proliferative and plateau phase cell cultures. *Radiology (Easton, Pa.)* **113,** 209–211.

Selawry, O. S., Carson, J. D., and Moore, G. E. (1958). Tumor responses to ionizing rays at elevated temperatures. *Am. J. Roentgenol. Radium Ther.* **80,** 833–839.

Shingleton, W. W., Bryan, F., O'Quinn, W., and Krueger, L. C. (1962). Selective heating and cooling of tissue in cancer chemotherapy. *Ann. Surg.* **156,** 408–416.

Song, C. W. (1978). Effect of hyperthermia on vascular functions of normal tissues and experimental tumors. *J. Natl. Cancer Inst. (US)* **60,** 711–713.

Song, C. W., Kang, M. S., Rhee, J. G., and Levitt, S. H. (1980). The effect of hyperthermia on vascular function, pH, and cell survival. *Radiology (Easton, Pa.)* **137,** 795–803.

Stehlin, J. S. (1980). Hyperthermic perfusion for melanoma of the extremities: experience with 165 patients, 1967 to 1979. *Ann. N.Y. Acad. Sci.* **335,** 352–355.

Stehlin, J. S., Giovanella, B. C., Ipolyi, P. D., Muenz, L. R., and Anderson, R. T. (1975). Results of hyperthermia perfusion for melanoma of the extremities. *Surg. Gynecol. Obstet.* **140,** 338–348.

Sternhagen, C. J., Doss, J. D., Day, P. W., Edwards, W. S., Doberneck, R. C., Herzon, F. S., Powell, T. D., O'Brien, F. F. G., and Larkin, J. M. (1978). Clinical use of radiofrequency current in oral cavity carcinoma and metastatic malignancies with continuous temperature control and monitoring. *In* "Cancer Therapy by Hyperthermia and Radiation (C. Streffer, D. von Beuningen, F. Dretzel, E. Röttinger, J. E. Robinson, E. Scherer, S. Seeber, and K.-R. Trott, eds.), pp. 831–834. Urban & Schwarzenberg, Baltimore, Maryland.

Stewart, F. A., and Denekamp, J. (1978). The therapeutic advantage of combined heat and X-rays on a mouse fibrosarcoma. *Br. J. Radiol.* **51,** 307–316.

Storm, F. K., Elliott, R. S., Harrison, W. H., and Morton, D. L. (1979). Normal tissue and solid tumor effects of hyperthermia in animal models and clinical trials. *Cancer Res.* **39,** 2245–2251.

Storm, F. K., Elliott, R. S., Harrison, W. H., and Morton, D. L. (1980). Hyperthermia therapy for human neoplasms: thermal death time. *Cancer (Philadelphia)* **46,** 1849–1854.

Suit, H. D., and Gerweck, L. E. (1979). Potential for hyperthermia and radiation therapy. *Cancer Res.* **39,** 2290–2298.

Suzuki, K. (1967). Application of heat to cancer chemotherapy. *Nagoya J. Med. Sci.* **30,** 1–21.

Thrall, D. E., Gillette, E. L., and Dewey, W. C. (1975). Effects of heat and radiation on normal and neoplastic tissue of the C3H mouse. *Radiat. Res.* **63,** 363–377.

Turano, C., Ferraro, A. Strom, R., Cavaliere, R., and Rossi-Fanelli, A. (1970). The biochemical mechanism of selective heat sensitivity of cancer cells. III. Studies on lysosomes. *Eur. J. Cancer* **6,** 67–72.

Twentyman, P. R., Morgan, J. E., and Donaldson, J. (1978). Enhancement by hyperthermia of the effect of BCNU against EMT6 mouse tumor. *Cancer Treat. Rep.* **62,** 439–443.

U, R., Noell, K. T., Woodward, K. T., Worde, B. T., Fishburn, R. I., and Miller, L. S. (1980). Microwave induced local hyperthermia in combination with radiotherapy of human malignant tumors. *Cancer* (*Philadelphia*) **45,** 638–646.

Vaupel, P. (1979). Oxygen supply to malignant tumors. *In* "Tumor Blood Circulation: Angiogenesis, Vascular Morphology, and Blood Flow of Experimental and Human Tumors" (H. I. Peterson, ed.), pp. 143–168. CRC Press, Boca Raton, Florida.

von Ardenne, M. (1978). On a new physical principle for selective local hyperthermia of tumor tissues. *In* "Cancer Therapy by Hyperthermia and Radiation" (C. Streffer, D. von Beuningen, F. Dretzel, E. Röttinger, J. E. Robinson, E. Scherer, S. Seeber, and K.-R. Trott, eds.), pp. 96–104. Urban & Schwarzenberg, Baltimore, Maryland.

von Ardenne, M., and Reitnauer, P. G. (1980). Selective occlusion of cancer tissue capillaries as the central mechanism of the cancer multistep therapy. *Jpn. J. Clin. Oncol.* **10,** 31–48.

Weinstein, J. N., Magin, R. L., Yatvin, M. B., and Zaharko, D. S. (1979). Liposomes and local hyperthermia: selective delivery of methotrexate to heated tumors. *Science* (*Washington, D. C.*) **204,** 188–191.

Weinstein, J. N., Magin, R. L., Cysyk, R. L., and Zaharko, D. S. (1980). Treatment of solid L1210 murine tumors with local hyperthermia and temperature-sensitive liposomes containing methotrexate. *Cancer Res.* **40,** 1388–1395.

Westra, A., and Dewey, W. C. (1971). Variation in sensitivity of heat shock during the cell-cycle of Chinese hamster cells *in vitro. Int. J. Radiat. Biol.* **19,** 467–477.

Witcofski, R. L., and Kremkau, F. W. (1978). Ultrasonic enhancement of cancer radiotherapy. *Radiology* (*Easton, Pa.*) **127,** 793–797.

Yatvin, M. B., Weinstein, J. N., Dennis, W. H., and Blumenthal, R. (1978). Design of liposomes for enhanced local release of drugs by hyperthermia. *Science* (*Washington, D.C.*) **202,** 1290–1293.

Yerushalmi, A. (1975). Cure of a solid tumor by simultaneous administration of microwave and X-ray irradiation. *Radiat. Res.* **64,** 602–610.

23 Effects of Hyperthermia on Cultured Mammalian Cells

Eiichi Kano
Shinji Yoshikawa
Michi Inui
Susumu Tsubouchi
Takashi Kondo

Department of Experimental Radiology and Health Physics
Fukui Medical University School of Medicine
Fukui 910-11, Japan

Junji Miyakoshi

Department of Radiation Biology
Kyoto College of Pharmacy
Kyoto 607, Japan

Masayo Furukawa

Department of Anatomy
School of Medicine, Osaka City University
Osaka 545, Japan

439

I. Introduction

Since 1970, numerous studies have evolved around hyperthermia for cancer treatment. We report herein findings in cell strains subjected to various culture systems in our laboratories.

II. Materials and Methods

A. Hyperthermia

A water bath (Tokyo Seisakusho, Model ET-45P) was used for the hyperthermic exposure. The temperatures were measured by an electrothermometer (Kyoto Keisokuki, Model LM-1S). The hyperthermia treatments at 40, 42, and 44°C were maintained within an error of ±0.05°C.

B. X Irradiation

Ionizing radiation was from a Toshiba X-ray generator (Model KXC-17). The physical conditions were 140 kVp, 5 mA, 2-mm Al filter, and exposure rate of 30 R/min. The dose rate was measured by a Radocon II dosimeter (Victoreen, Model 555).

C. Bleomycin (BLM) Treatment

Bleomycin in a 15-mg ampoule was diluted and added to the cell culture plate replenished with 4 ml of fresh MLN-3 to obtain the final concentration of 0.1 mg/ml for the treatments of cells.

The plates were incubated at 37°C for 24 h in the experiments of the BLM-resistant variant induction and at either 37 or 40°C for the graded periods of 0.5 to 6 h in the BLM treatment time–survival experiments, respectively.

D. Cell Lines

Lines used were murine L fibroblasts, Ehrlich's murine ascites tumor cells, Chinese hamster V-79 cells, and human HeLa S3 cells. These cell lines were colonially cloned and used throughout the present series of experiments *in vitro*.

E. Culture Media

All the cell lines were maintained in a growth medium MLN-15: an enriched MEM solution, 1 liter of which contained 730 ml of Eagle's MEM solution (Nissui), 20 ml of 2.5% w/v lactalbumin hydrolysate solution (Difco), 100 ml of NCTC-135 solution (Difco), 150 ml of inactivated bovine serum, and antibiotics. Numerals following MLN- represent volume/volume percentages of inactivated bovine serum in the medium.

F. Culture Conditions

Cells used in the experiments were obtained in cell suspension by trypsinizing those of farming cultures in the plastic plates. The control growth was monitored during the experiments, which were performed on successive days to that of the cell seeding.

In the experiments of water bath immersion, cells were trypsinized, suspended in plastic test tubes, and immersed. The cells after the treatments were seeded again in appropriate cell numbers per plate to yield pertinent numbers of colonies as the survivors and to estimate the precise number of surviving fractions (i.e., ~100 colonies/plate 6 cm in diameter). In other experiments, cells seeded beforehand on the plates were then treated on the successive day.

After the treatments, the plates were replenished with 8 ml of MLN-15, placed in a CO_2 incubator, and the colony formation observed.

For experimental procedures, see Section III.

G. Survival Criterion

After the final treatments, the cells on the plates, or otherwise cells seeded on the plates again, were incubated for 6 to 8 days to obtain colonies in macroscopic size and composed of 50 cells or more. The colonies were stained with methylene blue for 0.5 h at 37°C, and the number of colonies per plate was counted. The cell surviving fraction from each treatment was routinely estimated as the ratio of the number of colonies formed per plate divided by the number of inoculated cells per plate. The estimated fractions were corrected to the surviving fraction of the untreated control, plating efficiency. Three or more replicate plates were used for each survival point and replicate experiments were done two to four times, according to the consistency of the results obtained.

III. Results

A. Differential Sensitivities to Low and High Hyperthermia Temperatures and Different Sensitivities among Cell Lines[1]

Lines of cells in exponential phase (L, V-79, Ehrlich, and HeLa S3) were prepared in single-cell suspension, and the suspensions were immersed in the water bath for graded periods. Cells after the scheduled treatments were seeded and incubated in the plastic culture plates.

As shown in Figs. 1 and 2 and Table I, cell lines showed individual thermosensitivities. Only L cells among the assayed four lines were extraordinarily thermosensitive.

TABLE I

Parameters of Heat Treatment Time–Survival Curves

| | Parameters[a] | | | |
| | 42°C | | 44°C | |
Cell lines	T_0 (min)	T_q (min)	T_0 (min)	T_q (min)
V-79	248	−88.0	7.3	11.0
L	31	−2.4	2.8	5.9
EH	215	−77.0	7.7	11.0
HeLa S3	278	−96.0	7.3	11.0

[a] Defined similarly to D_0 in X-ray dose–survival curves, T_0 shows immersion time required for cell survival to be reduced to $1/e$ or 37%, and represents cellular heat sensitivity. Defined similarly to D_q, T_q represents the sublethal region expressed by treatment time. The negative value of T_q, mingled, represents upward concavity on the survival curve at 42°C.

[1] Westra and Dewey, 1971; Kano *et al.,* 1977, 1979, 1982; Bauer and Henle, 1979.

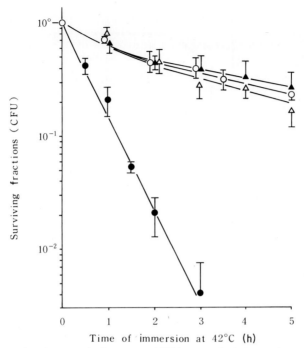

Fig. 1. Immersion time–survival curves at 42°C by water bath immersion. Vertical bars, ±SD. Cell lines: (○) V-79, (●) L, (△) EH, (▲) HeLa S3. From Kano *et al.* (1979).

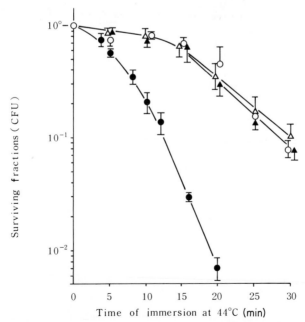

Fig. 2. Immersion time–survival curves at 44°C by water bath immersion. Cell lines: (○) V-79, (●) L, (△) EH, (▲) HeLa S3. Vertical bars, ±SD. From Kano *et al.* (1979).

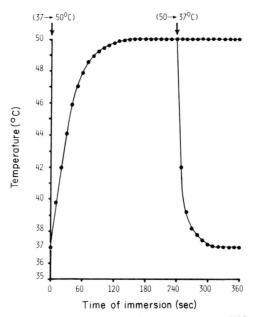

Fig. 3. Relationship of immersion time to medium temperature at 50°C. Ordinate: temperature of medium for cell suspension. Arrow marks indicate the time at which the medium was altered from 37 to 50°C or vice versa. From Kano *et al.* (1982).

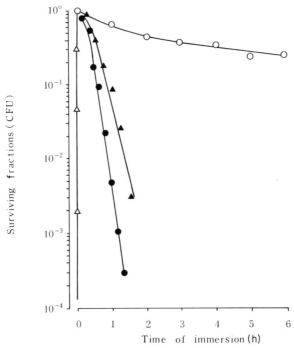

Fig. 4. Immersion time–survival curves for V-79 cells at various temperatures. (○) 42°C, (▲) 43°C, (●) 44°C, (△) 50°C. From Kano *et al.* (1982).

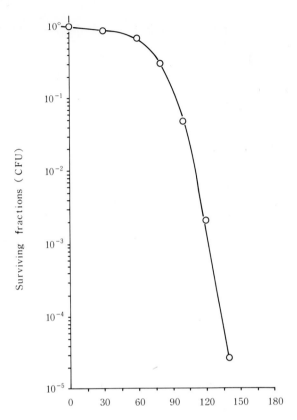

Time of immersion at 50°C (sec)

Fig. 5. Detailed 50°C immersion time–survival curve for V-79 cells. From Kano *et al.* (1982).

The 44°C heating time–survival curves were concaved downward with the initial shoulder region as in the radiation dose–survival curves, whereas the 42°C curves concaved upward. Cells subjected to 42°C of heat appeared to develop thermotolerance during the water bath immersion.

Hyperthermic immersion time–cell survival assays of V-79 cells at 50°C and the immersion time–temperature relationship are shown in Figs. 3–6. An Arrhenius plot was drawn with regard to temperatures of 42, 43, 44, and 50°C for a comparison with data in other reports. No additional bending in the curves was observed at temperatures between 43 and 50°C (Fig. 7). Parameters of the curves are shown in Table II.

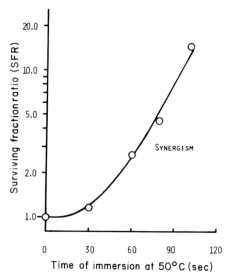

Fig. 6. Immersion time–surviving fraction ratio (SFR) for V-79 cells at 50°C.

$$SFR = \frac{SF\ (4.5\ Gy) \times SF\ (50°C,\ T)}{SF\ (4.5\ Gy + 50°C,\ T)}$$

From Kano *et al.* (1982).

TABLE II

Parameters of Hyperthermic Immersion Time–Cell Survival Curves of V-79 Cells

Temperature (°C)	$T_0{}^a$ (min)	$T_q{}^b$ (min)	n
42	384.0	−182.0	0.58
43	12.0	22.0	5.2
44	6.7	18.0	8.6
50	0.1	1.5	—

[a] T_0 is the time required to reduce survival by a factor of $1/e$ in the exponential region of the survival curve.

[b] T_q is the quasi-threshold time, at which a back extrapolare of the exponential region intersects the abscissa on 1.0 survival fraction.

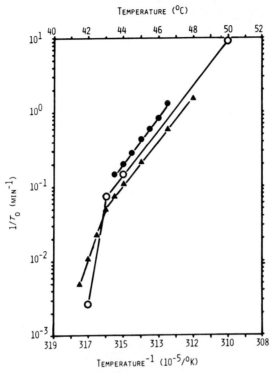

Fig. 7. Arrhenius plot. (○) Data obtained in the present experiments, V-79 cells. (●) Data of Westra and Dewey (1971), CHO cells. (▲) Data of Bauer and Henle (1979), CHO cells. See also Kano *et al.* (1982).

B. Step-up and Step-down Heating and Induction of Thermotolerance and Thermopotentiation[2]

Trypsinized V-79 cells in single-cell suspension in plastic test tubes were immersed in a water bath at 42 or 44°C for graded periods.

In the experiments of split-dose hyperthermia, cells were immersed at 42 or 44°C for a fixed period, at 37°C for graded interval periods, and 42 or 44°C for graded periods. In the case of intervals over 24 h, cells immersed in test tubes were seeded in plastic plates after the conditioning (first) hyperthermia and incubated at 37°C in the CO_2 incubator for the scheduled interval periods. Cells were retrypsinized and the single-cell suspensions in test tubes were immersed for exposure to the second hyperthermia. The procedures were simply expressed as shown here: (1) 42 → 44°C

[2] Miyakoshi *et al.*, 1979, 1983; Kano *et al.*, 1981.

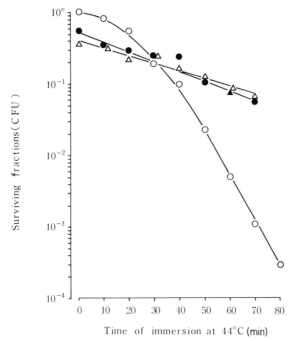

Fig. 8. Survival curves of cells exposed to 44°C hyperthermia alone and the step-up heating of 42 → 44°C sequence. Hamster V-79 cells were exposed to 42°C for 2 h (●) or 4 h (△), and then further exposed to 44°C for graded periods. Survival of cells exposed to 42°C for 2 h and 4 h was about 0.52 and 0.36, respectively. For the control experiment, cells were exposed to 44°C alone (○). From Miyakoshi *et al.* (1983).

and 42 → 37 → 44°C; (2) 44 → 42°C and 44 → 37 → 42°C; and (3) 44 → 37 → 44°C.

1. Step-up Heating without or with 37°C Interval

As shown in Figs. 8 and 9, conditioning exposure at 42°C induced a thermotolerance during the 42°C heating that was observed in the successive second heating at 44°C. The induced tolerance was maintained for about 3 h and was followed by a decrease through the 37°C interval time.

2. Step-down Heating without or with 37°C Interval

As shown in Fig. 10, conditioning exposure at 44°C induced a thermopotentiation during the 44°C heating that was observed in the successive second heating at 42°C. The induced potentiation decreased through the 37°C interval which continued for 6 h, as shown in Fig. 11.

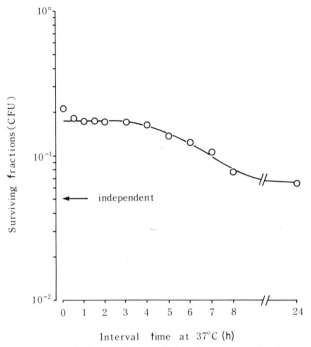

Fig. 9. Disappearance of thermotolerance induced by step-up heating. Hamster V-79 cells were exposed to 42°C for 2 h, immediately followed by transfer to 37°C for various intervals up to 24 h, and then further exposed to 44°C for 40 min. The arrow indicates the independent level of survival, which is the multiplication of two surviving fractions obtained from 42°C for 2 h and 44°C for 40-min treatments. From Miyakoshi *et al.* (1983).

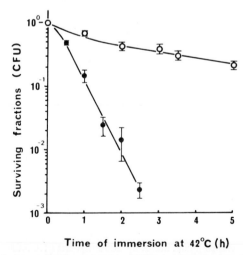

Fig. 10. Survival curves of cells exposed to 42°C hyperthermia alone (○) or after preheating for 15 min at 44°C (●). The curve for the combined treatment is corrected for the effect of the first exposure at 44°C. Vertical bars, ±SD. From Miyakoshi *et al.* (1979).

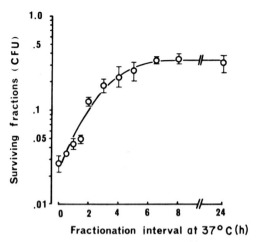

Fig. 11. Recovery kinetics of cells exposed to the combined 44 → 42°C hyperthermia treatment, as shown in Fig. 10. The cells were exposed to 44°C hyperthermia for 15 min followed by immersion at 37°C for various intervals up to 24 h and further exposed to 42°C hyperthermia for 90 min (○). Responses to two single hyperthermic treatments: (▲) 15 min at 44°C, (■) 90 min at 42°C. The additive surviving fraction from these two single hyperthermic treatments is approximately 0.4. Vertical vars, ±SD. From Miyakoshi *et al.* (1979).

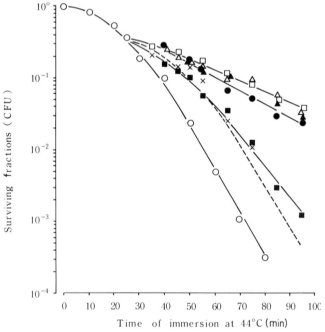

Fig. 12. Thermotolerance induction by split-dose hyperthermia at 44°C. Hamster V-79 cells were exposed to 44°C for 25 min, immediately followed by transfer to 37°C for various intervals up to 72 h, and then further exposed to 44°C for graded periods. Each symbol represents the interval time at 37°C as follows: zero (○), 3 h (●), 6 h (△), 18 h (▲), 24 h (□), 48 h (■), and 72 h (x). The independent curve (-----) represents the control curve of 44°C hyperthermia alone. From Miyakoshi *et al.* (1983).

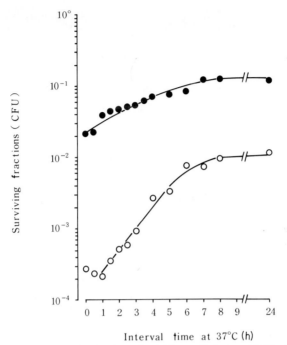

Interval time at 37°C (h)

Fig. 13. Thermotolerance induction by an equivalent split dose at 44°C for 25 min (●) and 40 min (○), immediately followed by transfer to 37°C for various intervals up to 24 h, and then further exposed to 44°C for 25 and 40 min, respectively. From Miyakoshi *et al.* (1983).

3. Induction of Thermotolerance in Fractionated 44°C Hyperthermia with 37°C Interval

As shown in Figs. 12 and 13, a thermotolerance was induced after the conditioning at 44°C heating that reached a maximum at about 6 h, continued for about 18 h, and finally decreased to a level slightly above the independent full recovery (broken line) at 48 h.

C. Effects of Combined Treatments of X Irradiation and Hyperthermia on Cell Survival[3]

Exponentially growing V-79 cells in monolayers were trypsinized in 0.03% trypsin solution to obtain single-cell suspensions in MLN-3. Cell concentrations of the suspensions were adopted for appropriate survival colonies per plate in the final incubations in the plates. Aliquots of 4 ml of

[3] Miyakoshi *et al.*, 1979; Kano *et al.*, 1981.

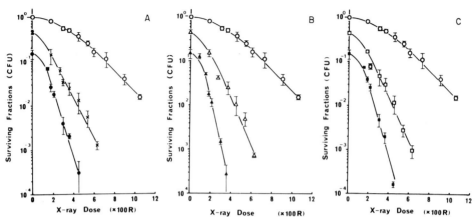

Fig. 14. X-Ray dose–survival curves of cells treated with X irradiation alone or in combination with 42 and 44°C hyperthermia. The cells were exposed to X irradiation alone or in combination with 42°C hyperthermia for 60 min and 44°C for 15 min. The sequences of the combined treatments are as follows: (A) X irradiation alone (○), X → 42 → 44°C (x), X → 44 → 42°C (●); (B) X irradiation alone (○), 42 → X → 44°C (△), 44 → X → 42°C (▲); (C) X irradiation alone (○), 42 → 44°C → X (□), and 44 → 42°C → X (■). Vertical bars, ±SD. From Miyakoshi *et al.* (1979).

each cell suspension were transferred into plastic tubes, which were then immersed in a water bath at 37°C 10 min prior to the scheduled treatments of hyperthermia and X irradiation.

Cells were successively exposed to the combined treatments of hyperthermia (42°C 60 min and 44°C 15 min) and X irradiation with graded doses, in the different sequences. In the control experiments, cells were

TABLE III

D_0 Values and Thermal Enhancement Ratios for Survival Curves of V-79 Cells Subjected to Combined Treatments with X irradiation, and 42 and 44°C Hyperthermia

First treatment	$(X)^a$	(X)	(X)	$(42)^b$	$(44)^c$	(42)	(44)
Second treatment	n.t.^{d}	(42)	(44)	(X)	(X)	(44)	(42)
Third treatment	n.t.	(44)	(42)	(44)	(X)	(X)	
D_0 value (R)	172	95	60	83	48	88	55
$\dfrac{D_0(\text{X irradiation alone})^e}{D_0(\text{combined treatment})}$	(1.00)	1.81	2.87	2.07	3.58	1.95	3.13

^{a} (X), X irradiation with various doses.
^{b} (42), 60-min treatment at 42°C.
^{c} (44), 15-min treatment at 44°C.
^{d} Not treated.
^{e} Thermal enhancement ratio (TER) for D_0.

immersed at 37°C for equivalent periods to those of the correspondingly treated groups. Under all the conditions, the extracellular pH, which was read on a pH meter (Hitachi-Horiba, Model M-7), varied from 7.4 to 7.8.

As shown in Fig. 14 and Table III, hyperthermic radioenhancement ratios in D_0 were compared in which (*a*)sequences of step-down heatings and X irradiation showed a greater enhancement than those of step-up heatings and X irradiation, and (*b*) the position of X irradiation in between the two hyperthermia treatments showed the greatest enhancement among the three possible forms of X irradiation.

D.   Recovery Kinetics from Damage by Hyperthermia and X Irradiation[4]

Single-cell suspensions in the exponential phase were placed in test tubes and were immersed in a water bath at 37°C for 10 min prior to the sequential treatments with hyperthermia (42°C 60 min and 44°C 15 min) and X irradiation (3 Gy), with the interval (37°C, graded periods) in all the possible sequences. In the control experiments, cells were only immersed at 37°C for the equivalent periods to those of the correspondingly treated groups. The pH of the medium was measured between 7.4 and 7.8 during the present hyperthermia.

Recoveries in survivals through the 37°C intervals for graded periods were assayed for the following sequences:

	Sequences	Thermal enhancement ratios (no interval)
(1-1)	(44°C + X) → Intervals → 42°C	3.58
(1-2)	42°C → Intervals → (44°C + X)	1.95
(2-1)	(X + 44°C) → Intervals → 42°C	2.87
(2-2)	42°C → Intervals → (X + 44°C)	2.07
(3-1)	44°C → Intervals → (42°C + X)	3.13
(3-2)	(42°C + X) → Intervals → 44°C	2.07
(4-1)	44°C → Intervals → (X + 42°C)	3.58
(4-2)	(X + 42°C) → Intervals → 44°C	1.81
(5-1)	(42°C + 44°C) → Intervals → X	1.95
(5-2)	X → Intervals → (42°C + 44°C)	1.81
(6-1)	(44°C + 42°C) → Intervals → X	3.13
(6-2)	X → Intervals → (44°C + 42°C)	2.87

[4] Miyakoshi *et al.,* 1982a,b.

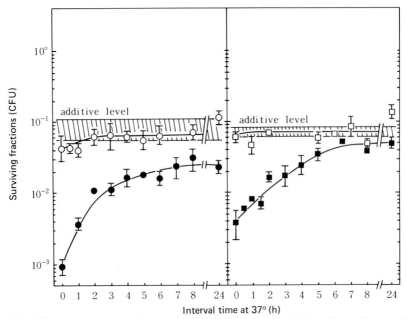

Fig. 15. Recovery kinetics from damage by hyperthermia and X irradiation. See text for details. Left: (●) sequence (1-1), (○) sequence (1-2). Right: (■) sequence (2-1), (□) sequence (2-2). Vertical bars, ±SD. From Miyakoshi *et al.* (1982a).

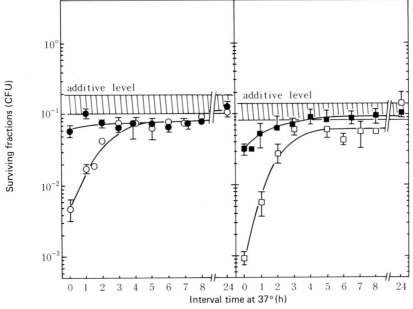

Fig. 16. Recovery kinetics from damage by hyperthermia and X irradiation. See text for details. Left: (○) sequence (3-1), (●) sequence (3-2). Right: (□) sequence (4-1), (■) sequence (4-2). Vertical bars, ±SD. From Miyakoshi *et al.* (1982a).

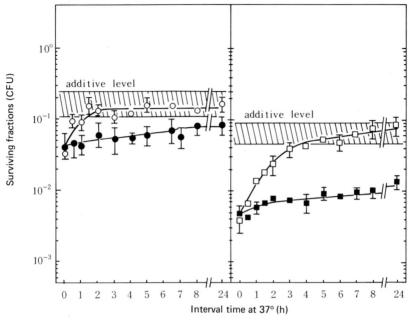

Fig. 17. Recovery kinetics from damage by hyperthermia and X irradiation. See text for details. Left: (●) sequence (5-1), (○) sequence (5-2). Right: (■) sequence (6-1), (□) sequence (6-2). Vertical bars, ±SD. From Miyakoshi *et al.* (1982a).

As shown in Fig. 15, sequence (1-1) produced fewer survivors through the interval periods up to 24 h (1-2). This result was not remarkably changed when the part of the sequence (44°C + X) was altered by (X + 44°C), that is, sequences (2-1) and (2-2).

In comparisons, regarding immediate survivals and those recovered, between sequences of the pair (1-1) and (1-2), and of all the other five pairs, respectively, there was no apparent change in the order in thermal enhancement ratios (TER) between sequences with and without 37°C intervals. Sequences (1-2) and (2-2) showed no apparent synergistic cell killing effect other than the additive effect. Intervals required to reach plateaus of the recovery curves varied slightly. Sequences (6-1) and (3-1) should be compared, in which intervals were interpolated as follows: in sequence (6-1), (44°C + 42°C) → Intervals → X, and in sequence (3-1), 44°C → Intervals → (42°C + X). The comparison showed that survivors without intervals were the same and that the interval required to reach the plateau of the recovery curve in sequence (3-1) was 4 h. The interval period required to reach the additive level was 24 h, whereas the interval in sequence (6-1) was unclear because of no leveling plateau and was over 24 h, respectively, as shown in Figs. 16 and 17.

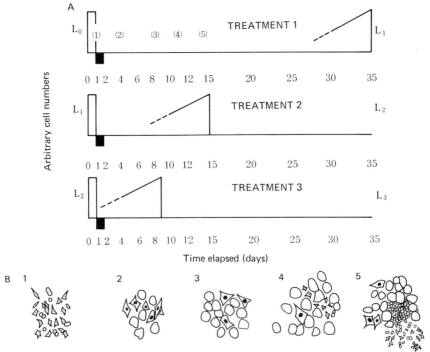

Fig. 18. (A) Schematic illustrations of histories of BLM-resistant L cells. (□, left side) Initial cell numbers; (---——) changes in cell numbers; (■) BLM treatment periods. Numerals in parentheses on treatment 1 represent schematic number of Fig. 18B. (B) Morphological illustration of surviving L cells after BLM treatment (0.1 mg/ml, 24 h). (1) Control; (2) 4, (3) 8, (4) 11, and (5) 14 days after BLM treatment. Incidence: 10^{-6} approximated. From Furukawa *et al.* (1983).

E. Thermochemopotentiation of Bleomycin-Resistant Variant Cells by Low Hyperthermia at 40°C[5]

L cells, a thermosensitive strain, were repeatedly treated with bleomycin, and the survivors with a reduced sensitivity to bleomycin were designated bleomycin-resistant L cells (L_1, L_2, and L_3) according to the frequencies of bleomycin treatment for 24 h, as shown in Fig. 18. Chinese hamster V-79 cells were also treated to obtain bleomycin-resistant strains (V_1, V_2, and V_3). Original V-79 cells showed a further reduced bleomycin sensitivity than did the original L cell.

As shown in Fig. 19, slopes of the time–survival curves for the strains of cells were steeper in the simultaneous 40°C hyperthermia than in the

[5] Furukawa *et al.*, 1983.

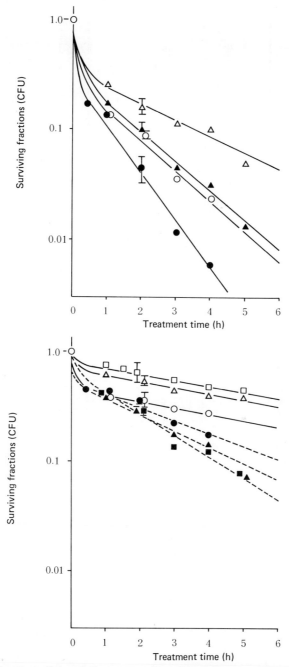

Fig. 19. Bleomycin (0.1 mg/ml) treatment time–survival relationships of original L_0 and L_2 (A) and V_0, V_2, and V_3 cells (B). Treatment at 37°C (open symbols); and at 40°C (closed symbols. Original L_0 cells (○, ●); L_2 cells (△, ▲). (B) Original V_0 cells (○, ●); V_2 cells (△, ▲); V_3 cells (□, ■). Vertical bars, ±SD. From Furukawa *et al.* (1983).

TABLE IV

Parameters of BLM Treatment Time–Survival Curves[a]

	L Cells		V-79 Cells		
	Original cells	Resistant variant two times screening by BLM	Original cells	Resistant variant two times screening by BLM	Resistant variant three times screening by BLM
	L_0	L_2	V_0	V_2	V_3
37°C T_0[b]	93 min	174 min	402 min	402 min	402 min
n[c]	0.28	0.35	0.45	0.69	0.80
40°C T_0	60 min	96 min	213 min	174 min	129 min
n	0.28	0.31	0.52	0.52	0.66
TER[d]	1.55	1.81	1.89	2.31	3.12
	HPG[e]	1.17	HPG	1.22	1.65

[a] Bleomycin (BLM) was treated in 0.1 mg/ml at 37 or 40°C.
[b] Bleomycin treatment time, for which surviving fraction in the resistant exponential portion of treatment time–survival curves were reduced by 1/e.
[c] Extrapolation number on the ordinate.
[d] Thermal enhancement ratio, (T_0 at 37°C)/(T_0 at 40°C).
[e] Hyperthermic potentiation gain at 40°C, (TER of variant cells)/(TER of the original cells).

37°C conventional bleomycin treatment. Parameters of the survival curves, T_0, and n values are shown in Table IV. Thermal enhancement ratio in T_0 of L_2 cells, which originated from bleomycin-sensitive L_0 cells, was 1.81, and that of L_0 cells was 1.55. Hyperthermic potentiation gain (HPG) was represented by TER of resistant variant cells/TER of the original cells and estimated as $1.81/1.55 = 1.17$. In contrast, TER values of V_2 and V_3 cells were 2.31 and 3.12, respectively, and HPG values were $2.31/1.89 = 1.22$ and $3.12/1.89 = 1.65$, respectively, as shown in Table IV.

References

Bauer, K. D., and Henle, K. J. (1979). Arrhenius analysis of heat survival curves from normal and thermotolerant CHO cells. *Radiat. Res.* **78**, 251–263.

Furukawa, M., Kano, E., Yoshikawa, S., Inui, M., Kamimoto, Y., Miyakoshi, J., and Heki, S. (1983). Hyperthermic resensitization of bleomycin-resistant variant strains of murine L-fibroblasts and Chinese hamster V-79 cells *in vitro*. *In* "Fundamentals of Cancer Therapy by Hyperthermia, Radiation and Chemicals" (E. Kano, J. Egawa, Y. Onoyama and R. U, eds.), pp. 171–180. MAG Bros. Inc., Tokyo.

Kano, E., Miyakoshi, J., and Sugahara, T. (1977). Difference in sensitivities to hyperthermia and ionizing radiation of various mammalian cell strains *in vitro*. *In* "Cancer Therapy by Hyperthermia and Radiation" (C. Streffer, D. von Beuninger, F. Dretzel, R. Röttinger, J. E. Robinson, E. Scherer, S. Seeber, and K.-R. Trott, eds.), pp. 188–190. Urban & Schwarzenberg, Baltimore and Munich.

Kano, E., Kato, H., Miyakoshi, J., Ikebuchi, M., Furukawa, M., and Sugahara, T. (1979). Difference in hyperthermia at forty-two and forty-four centigrade degrees and by water bath and high frequency. *Proc. Int. Congr. Radiat. Res. 6th,* pp. 841–846.

Kano, E., Miyakoshi, J., Furukawa, M., and Heki, S. (1981). The recurrent interest in the recent research in experimental hyperthermia for cancer therapy *in vitro. Proc. IAEA Semin. Kyoto 1981,* pp. 137–142.

Kano, E., Miyakoshi, J., Furukawa, M., Kato, H., Ohsaki, S., Nishida, T., and Heki, S. (1982). Effects of hyperthermia at 50°C on V-79 cells *in vitro. J. Radiat. Res.* **23**, 218–227.

Miyakoshi, J., Ikebuchi, M., Furukawa, M., Yamagata, K., Sugahara, T., and Kano, E. (1979). Combined effects of X-irradiation and hyperthermia (42 and 44°C) on Chinese hamster V-79 cells *in vitro. Radiat. Res.* **79**, 77–88.

Miyakoshi, J., Heki, S., Yamagata, K., Furukawa, M., and Kano, E. (1983). Induction of thermotolerance by hyperthermia (42°C and 44°C) in Chinese hamster cells. *In* "Fundamentals of Cancer Therapy by Hyperthermia, Radiation and Chemicals" (E. Kano, J. Egawa, Y. Onoyama and R. U, eds.), pp. 135–147. MAG Bros. Inc., Tokyo.

Miyakoshi, J., Heki, S., Furukawa, M., and Kano, E. (1982a). Recovery kinetics from the damage by step-up and step-down heatings in combination with radiation in Chinese hamster cells. *J. Radiat. Res.* **23**, 187–197.

Miyakoshi, J., Furukawa, M., and Kano, E. (1982b). Recovery kinetics from radiation and hyperthermia (42, 44°C) damages on cultured Chinese hamster V-79 cells. *Natl. Cancer Inst. Monogr.* **61**, 263–266.

Westra, A., and Dewey, W. C. (1971). Variation in sensitivity to heat shock during the cell-cycle of Chinese hamster cells *in vitro. Int. J. Radiat. Biol.* **19**, 467–477.

PART SIX

Cellular Radiosensitivity and Its Mechanisms

24 Radiosensitivity, DNA Repair, and DNA Replication in Cells Derived from Patients with Ataxia Telangiectasia

Osamu Nikaido
Masami Watanabe

Division of Radiation Biology
Faculty of Pharmaceutical Sciences
Kanazawa University, Kanazawa 920, Japan

Tsutomu Sugahara

Kyoto National Hospital
Kyoto 612, Japan

I. Introduction

Ataxia telangiectasia (AT) is a rare autosomal recessive disease, in which patients show characteristic features of immune deficiency, progressive degeneration of cerebellar tissues, ataxia, oculocutaneous telangiectasias, possible leukemia and malignant lymphoma, and a high risk for adverse reactions to therapeutic irradiation. Epidemiological surveys on the incidence among families with AT patients revealed that both patients with AT homozygotes and those with heterozygotes are at high risk for developing cancer (Swift *et al.*, 1976).

The results on radiosensitivity of cells derived from AT heterozygotes are controversial. An intermediate radiosensitivity between normal and AT homozygote cells was noted in cell strains derived from the heterozygotes (Paterson *et al.*, 1979). In contrast, there was a normal radiosensitivity in heterozygote cells when the cells were irradiated with X rays under both hypoxic and oxic conditions (Kinsella *et al.*, 1982).

Factors determining the radiosensitivity of AT cells revealed a deficient removal of γ-endonuclease-sensitive sites in the DNA of certain AT cells (Paterson *et al.*, 1976). However, the discovery of repair-proficient but radiosensitive AT cells ruled out the possibility of AT cells as an X-ray analog to xeroderma pigmentosum cells sensitive to ultraviolet light (Paterson, 1976). The low levels of AT cells in the priming activity of γ-irradiated DNA have been reported (Inoue *et al.*, 1977). It was also found that suppression of DNA synthesis after irradiation is less effective in AT cells (Houldsworth and Lavin, 1980; Painter and Young, 1980; de Wit *et al.*, 1981). How the enhanced rate of DNA synthesis in X-irradiated AT cells reflects the high radiosensitivity remains obscure.

This chapter deals with our preliminary studies on a survey of radiosensitivity among the Japanese population involving use of cells derived from skin biopsies. The cells derived from Japanese AT homozygotes were significantly sensitive to X irradiation, whereas cells from AT heterozygotes were not radiosensitive. The D_0 values of cells derived from apparently healthy individuals ranged from 148 to 166 R. We also analyzed the synthesis and repair of DNA in AT cells irradiated with X rays, by means of alkaline elution and host cell reactivation of γ-irradiated herpes simplex virus. Cells from AT patients showed a higher rate of DNA synthesis than control cells after 2 kR of X irradiation.

II. Materials and Methods

A. Establishment of Cell Strains and Culture Medium

The culture medium was composed of α-modified MEM (Flow Laboratories, McLean, Virginia) supplemented with 10% fetal bovine serum (M. A. Bioproducts, Walkersville, Maryland) and 50 μg/ml of kanamycin sulfate (Yamanouchi Pharmaceutical Co. Ltd., Kyoto, Japan).

Biopsy specimens were obtained from the skin of the upper inner arms of healthy volunteers. Skin specimens were aseptically minced with razor blades into fragments (0.5 × 0.5 mm) after removal of the fat tissues. Three to four pieces of these fragments were placed on a plastic dish onto which 0.5 ml of culture medium had been placed. The dishes were incubated in a humidified 5% CO_2 incubator at 37°C for 4 days, after which 4.5 ml of fresh culture medium were added to each dish. Thereafter the medium was replenished every 4 days. When actively growing fibroblastic cells occupied two-thirds of the culture surface, the cells were treated with 0.1% trypsin (Difco Laboratories, Detroit, Michigan) and 0.01% EDTA–Na_2 (Wako Pharmacy, Osaka, Japan) in Dulbecco's phosphate-buffered saline (PBS), then suspended in culture medium. At this time, the culture age was designated PDN (population doubling number) = 0. An aliquot of cell suspension (10^6 cells/15 ml) was poured into a 75-cm^2 culture flask. Three flasks of cells were successively cultured. Fresh medium was then added biweekly and subcultures carried out from the fourth to the seventh days, just prior to reaching confluency. The PDN attained with each cell strain was calculated by the method described previously (Ban *et al.*, 1980). Cells derived from skin biopsies were assayed for their radiosensitivity at 5 to 14 PDNs.

B. Colony-Forming Method

Cellular radiosensitivity was determined by the colony-forming method. Cells at the exponentially growing phase were trypsinized and resuspended in the culture medium. Each 6 ml of cell suspension was poured into a plastic tube and the preparation irradiated with various doses of X rays. After serial dilution of the irradiated cell suspension with culture medium, 1 ml of the cell suspension (5×10^2–1×10^4 cells/ml) was put into a plastic dish (9 cm diameter) that had been filled with 9 ml of fresh medium. The cells were then incubated in a humidified 5% CO_2 incubator at 37°C for 14 days. The dishes were then rinsed twice with PBS, fixed with ethanol, stained with Giemsa, and examined under a dissecting microscope. Only colonies of over 50 cells were counted.

C. Host Cell Reactivation of γ-Irradiated Herpes Simplex Virus

The procedures for host cell reactivation of virus were the same as previously reported (Nikaido *et al.*, 1980). The stock suspension of herpes simplex virus (HSV), having a titer of 1.5 to 1.7×10^7 pfu/ml against

human amnion F1 cells, was used. This suspension was irradiated with
^{60}Co γ-cell type in a dose of 7.1×10^3 rads at $-75°C$. Each 0.5 ml of γ-
irradiated virus suspension was poured onto freshly confluent cells in a
plastic dish (6 cm diameter) that had been washed with PBS immediately
before virus infection. The cells were incubated at 37°C for 90 min. Virus
adsorption was terminated by adding 4.5 ml of complete medium containing 0.25% human γ globulin (human immunoglobulin: Midori Juji Co.
Ltd., Osaka, Japan). Plaques were scored on the third day of incubation
under a dissecting microscope, and survival curves were depicted as a
function of the γ-ray doses.

D. Cell Labeling and Alkaline Elution Method

Exponentially growing cells were labeled with 0.01 μCi/ml of [*methyl-*
^{14}C]thymidine ([^{14}C]TdR, 50–60 mCi/mmol: Amersham International,
Amersham, United Kingdom) for 8 h. After incubation in fresh medium
for 18 h, cells were irradiated with various doses of X ray at 0°C. These X-
irradiated cells were analyzed in terms of DNA single-strand breaks and
rejoining, using the alkaline elution method. In case of the chase experiment, cells were again labeled with 10 μCi/ml of [*methyl-*^{3}H]thymidine
([^{3}H]TdR, 25 Ci/mmol: Amersham International, Amersham, United
Kingdom) for 10 min after X irradiation and then were incubated at 37°C
in fresh medium containing 5 μg/ml of thymidine (TdR, Wako Pharmacy,
Osaka, Japan) for various periods. Immediately after or at various intervals up to 4 h after [^{3}H]TdR labeling, approximately 5×10^5 to 1×10^6
cells were analyzed using the alkaline elution method.

The alkaline elution method used was the same as that described by
Watanabe *et al.* (Chapter 19, this volume). Cells treated in turn with
[^{14}C]TdR, X ray, and [^{3}H]TdR, and incubated for various periods in the
presence of TdR were trapped on a polyvinyl chloride filter of 2 μm pore
size, washed three times with PBS, and lysed in a lysis solution at 30°C.
These cells were then washed with Na$_3$–EDTA solution to remove the
lysis solution, after which DNA was eluted with alkaline solution in the
dark at a pump speed of 0.07 ml/min. Ten fractions collected at 60-min
intervals were neutralized by adding 2 N HCl. Radioactivity of each fraction was counted in a liquid scintillation counter using Triton X-100 toluene scintillant. Radioactivity remaining on the filter after elution was
estimated by subtracting the total radioactivity of fractions eluted from
the radioactivity on the filter before the elution. This value was confirmed
by the direct measurement of radioactivity remaining on the filter after
and before elution by soaking the filters in 5 ml of the scintillant and
counting in a liquid scintillation counter. The radioactivity remaining on

the filter after elution was shown as a percentage of the radioactivity on the filter before elution. Percentage ^{14}C radioactivity remaining on the filters after elution of X-irradiated cells was normalized against that remaining on the filter after elution of unirradiated control cells. In contrast, percentage ^{3}H radioactivity remaining on the filters after elution of [^{3}H]TdR-labeled cells chased for various hours was normalized against percentage ^{14}C radioactivity on the filters after elution of unirradiated control cells.

E. X Irradiation

Cells were irradiated using Shimadzu Shin-Ai-Go (Shimadzu Mfg. Co., Kyoto, Japan) operating at 182 kVp and 15 mA with 0.9 Cu + 0.5 Al filter, at a dose rate in air of 75 R/min, as measured with a Victoreen condenser chamber before and after the irradiation.

III. Results

A. Assay of Radiosensitivity in Various Cells

Six cell strains derived from normal donors, five from AT homozygotes, and one from AT heterozygotes were examined for radiosensitivity. The survival curves for six normal cell strains exhibited a shoulder region at X-ray doses less than 200 R and declined exponentially with doses of over 200 R. The dose–survival curves for five cell strains derived from AT homozygotes declined exponentially with dose, and AT cell strains are significantly sensitive compared with normal cells, as shown in Fig. 1. However, the cell strain derived from AT heterozygote (AT4M) showed the same radiosensitivity as that of normal cells. The results are summarized in Table I. It is apparent from the table that AT cells derived from Japanese patients show the same levels of radiosensitivity as AT3BI and AT5BI. The D_0 values of normal cell strains were distributed from 148 to 166 R.

B. Repair of DNA Revealed by Host Cell Reactivation of Virus

Various cells were assayed for γ-ray survival of herpes simplex virus. Normal and AT cells did not differ with regard to host cell reactivation of γ-irradiated virus, as shown in Fig. 2.

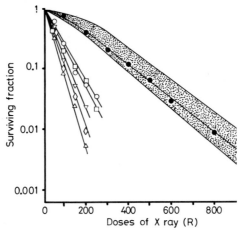

Fig. 1. Dose–survival curves for various cells derived from AT homozygotes (open symbols) and an AT heterozygote (●). Dotted area is delineated by the extremes of the means of the six strains shown in Table I.

TABLE I

Cell Survival after X Irradiation of Various Cell Strains

Strain	Description	Sex	Age at biopsy	Number of experiments	Plating efficiency	D_0(R)
A.H.	Normal	F	1.8	4	20.3	162 ± 7[a]
T.H.	Normal	F	32	3	6.9	148 ± 15
J.N.	Normal	F	30	3	8.3	163 ± 12
H.I.	Normal	M	20	2	20.0	166 ± 8
K.W.	Normal	M	24	2	8.5	157 ± 12
Y.O.	Normal	F	33	3	6.7	152 ± 5
AT1OS[b]	AT homozygote	M	10	2	9.3	45 ± 10
AT14OT[c]	AT homozygote	M	7	3	14.7	70 ± 6
AT4TO[d]	AT homozygote	F	11	2	1.8	40 ± 12
AT3BI[e]	AT homozygote	M	4	2	5.2	52 ± 15
AT5BI[e]	AT homozygote	M	18	2	17.1	63 ± 7
AT4MTO[d]	AT heterozygote, mother of AT4TO	F	—[f]	3	12.3	157 ± 15

[a] Mean ±SE.
[b] From Dr. M. Ikenaga, Osaka, Japan.
[c] From Dr. A. Shima, Ohtsu, Japan.
[d] From Dr. M. S. Sasaki, Kyoto, Japan.
[e] From Dr. D. G. Harden, Birmingham, United Kingdom.
[f] Unknown.

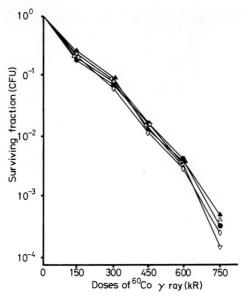

Fig. 2. Host cell reactivation of γ-irradiated herpes simplex virus in cells derived from normal donors, A.H. (●) and K.W. (▲); and AT homozygotes AT1OS (◊), AT3BI (▽), and AT5BI (△).

Both AT3BI cells defined as repair deficient and AT5BI cells as repair proficient (Paterson, 1976) showed the same repairability to γ-damage of DNA as normal cells, as revealed by host cell reactivation of the virus. Zamansky and Little (1982) reported much the same observation.

C.   Single-Strand Breaks and Rejoining in DNA

Exponentially growing cells were labeled with [^{14}C]TdR for 8 h, incubated at 37°C for 18 h without labeling, and then irradiated with various doses of X ray at 0°C. Alkaline elution of ^{14}C-labeled DNA was carried out immediately after irradiation. Elution patterns of DNA from X-irradiated normal cells are shown in Fig. 3. Percentage of radioactivity remaining on the filter declined exponentially with increasing fraction numbers when the cells were irradiated with X-ray doses up to 0.5 kR. However, elution patterns became biphasic in cells irradiated with doses of over 1.0 kR. Percentage of radioactivity remaining on the filter at the tenth fraction in irradiated cells was normalized to that in unirradiated cells, as described in Section II. These normalized values of radioactivity (percentage of control) in both normal and AT cells immediately and at 2 h incuba-

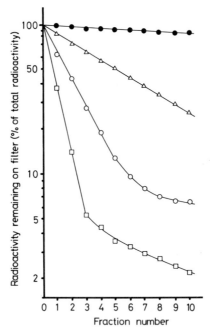

Fig. 3. Alkaline elution profiles for ¹⁴C-labeled DNA in normal cells irradiated with various doses of X ray. Cells were irradiated with 0 (●), 0.5 (△), 1.0 (○), and 1.5 kR (□).

tion after X irradiation were plotted as a function of X-ray doses, as shown in Fig. 4. The normalized radioactivity on the filter in both normal and AT cells declined exponentially with increasing doses of X ray. There were no significant differences in the trend of decline of normalized radioactivity remaining on the filters, between normal and AT cells. The retention of radioactivity appeared to recover to the level of the unirradiated controls, within 2 h incubation after 0.5 kR of X irradiation. In contrast, this recovery in cells irradiated with high doses of over 1.0 kR was not completed within 2 h incubation. Again there were no significant differences in the rate of the recovery between normal and AT cells incubated for 2 h after irradiation. These results suggest that induction and rejoining of DNA single-strand breaks in AT cells take place in the same manner as in normal cells.

D. Retention of ³H-Labeled Cellular DNA on the Filters at Various Incubation Times

Cells template labeled with [¹⁴C]TdR were irradiated with 0 or 2 kR of X ray and labeled with a high concentration of [³H]TdR for 10 min. After

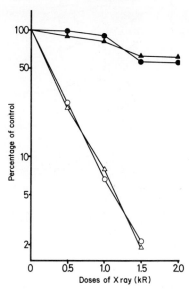

Fig. 4. The relationship between X-ray doses and radioactivity remaining on the filter, and the recovery of radioactivity at 2 h incubation after 0.5-kR X-ray. Open symbols indicate cells eluted immediately after X irradiation; closed symbols show that the cells were incubated at 37°C for 2 h after X ray and then eluted. Normal A.H. cells (○, ●); AT10S cells (△, ▲).

various numbers of hours of chase incubation at 37°C in the presence of TdR, the cells were examined by the alkaline elution method. Elution patterns of both ^{14}C- and ^{3}H-labeled DNA in unirradiated normal cells incubated for various times after [^{3}H]TdR labeling are shown in Fig. 5. Percentage ^{3}H radioactivity remaining on the filters declined biphasically when cellular DNA was eluted immediately after the labeling (0 h). Percentages of ^{3}H radioactivity remaining on the filters increased with increasing chase time and reached the same level as those of ^{14}C radioactivity with 8 h incubation (data not shown).

Figure 6 shows the normalized radioactivity of both ^{14}C and ^{3}H remaining on the filters at various chase times after 2 kR of X irradiation followed by [^{3}H]TdR pulse labeling. Normalized ^{14}C radioactivity remaining on the filter in X-irradiated normal and AT cells increased with increasing chase time up to 1 h and decreased thereafter. In contrast, normalized ^{3}H radioactivity retained on the filters increased in both X-irradiated normal and AT cells up to 4 h. However, a significant retardation of normalized ^{3}H radioactivity on the filters in X-irradiated normal cells is appearent compared to that in unirradiated normal cells. X-Irradiated AT cells seem to retain more normalized ^{3}H radioactivity on the filters than X-irradiated normal cells after 4 h incubation. Nevertheless, a significant retardation in

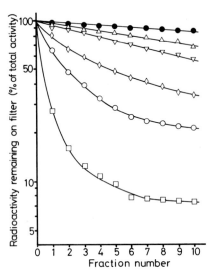

Fig. 5. Changes of ³H radioactivity remaining on filter in cells at various chase times. Elution profiles for ³H-labeled DNA were obtained from normal A.H. cells immediately after (□), 1 h (○), 2 h (◇), 4 h (▽), and 6 h (△) after [³H]TdR labeling. Closed symbols show the profile for ¹⁴C-labeled DNA.

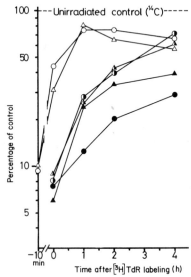

Fig. 6. Changes of retention of both ¹⁴C-labeled and ³H-labeled DNA on filters in cells chased for various numbers of hours. Template-labeled cells with [¹⁴C]TdR were irradiated with 2 kR of X ray at −10 min followed by a 10-min pulse labeling with [³H]TdR. Percentage of ¹⁴C and ³H radioactivity remaining on filters in irradiated cells was normalized to ¹⁴C radioactivity in unirradiated cells. For details, see Section II. AT1OS cells (△, ▲, ▲); normal A.H. cells (○, ◐, ○). Open symbols show the retention of ¹⁴C-labeled DNA in cells chased for various numbers of hours after X ray (2 kR). Half-closed symbols show the retention of ³H-labeled DNA in unirradiated cells chased for various numbers of hours. Closed symbols show the retention of ³H-labeled DNA in cells chased for various numbers of hours after X irradiation (2 kR).

normalized ^{3}H radioactivity at the fourth hour of incubation was observed in X-irradiated AT cells in comparison with that in unirradiated AT cells.

IV. Discussion

The results obtained in this study show that radiosensitivity, defined as the D_0 of cells from the Japanese normal population, varies widely, and that Japanese AT cells are highly sensitive to X irradiation (Fig. 1 and Table I). However, radiosensitivity of one cell strain derived from an AT heterozygote was categorized into the range of the normal cells.

We attempted to detect repair deficiency in AT cells by means of host cell reactivation of γ-irradiated herpes simplex virus. However, none of the AT cells showed retarded levels of host cell reactivation (Fig. 2). These results are in good agreement with the data of Zamansky and Little (1982). Furthermore, AT3BI cells defined as deficient in repairability to γ-endonuclease-sensitive sites showed the same ability in host cell reactivation as repair-proficient AT5BI cells. Host cell reactivation of ultraviolet light-irradiated herpes simplex virus has been frequently used as a probe to detect deficient repairability in various xeroderma pigmentosum cells (Lytle *et al.*, 1982). Other investigators found a lesser degree of suppression of DNA synthesis in AT cells after irradiation with ionizing radiation (Houldsworth and Lavin, 1980; Painter and Young, 1980; de Wit *et al.*, 1981). We also investigated DNA synthesis in AT cells after irradiation with various doses of X ray and found that the normal rate of DNA synthesis was preserved, even after 4 kR of X irradiation (data not shown). This radiotolerant DNA synthesis in AT cells was attributed to a diminished suppression of DNA initiation (Painter and Young, 1980).

The alkaline elution method has been used to detect DNA single-strand breaks and their rejoining in mammalian cells (Formace and Little, 1980). In this study, the extent of DNA single-strand breaks induced by X irradiation up to 2 kR and their rejoining during subsequent incubation for 2 h were not significantly different in normal and AT cells, as shown in Fig. 4. These results are consistent with the findings of Fornace and Little (1980) and Taylor *et al.* (1975).

As shown in Fig. 5, when chase incubation time was not over 2 h, the elution profiles for ^{3}H-labeled DNA were biphasic. However, by prolonging the chase time to 4 h, the elution profiles for DNA became linear and resembled those for ^{14}C-labeled DNA irradiated with X-ray doses less than 0.5 kR. These results clearly indicate that the retention of ^{3}H-labeled DNA on filters increased with increasing chase time and suggest chain elongation of the newly synthesized DNA during chase incubation. The biphasic nature of the profiles for ^{3}H-labeled DNA from pulse-labeled cells were interpreted as a rapidly eluting component composed of relatively small DNA molecules, and a slowly eluting component representing labels attached to preexisting larger DNA molecules (Meyn and Fletcher, 1981). In this experiment, percentage radioactivity remaining on the filters from the tenth fraction was taken as a value representing the fraction of the slowly eluting component in total radioactivity retained on the filters before elution. However, neither actual rates of chain elongation of newly synthesized DNA nor molecular weight of single-stranded DNA could be obtained in this study because of the qualitative nature of the alkaline elution method.

The retention of ^{3}H radioactivity in both normal and AT X-irradiated cells was compared with their unirradiated counterparts at various chase times. The results shown in Fig. 6 suggest that the normalized ^{3}H radioactivity remaining on the filter in X-irradiated AT cells was higher than that in X-irradiated normal cells and comparable to that in unirradiated AT and normal cells 2 h after chase incubation. Thus, the suppression effect of 2 kR of X ray on DNA chain elongation was evident only in normal cells. Incorporation of [^{3}H]TdR into DNA during a 10-min pulse-labeling period after X irradiation was slightly lower in normal cells than in AT cells, indicating that the suppression of DNA synthesis after X irradiation was more pronounced in normal cells (data not shown). In contrast, normalized ^{14}C radioactivity remaining on the filters in X-irradiated normal and AT cells increased within 1 h but never reached the level in unirradiated control cells, and it decreased thereafter. The latter result may indicate the degradation of DNA in cells irradiated with high doses of X ray.

In conclusion, we examined the radiosensitivity of cells derived from not only healthy donors and AT homozygotes but AT heterozygotes, in a Japanese population. Radiosensitivity of normal human cells, defined as D_0, was distributed widely from 148 to 166 R. Japanese AT cells were sensitive to X ray and showed comparable radiosensitivity with AT3BI and AT5BI cells. The results of host cell reactivation of γ-irradiated virus infecting AT cells did not confirm a deficient repairability to γ-damaged DNA. Furthermore, application of the alkaline elution method to detect the extent of ^{3}H radioactivity retained on the filters revealed a lesser suppression of DNA synthesis in AT cells after X irradiation.

Acknowledgments

We are grateful to Drs. M. S. Sasaki, M. Ikenaga, A. Shima, and D. G. Harnden for kind donations of various cells and skin biopsies derived from AT homozygotes and heterozygotes. This work was supported in part by a Grant-in-Aid from the Ministry of Education, Science and Culture, Japan.

References

Ban, S., Nikaido, O., and Sugahara, T. (1980). Acute and late effects of a single exposure of ionizing radiation on cultured human diploid cell populations. *Radiat. Res.* **81,** 120–130.

de Wit, J., Jaspers, N. G. J., and Bootsma, D. (1981). The rate of DNA synthesis in normal human and ataxia telangiectasia cells after exposure to X-irradiation. *Mutat. Res.* **80,** 221–226.

Formace, A. J., Jr., and Little, J. B. (1980). Normal repair of DNA single strand breaks in patients with ataxia telangiectasia. *Biochim. Biophys. Acta* **607,** 432–437.

Houldsworth, J., and Lavin, M. F. (1980). Effect of ionizing radiation on DNA synthesis in ataxia telangiectasia cells. *Nucleic Acids Res.* **8,** 3709–3720.

Inoue, T., Hirano, K., Yokoiyama, A., Kada, T., and Kato, H. (1977). DNA repair enzymes in ataxia telangiectasia and Bloom's syndrome fibroblasts. *Biochim. Biophys. Acta* **479,** 497–500.

Kinsella, T. J., Mitchell, J. B., McPherson, S., Russo, A., and Tietze, F. (1982). *In vitro* X-ray sensitivity in ataxia telangiectasia homozygote and heterozygote skin fibroblasts under oxic and hypoxic conditions. *Cancer Res.* **42,** 3950–3956.

Lytle, C. D., Nikaido, O., Hitchins, V. M., and Jacobson, E. D. (1982). Host cell reactivation by excision repair is error-free in human cells. *Mutat. Res.* **94,** 405–412.

Meyn, R. E., and Fletcher, S. E. (1981). Measurement of postreplication repair by alkaline elution. *In* "DNA Repair: A Laboratory Manual of Research Procedures" (E. C. Friedberg and P. C. Hanawalt, eds.), pp. 487–492. Dekker, New York.

Nikaido, O., Ban, S., and Sugahara, T. (1980). Population doubling numbers in cells with genetic disorders. *Adv. Exp. Med. Biol.* **129,** 303–311.

Painter, R. B., and Young, B. R. (1980). Radiosensitivity in ataxia-telangiectasia: a new explanation. *Proc. Natl. Acad. Sci. USA* **77,** 7315–7317.

Paterson, M. C. (1976). Ataxia telangiectasia: an inherited human disease involving radiosensitivity, malignancy and defective DNA repair. *In* "Research in Photobiology" (A. Castellani, ed.), pp. 207–218. Plenum, New York.

Paterson, M. C., Smith, B. P., Lohman, P. H. M., Anderson, A. K., and Fishman, L. (1976). Defective excision repair of γ-ray-damaged DNA in human (ataxia telangiectasia) fibroblasts. *Nature (London)* **260,** 444–447.

Paterson, M. C., Anderson, A. K., Smith, B. P., and Smith, P. J. (1979). Enhanced radiosensitivity of cultured fibroblasts from ataxia telangiectasia heterozygotes manifested by defective colony-forming ability and reduced DNA repair replication after hypoxic-irradiation. *Cancer Res.* **39,** 3725–3734.

Swift, M., Shalman, L., Perry, M., and Chase, C. (1976). Malignant neoplasms in the families of patients with ataxia telangiectasia. *Cancer Res.* **36,** 209–215.

Taylor, A. M. R., Harden, D. G., Arlett, C. F., Harcourt, S. A., Lehmann, A. R., Stevens, S., and Bridges, B. A. (1975). Ataxia telangiectasia: a human mutation with abnormal radiation sensitivity. *Nature (London)* **258,** 427–429.

Zamansky, G. B., and Little, J. B. (1982). Survival of ^{60}Co-irradiated herpes simplex virus in 15 human diploid fibroblast cell strains. *Mutat. Res.* **94,** 245–255.

25 Physical Modification of Thermal Neutron-Induced Biological Effects

Yowri Ujeno

Department of Experimental Radiology,
Faculty of Medicine, Kyoto University
Kyoto 606, Japan

I. Introduction

The biological effects and/or clinical application of various kinds of high-LET (linear energy transfer) radiation, including neutrons, protons, heavy particles, and pions, have been studied. The fast neutrons have been associated with biological and clinical research, but little is known of the biological effects of thermal neutrons, the final form of fast neutrons that lose energy in the materials. It is difficult to acquire massive thermal neutrons unless a nuclear reactor is available. In this chapter the thermal neutrons are considered as those with energies of 0.250 E-7 MeV. In International Commission on Radiation Units and Measurements (1969),

Modification of Radiosensitivity in Cancer Treatment

477

the thermal neutrons are defined as the neutrons with energies with an effective cadmium cutoff of less than about 0.5 eV.

Factors regarding thermal neutrons studied in radiation biology can be classified into two categories.

1. Physicotechnological factors
   a. The complexity of nuclear reactions in tissues by thermal neutrons
   b. The contaminations of γ rays and other neutrons in the thermal neutron beam, or difficulty in acquiring practically pure thermal neutron fluence
   c. $^{10}B(n,\alpha)^7Li$ nuclear reaction
   d. $^{31}P(n,\gamma)^{32}P$ nuclear reaction
   e. Others
2. Biological factors
   a. Comparative radiosensitivity of normal and malignant cells to thermal neutrons
   b. Distributions of elements, especially, ^1H, ^{10}B, ^{14}N, ^{23}Na, or ^{31}P, in cells
   c. The volume and the shape of subjects irradiated with thermal neutrons
   d. The biological effects of mixed radiation
   e. The characteristics of biological effects induced by high-LET radiation

These factors are mainly discussed with reference to the radiobiological experiments.

II. Technological Problems

One of the most important requirements for experiments in radiation biology of thermal neutrons is to have a radiation field that will ensure a massive and practically pure thermal neutron beam, contaminated little with primary γ rays and other neutrons. It is all but impossible to eliminate primary γ rays and neutrons completely, except thermal neutrons, from the nuclear reactor beam. The primary γ rays referred to herein are those occurring not only in the core of the nuclear reactor but also in the wall of the reactor. Of considerable importance is how the radiation field (of thermal neutrons) is set with a low γ : thermal neutrons ratio and a low cadmium (Cd) ratio.

In the Research Reactor Institute of Kyoto University (KUR), the field is constructed according to the bismuth scatter method (Kanda *et al.,*

1975). When there is no material that will induce secondary γ rays in the radiation field, the γ : thermal neutron ratio is about 0.005 at 15 cm from the window surface of the bismuth block set into the lead wall of the reactor. In this case, the thermal neutron fluence of 0.96×10^9 n/cm² is assumed to be 1 rem unit, and the exposure in R units of primary γ rays is divided by the rem value of thermal neutrons. The ratio is about one order less than the values of other institutions in the world (Kanda et al., 1975; Aizawa et al., 1980).

III. Induction of Secondary γ Rays

The biological materials—that is, cells, culture medium, mammalian body, or experimental equipment—induce various energies of γ rays when irradiated with thermal neutrons. In such cases, γ rays due to $^1H(n,\gamma)^2H$ reaction should be taken into account in biological experiments because of the large amount of hydrogen element and the comparatively high energy of 2.22 MeV of γ rays. For this reason, the volume of culture medium should be kept at a minimum to decrease the secondary γ rays induced in the medium. The secondary γ rays induced in the experimental equipment are large in comparison with the kerma value of thermal neutrons or primary γ rays and increases the total absorbed dose in cells. For example, the ratio of thermal neutron fluence: γ rays (n/cm²/R) is about 60 times higher in the most suitable experimental condition than in the most unsuitable condition (Ujeno et al., 1980). In our experiment, a thin Teflon box, dry circulating air to maintain constant the temperature in the box, a Teflon cell container, and a special para-γ wagon constructed with Teflon, bismuth, and a small amount of aluminum, are used. Using these materials, few secondary γ rays are induced (Ujeno et al., 1980).

IV. Elements in Cells

To estimate the absorbed dose of thermal neutrons, it is necessary to know both the macro- and microscopic distributions of elements that induce deleterious nuclear reactions due to thermal neutrons. In this case, the distributions of molecules need not be taken into account, because molecular structures are independent of nuclear reactions.

Considering the amount of elements in tissues, the released energy, and the cross section to thermal neutrons, ^1H, ^{10}B, and ^{14}N are the most important elements that induce reactions of $^1H(n,\gamma)^2H$, $^{14}N(n,p)^{14}C$, $^{10}B(n,\alpha)^7Li$, and $^{10}B(n,\alpha)^7Li^*$. The nuclear reaction of $^{31}P(n,\alpha)^{32}P$ plays a definite role in the cell killing, if ^{31}P in the DNA molecules transmutates to ^{32}P. The actual killing effect of thermal neutrons to amoebae is higher than the killing effect estimated with the absorbed doses of induced γ rays in the nuclear reaction because of the transmutation (Kawai *et al.*, 1977). The nuclear reaction of ^{23}Na(n,γ)^{24}Na is also evident because of a certain amount of ^{23}Na included in the culture medium. The transmutant ^{24}Na releases energy with 2.75 MeV (maximum), but its physical half-life is short, that is, 14.96 h. Details on the macroscopic distribution of elements in various tissues of the reference materials, including human, animals, and plants, have been documented (Ujeno, 1982). The amount of ^{10}B is negligible in mammalian tissues. The amount of hydrogen in cells has to be measured in order to estimate the dose of thermal neutrons. It should also be pointed out that the amount of hydrogen varies, depending on phase of the cell cycle. Hydrogen is present in larger amounts in the M phase than in the S phase (Beall *et al.*, 1976).

V. Dose Estimation

The experimental equipment and geometrical positions of the equipment in the field also modify the thermal neutron fluence and the absorbed doses of primary and secondary γ rays. For these reasons, it is necessary to measure the thermal neutron fluence and the absorbed doses of γ rays at each position of the equipment and at each irradiation. The thermal neutron fluence is measured with a gold foil, and γ rays are measured with TLD (thermal luminescence dosimeter) powder, in special small Teflon tube containers in order to avoid the induction of secondary γ rays in the containers of the TLD power.

A. Dose of Thermal Neutrons

With regard to conversion of the absorbed dose from the fluence, the conversion factor of 9.36×10^8 n/cm^2 to 1 rem published in International Commission on Radiation Protection (ICRP) (1971) is the value proper for the field of health physics but not for the field of radiation biology. A value, 0.272 E-01 to $10^7 \times (\mu\kappa/\rho)$E in erg/cm^2/g for tissue approximation is reported in ICRU (1969), although the kerma factor of thermal neutrons is not given to tissue approximation in ICRU (1977). The relationship of kerma to fluence is given in a graph (Snyder, 1958). The kerma values were calculated by Bach and Caswell (1968). These values vary slightly, however, depending on the data used for calculation. For this reason, the equations related to each material should be part of each experiment. The conversion equations from thermal neutron fluence to absorbed dose have been described in detail (Brownell *et al.*, 1963; Kobayashi and Kanda, 1977).

The following equation is used in our experiments, where E_ι is the

$$D(\text{rads}) = \sum_\iota E_\iota(\text{rads/cm}^2/\text{n})\rho_\iota\Phi(\text{cm}^2) + 1.77 \times 10^{-10}(\text{rads/cm/n})P_\text{H}(\text{g})\rho_\iota\Phi(\text{cm}^{-2})\Delta t(\text{cm})$$

kerma value in rads of element ι, ρ_ι is the abundance of element ι, P_H is the weight of hydrogen in 1 g of material, Φ is the thermal neutron fluence, and Δt is the thickness of material. In this calculation, ι means only ^{14}N approximately.

If neutrons with various energies are included in the nuclear reactor beams, we have to calculate the absorbed dose of neutrons with each energy. For example, Zamenhof *et al.* (1975) calculated these values using the program code LASL 42 of Sandmeir *et al.* (1974), which is constructed with Harris' (1970) code of ANDY and Engle's (1967) data of ANISN. It should be pointed out that other data cannot directly be used to calculate the absorbed dose as there are differences in data, including constants.

B. The Volume and Shape of Subject

As shown in the equation just given, the absorbed dose of γ rays of ^{1}H(n,γ)^{2}H depends on the Δt value. For example, this is about 5×10^{-4} cm for a cell, but the values listed in the table of Loevinger *et al.* (1956) with regard to the average geometrical factors are used for tumors or bodies. The difference in Δt values of cells and whole bodies is over several orders. The value is 0.89 cm for our Teflon tubes containing the cells used in our experiments.

C. The Dose Delivered with ^{10}B(n,α)^{7}Li Reaction

This is the most important reaction with regard to neutron capture therapy. The energy of α or ^{7}Li is 1.492 MeV or 0.852 MeV, and the average track length of both particles is about 8.96 or 4.81 μm in water, respectively. For the track length, the reactions occurring not only in the cell nucleus but also in the cell plasma or even on the cell surface can destroy the DNA molecules in the cell nuclei. However, if the reaction occurs more than 9 μm distant from the surface of cells in the culture medium, these particles cannot destroy the cells. Thus, the dose in the cells does not correspond to that in the culture medium. The details of dose calculation of the reaction in a microscopic region were reported by Kitao (1975); that is, the absorbed dose of α and ^7Li in the model tumors and in the wall of fine blood vessels can be estimated with his "combined LET" method and geometrical factors. This calculating method is useful for neutron capture therapy against brain tumors. Estimation of the dose using the length of track relative to the radius of cell nucleus has most recently been reported (Kobayashi and Kanda, 1982).

It is most difficult to estimate quantitatively the contribution of this reaction in biological effects. Some authors expressed it as a RBE (relative biological effectiveness) value (Matsumura *et al.,* 1962; Davis *et al.,* 1969, 1970; Saigusa and Ueno, 1978), a maximum usable depth (MUD) (Zamenhof *et al.,* 1975), a boron accumulation effect (BAE) (Kobayashi and Kanda, 1977), or the boron selective dose ratio (BSDR) (Kobayashi and Kanda, 1982). However, this can probably be simply and adequately expressed as an absorbed dose (rads or Gy). However, if the data calculated with the track structure theory (Butts and Katz, 1967; Saigusa and Ueno, 1978) are compared with those calculated with the relative track length method (Kobayashi and Kanda, 1982), despite differences in the processes of calculation, the doses related to a low survival of cells *in vitro* are similar (Ujeno, 1982).

VI. Characteristics of Biological Effects of Mixed Radiation and Modifications of the Effects

The nuclear reactor beams are a typical form of mixed radiation. Whether the biological effects of mixed radiation are simply the added effects of each component has to be given attention. Akaboshi *et al.* (1973) showed that the biological effects of nuclear beams followed with γ rays are different from those of irradiations in the reversed order, thereby suggesting that the repair processes of damage due to thermal neutrons differ from those related to γ-ray damages, qualitatively and/or quantitatively.

Characteristics of nuclear reactor beams can also be observed in chromosomal aberration. Multitype and isochromatid aberrations are most evident after irradiation of nuclear reactor beams. Irradiation with 97.8 cGy induced a 10% multitype aberration in cells of *Muntiacus muntjak* (Ujeno, 1982).

The total absorbed dose given with thermal neutrons is enhanced with increases in the amount of hydrogen element in the materials. If some of the hydrogen in materials is replaced by deuterium, the absorbed dose decreases; thus the biological effect decreases necessarily, and this was verified with inactivation of DNase I (Akaboshi *et al.,* 1980). However, the killing effect of thermal neutrons on mammalian cells increased in culture medium containing D_2O (Ujeno and Takimoto, 1980). This result suggests that the deuterium element interferes with biological processes, probably those related to repair of radiation-induced damage in mammalian cells. The enhancement by deuterium is observed in the cell killing due to a low-LET radiation (Ben-Hur and Riklis, 1980; Ben-Hur *et al.,* 1980; Utsumi *et al.,* 1981). The deuterium enhancement ratio (der) was higher in irradiation of X rays with low LET value than of nuclear reactor beams with a comparatively high LET value (Ujeno and Takimoto, 1980).

VII. The Theoretical Estimations of Dose and RBE of Thermal Neutrons

The estimations of dose–survival curves using the track structure theory (Butts and Katz, 1967) were reported from our laboratory (Saigusa and Ueno, 1978). As the four parameters necessary to estimate the curves by this theory, the following values were used: E_0 (D_0 value) = 190 rads, m (an extrapolation number) = 2.5, δ_0 (a plateau value of the extrapolated cross section) = 4.6×10^{-7} cm^2, and K ($Z^2/\beta^2 \times \frac{1}{4}$ where Z is an effective charge number and β is a relative speed) = 1400. The calculated RBE value of thermal neutron beams with a γ-ray contamination of 0.005 was about 3.0 in the 10^{-8} surviving fraction.

The RBE values of thermal neutrons on the tumor level (Ujeno *et al.,* 1981) were slightly smaller than those of the cellular level (Ujeno *et al.,* 1980). This is because the contributions of γ rays on the tumor-bearing mouse body is not taken into account in the calculation. These data also were smaller than the theoretically estimated data (Saigusa and Ueno, 1978), as the contamination of γ rays in practical experimental conditions is greater than that estimated theoretically, in air. These results are given in Table I.

VIII. Conclusion

Problems remain with regard to the biological effects of thermal neutrons. Our results presented herein are the findings obtained after close cooperation with biologists, chemists, physicists, and technologists. The macro- and microscopic doses, the quality of radiation, and physical fac-

TABLE I

The RBE Values on Nuclear Reactor Beams

Experimental conditions	RBE	References
Seeds of *Triticum monococcum flavescens*		Matsumura *et al.* (1962)
Chromosome aberration, α and ^{7}Li	23 ± 10	
Chlorophyll mutation, α ^{7}Li	29 ± 10	
Cell killing		Davis *et al.* (1969)
MTTR (M.I.T. Nuclear Reactor) beam	1.51	
Neutrons	2.2	
γ	0.8	
Cell killing		Davis *et al.* (1970)
α	3.7	
Tissue, >2 Gy		Zamenhof *et al.* (1975)
Thermal neutrons	2.2	
γ	1.0	
α and ^{7}Li	3.7	
Tissue		Kanda *et al.* (1975)
p and α	5	
Cell killing, >2 Gy, calculated values		Saigusa and Ueno (1978)
p and α	3.2	
Cell killing, >2 Gy		Ujeno *et al.* (1980)
KUR (Kyoto University Reactor) beam	1.44	
Thermal neutrons	2.17	
Mouse tumor		Ujeno *et al.* (1981)
KUR (Kyoto University Reactor) beam	1.32	
Thermal neutrons	1.80	

tors such as the amount of elements, volume, or shape of the subject can readily be altered, thus making feasible various experimental projects. Chemical substances carrying a large amount of ^{10}B in the tumor have to be improved, and chemical, pharmacological, and pharmaceutical studies on ^{10}B and boron chemistry remain to be done. Some clinical data on neutron capture therapy in Japan have been reported (Hatanaka, 1983).

References

Aizawa, O., Kanda, K., Nozaki, T., and Matsumoto, T. (1980). Remodeling and dosimetry on the neutron irradiation facility of the Musashi Institute of Technology reactor for boron neutron capture therapy. *Nucl. Technol.* **48**, 150–163.

Akaboshi, M., Kawai, K., Maeda, T., and Shimizu, A. (1973). Effects of thermal neutrons on living cells. I. Lethal effects of thermal neutrons on amoeba. *J. Radiat. Res.* **14**, 411–416.

Akaboshi, M., Kawai, K., Maki, H., and Honda, Y. (1980). Inactivation of deoxyribonuclease I in aqueous solution. *Int. J. Radiat. Biol.* **37,** 677–683.

Bach, R. L., and Caswell, R. S. (1968). Energy transfer to matter by neutrons. *Radiat. Res.* **35,** 1–25.

Beall, P. T., Hazlewood, C. F., and Rao, P. N. (1976). Nuclear magnetic resonance patterns of intracellular water as a function of HeLa cell cycle. *Science (Washington, D.C.)* **192,** 904–907.

Ben-Hur, E., and Riklis, E. (1980). Deuterium oxide enhancement of Chinese hamster cell response to γ radiation. *Radiat. Res.* **81,** 224–235.

Ben-Hur, E., Utsumi, H., and Elkind, M. M. (1980). Potentially lethal and DNA radiation damage: similarities in inhibition of repair by medium containing D_2O and hypertonic buffer. *Radiat. Res.* **84,** 25–34.

Brownell, G. L., Raju, M. R., Rydin, R. A., and Schermer, R. I. (1963). Neutron spectroscopy and dosimetry at the medical-therapy facility of the Massachusetts Institute of Technology reactor. *In* "Neutron Dosimetry" (Vol. 1, pp. 51–70). IAEA, Vienna.

Butts, J. J., and Katz, R. (1967). Theory of RBE for heavy ion bombardment of dry enzymes and viruses. *Radiat. Res.* **30,** 855–871.

Davis, M. A., Little, J. B., Reddy, A. R., and Ayyangar, K. (1969). RBE of the M.I.T. medical therapy neutron beam in monolayer cultures of HeLa cells. *Health Phys.* **16,** 469–473.

Davis, M. A., Little, J. B., Ayyangar, K. M. M. S., and Reddy, A. R. (1970). Relative biological effectiveness of the $^{10}B(n,\alpha)^7Li$ reaction in HeLa cells. *Radiat. Res.* **43,** 534–553.

Engle, W. W. (1967). Union Carbide Corp. Rep. No. K–1963.

Harris. D. R. (1970). LASL Rep. No. LA–4539.

Hatanaka, H. (1983). Clinical experience of boron-10 slow neutron capture therapy. *In* "Synthesis and Applications of Isotopically Labeled Compounds" (W. P. Duncan and A. B. Susan, eds.), pp. 167–174. Elsevier, Amsterdam.

International Commission on Radiation Protection (1973). "Data for protection against ionizing radiation from external sources, supplement to ICRP Publication 15, A report of ICRP Committee 3," International Commission on Radiation Protection, Pergamon Press, Oxford. (ICRP Publ. 21).

International Commission on Radiation Units and Measurements (1969). "Neutron fluence, neutron spectra and kerma," International Commission on Radiation Units and Measurements, Washington, D.C. (ICRU Publ. 13).

International Commission on Radiation Units and Measurements (1977). "Neutron dosimetry for biology and medicine," International Commission on Radiation Units and Measurements, Washington, D.C. (ICRU Publ. 26).

Kanda, K., Kobayashi, T., Ono, K., Sato, T., Shibata, T., Ueno, Y., Mishima, Y., Hatanaka, H., and Nishiwaki, Y. (1975). Elimination of gamma rays from a thermal neutron field for medical and biological irradiation purposes. *In* "Biomedical Dosimetry" (pp. 205–223). IAEA, Vienna.

Kawai, K., Maki, H., and Akaboshi, M. (1977). Effects of thermal neutrons on living cells. III. Estimation of absorbed dose in amoeba irradiated by thermal neutrons. *J. Radiat. Res.* **18,** 268–274.

Kitao, K. (1975). A method for calculation of the absorbed dose near interface from $^{10}B(n,\alpha)^7Li$ reaction. *Radiat. Res.* **61,** 304–314.

Kobayashi, T., and Kanda, K. (1977). "Estimation of Absorbed Energy in Cell Nucleus for Neutron Capture Therapy" (Rep. No. KURRI-TR-158). Kyoto Univ. Res. Reactor Inst., Kyoto.

Kobayashi, T., and Kanda, K. (1982). Analytical calculation of boron-10 dosage in cell nucleus for neutron capture therapy. *Radiat. Res.* **91,** 77–94.

Loevinger, R., Holt, J. G., and Hine, G. J. (1956). Internally administered radioisotopes. *In* "Radiation Dosimetry" (G. J. Hine and G. L. Brownell, eds.), pp. 801–873. Academic Press, New York.

Matsumura, S., Kondo, S., and Mabuchi, T. (1962). Boron effects upon gamma-ray and thermal neutron irradiation in einkorn wheat; RBE of heavy particles from $^{10}B(n,\alpha)^7Li$ reaction. *Seiken Jiho* **14,** 86–92.

Saigusa, T., and Ueno, Y. (1978). Calculated responses to a thermal neutron beam for hamster and HeLa cells containing boron-10 at different concentrations. *Phys. Med. Biol.* **23,** 738–752.

Sandmeir, H. A., Hansen, G. E., Seaman, R. E., Hirons, T. J., and Marshall, A. H. (1974). LASL Rep. No. LA-5137.

Snyder, W. S. (1958). Calculation of radiation dose. *Health Phys.* **1,** 51–55.

Ujeno, Y.(1982). The biological effects and RBE of thermal neutrons. *Zagadnienia Biofiz. Wspolczesnej* **7,** 73–89.

Ujeno, Y., and Takimoto, K. (1980). Deuterium isotope effect on radiation damages to mammalian cells. *Annu. Rep. Res. React. Inst. Kyoto Univ.* **13,** 62–66.

Ujeno, Y., Niwa, O., Takimoto, K., Kobayashi, T., and Kanda, K. (1980). Estimation of RBEs of thermal neutrons and reactor beam. *Strahlentherapie* **156,** 201–204.

Ujeno, Y., Takimoto, K., Kanda, K., Kobayashi, T., and Ono, K. (1981). RBEs of nuclear reactor beams and thermal neutrons in responses of B-16 melanoma. *Strahlentherapie* **157,** 682–684.

Utsumi, H., Hill, C. K., Ben-Hur, E., and Elkind, M. M. (1981). "Single-hit" potentially lethal damage: evidence of its repair in mammalian cells. *Radiat. Res.* **87,** 576–591.

Zamenhof, R. G., Murray, B. W., Brownell, G. L., Wellum, E. R., and Tolpin, E. I. (1975). Boron neutron capture therapy for the treatment of cerebral gliomas. I. Theoretical evaluation of efficiency of various neutron beams. *Med. Phys.* **2,** 47–60.

26 Radiosensitivities in Acute and Late Effects on Human Cells

Sadayuki Ban

Department of Pathology and Clinical Laboratories
Radiation Effects Research Foundation
Hiroshima 730, Japan

I. Introduction

The risk of cancer in various organs and mutation or malformation in the offspring, increases in organisms exposed to radiation, as an effect other than acute death. Another important effect of radiation is a nonspecific shortening of life span in organisms, although this postulation remains controversial. Storer (1965) studied the survival rate of mice exposed to X rays (100–500 R) and noted only a small number of acute deaths. However, the survival time of the exposed mice showed a dose-dependent decrease; that is, a shorter life span was associated with a greater exposure to radiation.

Warren's study (1956) of American radiologists suggested that shortening of the life span with radiation exposure probably also applied to humans. Many later studies of radiologists did not demonstrate a nonspecific shortening of life span by radiation (Court-Brown and Doll, 1958; Seltser and Sartwell, 1965; Matanoski *et al.*, 1975). Another extensive study on humans concerns follow-up of the atomic bomb survivors of Hiroshima and Nagasaki (Jablon and Kato, 1972; Beebe *et al.*, 1975; Kato *et al.*,

1982). These investigations to date revealed no nonspecific shortening of life span in the atomic bomb survivors.

This chapter is concerned with the effects of radiation on the proliferating ability of human-derived fibroblasts.

II. Radiosensitivity of Cultured Human-Derived Cells

Radiosensitivity of mammalian cells differs with the type and condition of cells. The dose causing death in half the number of humans or laboratory animals 30 days after a single whole-body irradiation is called the semilethal dose, expressed as $LD_{50/30}$. When animals are exposed to single lethal, massive (300–1000 R) whole-body irradiation, deaths occur from the fifth day. The cause of death at this time is myelophthisis, leukocytopenia, or hemorrhage due to thrombocytopenia, or disturbance of hematopoietic cells, and infection. Thus the highly proliferative cells of hematopoietic organs appear to be most sensitive to radiation. If the effect of radiation on cells can be estimated as the effect on the proliferating potential of cultured cells, this would provide a useful estimation for radiation effects in proliferating cell systems *in vivo*.

Puck and Harcus (1955) cultured human cell colonies and succeeded in quantitating the proliferating ability of cells. These cells were obtained from a black patient with uterine cervix cancer by Gey *et al.* (1952) and are known as HeLa cells, the oldest established cell line. Using this colony formation method, Puck and Marcus (1956) succeeded in determining survival rates following exposure to various doses of X ray. The dose–survival curve on a semilogarithmic graph was very distinctive. In a low dose range there is a shoulder, and the curve gradually forms a straight line. This dose–survival curve can generally be determined with two parameters. The first is the dose that causes the straight-line portion of the survival curve to decrease to 37% and is expressed as D_0. The second is the point where the straight-line portion of the curve intersects the survival probability axis (longitudinal axis) on extrapolation, expressed as n. According to the report of Puck and Marcus (1956), n in the dose–survival curve of HeLa cells was 2, and D_0 was 96 R. Data have accumulated on the survival curve of cultured mammalian cells following X irradiation. Regardless of the species and whether the cells were normal or malignant, all survival curves after X irradiation closely resembled those reported by Puck and Marcus (1956). With a few exceptions, n is in the range of 1 to 10 and D_0, in the range of 90 to 200 rads.

The relationship between the radiosensitivity of cultured cells obtained in the manner just described and the radiosensitivity of cells proliferating *in vivo* has to be considered. Till and McCulloch (1961) injected iv nucleated mouse bone marrow cells into another mouse of the same strain, which was previously subjected to whole-body irradiation of 900 R. When they removed the spleen 9 or 10 days later, they found that a number of the colonies formed from the transplanted bone marrow cells had been retained. They determined the percentage survival of bone marrow cells by transplanting ^{60}Co γ-ray-irradiated bone marrow cells and counting the colonies formed in the spleen. Their results were in close accord with those obtained by Puck and Marcus (1956), who used cultured cells. The value of D_0 was 115 ± 8 rads.

In contrast, by determining the percentage survival by colony formation, DNA repair-deficient mutants have been found in humans. Cleaver (1968) demonstrated that cells from patients with xeroderma pigmentosum (XP), an autosomal recessive hereditary disease, are extremely sensitive to ultraviolet rays (UV), and that this is attributable to a repair deficiency of UV-induced DNA damage. Because almost all XP patients develop skin cancer, Cleaver suggested that decreased or deficient repairability of UV-induced DNA damage may be involved in the carcinogenesis.

Ataxia telangiectasia (Louis-Bar syndrome, AT), also an autosomal recessive hereditary disease, is a highly cancer-prone disease associated with reduced immune function; it frequently develops into leukemia or malignant lymphoma, in young persons. The cells of patients with this disease (AT cells) have a very high sensitivity to ionizing radiation (Taylor *et al.*, 1975). It is assumed that AT cells are deficient in the capability to repair ionizing radiation-induced damage (Paterson *et al.*, 1976).

Figure 1 shows the dose–survival curve for normal human fibroblasts exposed to ionizing radiation of different energies (S. Ban, unpublished). The cells were irradiated with low-energy X rays [40 kVp, 5 mA, 0.2 Al filter, 0.23 mm Al half-value layer, (HVL)] at a dose of 200 R/min (Fig. 1A) and high-energy X rays (200 kVp, 20 mA, 0.3 Cu + 0.5 Al filter, 1.2 mm Cu HVL), at a dose of 60 R/min (Fig. 1B). The energy difference between the two types of radiation is considerable, but the dose–survival curves are fairly equal.

Dose–survival curves of X-irradiated AT cells are shown in Fig. 2 (S. Ban, unpublished). The AT cells (AT3BI, AT5BI) were established by Taylor *et al.* (1975) and Taylor (1978) and obtained from Professor Osamu Nikaido. The *n* values of both these cells approximated 1, and D_0 was in the range of 40 to 50 R. This was consistent with the D_0 value (approximately 50 rads) of ^{60}Co γ exposures made by Taylor *et al.* (1975) and the D_0 value (30.5 rads) reported by Lavin *et al.* (1978).

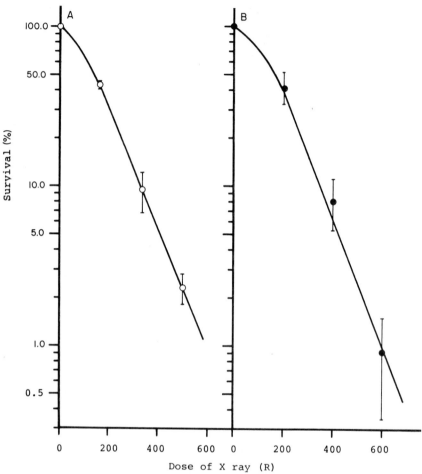

Fig. 1. Dose–survival curves obtained by colony formation after irradiation with low-dose X rays at various rates (A) and deep-therapy X rays (B). Vertical bars indicate the means and standard deviations obtained from experiments repeated four times or more. (A) Low-energy X rays (0.23 mm Al HVL) are irradiated at 40 kVp, 5 mA, and 0.2 Al filter, and the dose is 200 R/min ($n = 1.8$, $D_0 = 120$ R). (B) Deep-therapy X rays (1.2 mm Cu HVL) are irradiated at 200 kVp, 20 mA, and 0.3 Cu + 0.5 Al filter, and the dose is 60 R/min ($n = 2.5$, $D_0 = 110$ R).

The deleterious effects of ionizing radiation on cells are membrane damage, chromosome aberrations, and intracellular macromolecular damage. Damage to DNA carrying genetic information and its repair are particularly interesting subjects for study. McGrath and Williams (1966) developed an alkaline–sucrose density gradient centrifugation method to

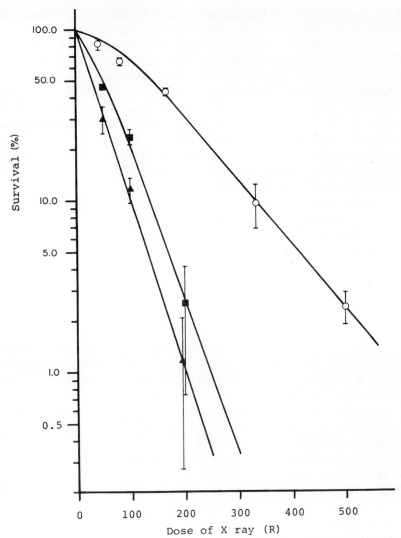

Fig. 2. Dose–survival curves of normal human lung fibroblasts (○) and fibroblasts derived from the skin of AT patients (▲, ■) after X-ray irradiations at 40 kVp, 5 mA, and 0.2 Al filter, at a dose rate of 200 R/min. Vertical bars indicate the means and standard deviations obtained from experiments repeated four times or more.

detect intracellular DNA single-strand breakage induced by X irradiation. The mean molecular weight of single-stranded DNA can easily be calculated by this method. However, the sensitivity for detection of DNA strand breakage is low, and for detection it is necessary to irradiate with X rays in excess of several kiloroentgens. Such a large dose of radiation is not biologically meaningful, as is evident from Figs. 1 and 2.

For efficient detection of DNA single-strand breakage, Kohn *et al.* (1974, 1981) developed an alkaline elution method. Cells in the logarithmic growth phase are labeled with [^{14}C]thymidine (0.02 μCi/ml), exposed to various doses of radiation, placed on a polyvinyl chloride filter, and then treated with an alkaline cell-lysing solution (pH 9.7). An alkaline solution (pH 12.1), containing EDTA and tetrapropylammonium hydroxide, is allowed to flow continuously over the DNA on the filter. Short DNA fragments produced by X-ray-induced DNA strand breakages now easily pass through the filter owing to their small molecular size. The eluate from the filter is gathered from time to time, and the amount of DNA in the eluate and on the filter is measured. Thus, the relationship between exposure dose and single-strand DNA elution pattern can be determined. Kohn *et al.* detected DNA single-strand breakages caused by X irradiation of 100 rads using this method. The sensitivity of the alkaline elution method becomes evident in that a massive radiation dose in excess of 5 krads is necessary when the aforementioned alkaline–sucrose density gradient centrifugation is used.

Figure 3 shows DNA elution patterns by the alkaline elution method following ^{60}Co-γ irradiation (dose rate 180 rads/min) of HeLa cells (S. Ban, unpublished). Both elution speed and elution volume of single-strand DNA increase with elevation of the γ-ray dose. When the cells are cultured at 37°C following irradiation, the DNA single-strand breakages rejoin within a very short time. Figure 4 shows the DNA elution pattern following incubation of γ-irradiated cells for 1 h at 37°C (S. Ban, unpublished). Because almost all breakages rejoin, the amount of eluted DNA of the irradiated cells is minute.

Compounds containing sulfhydryls (SH) such as cysteine, cysteamine, and MPG (2-mercaptopropionylglycine) have a protective effect against radiation (Mori *et al.*, 1978). Figure 5 shows the DNA elution pattern when cells in the presence of 60 mM cysteamine are irradiated with γ rays (S. Ban, unpublished). Compared with Fig. 3, there appears to be much less DNA breakage following exposure to the same dose.

III. Have Cultured Animal Cells a Finite Life Span?

When fibroblasts isolated from human fetal or embryonic lung are cultured *in vitro,* the cells die after the cell population has undergone doublings 40–60 times. The discovery by Hayflick and Moorhead (1961) that

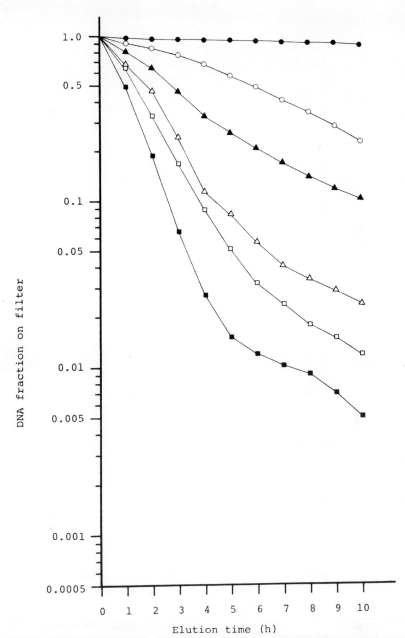

Fig. 3. Alkaline elution patterns of HeLa S3 cell DNA irradiated by various doses of ^{60}Co γ rays. The dose rate of γ rays is 180 rads/min. Dose amounts given: (●) 0, (○) 200, (▲) 400, (△) 600, (□) 800, and (■) 1000 rads.

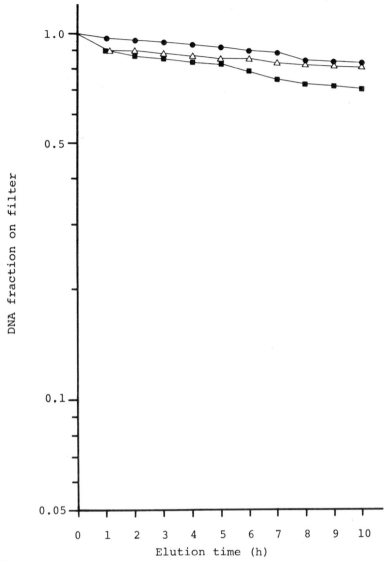

Fig. 4. Elution patterns of intracellular DNA of HeLa S3 cells irradiated with ^{60}Co γ rays and cultured at 37°C for 1 h. Dose amounts given: (●) 0, (△) 600, and (■) 1000 rads.

cultured human fetus-derived cells have life spans was an epochal achievement. The significance of the finite life span of such cells cultured *in vitro* remains unknown, and to what extent this reflects the aging life span of *in vivo* cells is conjectural. However, if cultured cells isolated

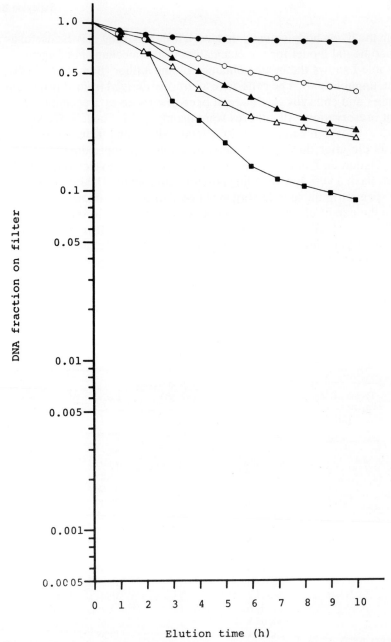

Fig. 5. Protective effect of cysteamine (60 mM) against DNA single-strand breakages, detected by alkaline elution method. Cysteamine was given 20 min prior to irradiation, and γ rays were applied in the presence of the chemical. Symbols for radiation dose amounts as in Fig. 3.

from the living body actually do have a life span, they may be useful as an experimental model for the elucidation of the mechanism of aging.

Table I shows the results obtained by the author (Ban *et al.*, 1980a; S. Ban, unpublished). The cells were all freshly derived from aborted human fetuses and embryos that had not been processed by freezing for permanent preservation. All cultures were maintained in Eagle's MEM culture medium supplemented with 10% fetal calf serum. Lung-derived fibroblasts die after they have undergone doublings approximately 50 times (population-doubling number, PDN). Liver- and heart-derived cells, however, have a very low doubling potential (life span). The difference in cell life span attributable to the organ of origin raises the important question of how the extent of differentiation of cells is involved in the life span.

Further, Hayflick (1974) demonstrated that the *in vitro* life span of cells obtained from different species correlates with the life span of the species from which the cells are derived. The *in vitro* life span of cells derived

TABLE I

Comparison of Life Spans of Human Diploid Cell Strains
Derived from Various Embryonic Tissues

Tissue of origin	Strain	Period in gestation (weeks)	PDN[a]	Mean $\pm$ SD
Lung	SK-LU 2	7	54.40	46.49 $\pm$ 5.66
	SK-LU 3	7	38.45	
	SK-LU 4	20	49.75	
	SK-LU 8	7	44.00	
	SK-LU 10	6.5	41.25	
	SK-LU 13	20	51.08	
Liver	SK-LI 2	7	21.00	19.75 $\pm$ 5.04
	SK-LI 4	20	16.32	
	SK-LI 6	6.5	21.41	
	SK-LI 8	7	27.82	
	SK-LI 10	6.5	24.36	
	SK-LI 11	6	14.42	
	SK-LI 12	7	12.89	
Heart	SK-H 2	7	10.04	9.85 $\pm$ 2.31
	SK-H 6	6.5	7.56	
	SK-H 8	7	7.62	
	SK-H 11	6	13.88	
	SK-H 12	7	10.17	

[a] PDN, population doubling number.

from the Galapagos tortoise, which has a long life span, is equivalent to a doubling frequency of as high as 72 to 114 times. The cells of humans, with a life span of 110 years, are able to double 40–60 times, and the cells of the chicken, with a life span of 30 years, 15–35 times. The cells of mice, having a life span of only 3.5 years, double only 14–28 times.

However, Stanley et al. (1975) investigated the in vitro life span of cells derived from horses, monkeys, cats, rabbits, and marsupial animals and reported the lack of a relationship between the life span of the donor animal and the frequency of doubling in vitro; hence, the assertion that the in vitro life span of an animal's cells, in terms of the PDN of cells related to the life span of the animal itself, may not be totally valid.

For each species of animals or cells used, the aging mechanisms are probably subject to various qualifications, by certain unknown factors. For example, when mouse cells are cultured in vitro, cells with an unlimited life span (established cells) appear at a rather high frequency. As shown in Fig. 6, fetal cells of golden hamsters and C57BL, CF1 strain mice can be divided into clones dying after doubling 10–13 times and clones acquiring infinite proliferative capabilities (D. Nikaido and S. Ban, unpublished). However, we never observed the spontaneous establishment of infinitely proliferating normal human diploid cells. Although we have no adequate explanation, an important key in considering carcinogenesis or life span has yet to be found.

As with fetal cells, the in vitro life span of adult-derived cells has been studied by such authors as Hayflick (1965), Goldstein (1971), Goldstein et al. (1969), Martin et al. (1970), and Guilly et al. (1973). All report finding an inverse correlation between cell donor age and cell life span, the latter shortening as the former increases. That is, aging of the living body is accumulated or copied in the individual cells, and the cells do not rejuvenate even if they are separated from the living body and placed under culture conditions in vitro. The finding that adult-derived fibroblasts are older than fetus-derived fibroblasts has been clearly demonstrated in vitro.

Evidence supporting the aging model at the human cell level was also obtained using the skin cells from progeria patients. In the skin fibroblasts of patients with Hutchinson–Gilford type progeria syndrome or Werner's syndrome, both autosomal recessive hereditary diseases (hereinafter referred to as progeria cells and Werner cells, respectively), are cultured, the former have a life span corresponding to a PDN of about 10 and Werner cells, 10–20 (Goldstein, 1969; Martin et al., 1965, 1970; Danes, 1971). Premature senility of the living body is thus reflected in culture as a short life span at the cellular level.

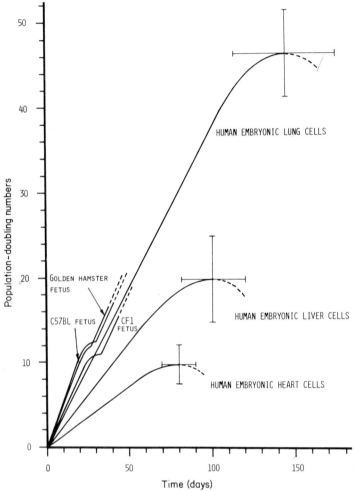

Fig. 6. Comparison of the *in vitro* life span of cultured fibroblasts obtained from embryos of human, golden hamster, CF1 mice, or C57BL mice.

The results obtained so far can be summed up as follows:

1. Normal tissue-derived cells of humans have finite proliferating potential in culture.
2. The *in vitro* PDN of cells derived from humans of various ages inversely correlates with cell donor age.
3. The *in vitro* PDN of cells derived from patients with hereditary premature aging is less than that in cells from disease-free individuals. Thus

the normal human diploid cells are useful as *in vitro* model (known as Hayflick's aging model) for the study of aging.

IV. Effect of Radiation on the Life Span of Human Normal Diploid Cells

If human diploid cells are indeed useful for the study of aging, will there be, as in the case of experimental animals, a radiation-induced life shortening at the cellular level? Macieira-Coelho *et al.* (1976, 1977) irradiated fibroblasts derived from normal human fetal lung with γ doses of 100 rads, several times at the rate of 0.28 rads/min, and observed changes in the cell life span. Definite shortening of the life span was observed with 100 rads exposure, but on exposure to 200, 300, and 500 rads, the life span was comparable to that of nonexposed cells. On the contrary, an extension of life span was observed on 400 rads exposure. However, when by the same method, γ rays were used to irradiate chicken-derived fibroblasts, shortening of life span in proportion to dose was observed. When mouse-derived fibroblasts were irradiated by γ rays, the time of entry into the infinite proliferation phase was earlier and dose dependent. Macieira-Coelho *et al.* suggested that the difference in the effect of radiation on the life span of these three cell lines was related to the probability of acquiring the capacity for infinite proliferation. Mouse cells readily become established, and transformation to an unlimited life span is further heightened by carcinogenic chemicals or tumor viruses. Shortening of life span by γ irradiation is not observed in mouse cells, but the acquisition of ability to proliferate infinitely is enhanced. It is almost impossible to establish chicken cell lines with an infinite doubling of potential, even when treated with carcinogenic chemicals or tumor viruses. In such cells, a definite shortening of life span by γ irradiation has been observed. However, the probability of human cells becoming established ranges between that of mouse and chicken cells. Establishment of lines of human cells is difficult using carcinogenic chemicals but can be done using tumor viruses. The effects of γ rays on the life span of such human cells seem to be nil.

Macieira-Coelho *et al.* (1978) reported that dose-dependent shortening of the life span was observed when adult lung-derived fibroblasts were exposed to γ rays; however, further investigations are required. Figure 7 shows the results of our study (Ban *et al.*, 1980a). Proliferation and life span of SK-LU 2 cells, fibroblasts derived from the lung of a normal human fetus, were observed following 50 or 100 R X irradiation. The half-value layer (HVL) of X rays (200 kVp, 20 mA, 0.3 Cu + 0.5 Al filter) was equivalent to 1.2 mm Cu, and irradiation was at a dose rate of 60 R/min.

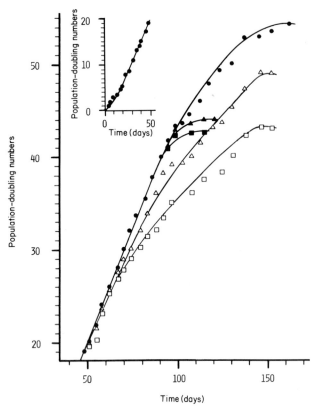

Fig. 7. Effect of low-level X irradiation on the life span of human diploid lung cells (SK-LU 2 strain) *in vivo*. SK-LU 2 cells were exposed to X rays (at times indicated by arrows) at 19 or 40 population-doubling numbers (PDN) as follows: (△) 50 R at 19 PDN, (□) 100 R at 19 PDN, (▲) 50 R at 40 PDN, (■) 100 R at 40 PDN. (●) Controls.

Compared with the nonirradiated group, a definite shortening of cell life span was observed in the irradiated group. Moreover, the life span-shortening rate was greater when exposure was made at a time when cells were older (40 PDN), as compared to younger cells (19 PDN).

Figure 8 shows a comparison of dose–survival (acute effect) and dose–life span shortening (late effect) following high-dose-range X irradiation of SK-LU 13 cells. Acute effects are expressed in percentage survival as determined by the colony formation method following X irradiation of 10 to 15-PDN cells. Late effects in the same dose range were evaluated by the percentage life span shortening following X irradiation. In the dose–life span shortening curves, the percentage of the remaining life span of the irradiated cell population against the remaining life span of the nonirradiated cell population is plotted according to the respective doses. The

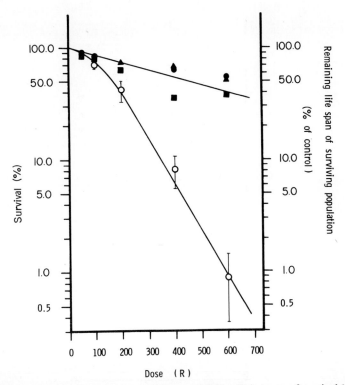

Fig. 8. Dose–response curve of normal human diploid cells in terms of survival (O——O) and shortening of the remaining life span of the surviving cell population (closed symbols). Vertical bars indicate the standard deviation of the mean for six independent experiments. The survival curve was evaluated from the colony-forming ability of SK-LU 13 cells at various ages. In the experiments with life shortening, cells were exposed to X rays at three active proliferating stages of the control cells: 19.00 PDN (●), 22.53 PDN (▲), or 26.76 PDN (■). The dose–life span curve shows the percentage of remaining life span of the surviving population against that of the unirradiated control.

cells were irradiated at 19.00, 22.53, and 26.76 PDN, when the proliferation activity was very high. The curve for dose–survival has a shoulder with an extrapolation number (n) of 2.5 and an exponential slope (D_0) of 110 R, but the dose–life span shortening curve has no shoulder ($n = 1$); rather it forms a straight line with a D_0 of 600 R. As the curves of the two are altogether different, different mechanisms or targets in acute and late effects may be involved. Of more importance is the suggestion of the presence of dose dependency in shortening of the cell life span and the absence of a threshold value in the life span-shortening effect of X rays.

Figure 9 shows life span shortening following 50 or 100 R of X irradiation at various points in time in the progress of aging *in vitro*. The horizontal axis shows the relative time of X irradiation, and 0 corresponds to 0

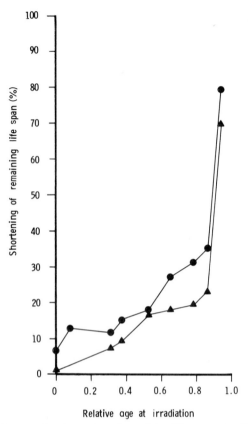

Fig. 9. Effect of age on the shortening of remaining life span using SK-LU 13 strain. X Rays, 50 (▲) or 100 R (●) were delivered at various ages in culture.

PDN and 1.0, to the time of the cell population's final doubling. The sensitivity to life span (remaining life span) shortening increases with aging. However, the dose–survival curves shown in Fig. 8 do not change with aging of cells, and in general the same results were obtained for all human fetal lung-derived fibroblasts that we have established (data not shown).

The rate of life span shortening in three different types of cells irradiated with 50 or 100 R of X rays at about the same time (19 or 20 PDN) is summarized in Table II. Although Eagle's MEM culture medium supplemented with the same lot of fetal calf serum was used, the life span shortening differs with the cell. This suggests that the sensitivity for late effect also differs with the cell.

If fibroblasts derived from human fetal lung do provide a useful model

TABLE II

Comparison of the Long-Term Effects of X Irradiation on the Three Human Diploid Cell Strains

Strain	Life span of control (PDN)[a]	Dose (R)	Age at which irradiated (PDN)	Shortening of life span	(%)	Percentage shortening of remaining life span
SMT-LU 2	54.40	50	19	5.30 PDN	(9.74)	14.97
		100	19	11.27	(20.72)	31.84
SMT-LU 8	44.40	50	20	5.10	(11.59)	20.90
		100	20	7.93	(17.86)	32.05
SMT-LU 13	51.08	50	19	2.97	(5.81)	9.26
		100	19	4.68	(9.16)	14.59

[a] PDN, population doubling numbers.

for evaluating X-ray-induced late effects, studies of late effects of other types of radiation, especially high-LET radiation, have to be done. We irradiated human fetal lung fibroblasts with radiation generated by a D_2O nuclear reactor, a KUR reactor (Research Reactor Institute, Kyoto University, 5000 kW), and compared the acute and late effects on the cells (Ban *et al.*, 1981). Thermal neutron fluence was measured by radioactivation of gold leaf. The adsorbed dose is expressed as the sum of thermal neutron and γ doses (nuclear reactor radiation dose). The absorbed dose rate was 1.4–4.0 rads/min, and the ratio of contaminated γ rays to neutrons was 0.55.

Figure 10 shows the dose–survival response, as determined by the colony formation method. A linear relationship of $n = 1$, $D_0 = 55$ rads was obtained. There was no threshold value in the lethal effect of thermal neutrons on human diploid cells *in vitro*. The dotted line in the figure shows the percentage survival (Fig. 8) following X irradiation.

Figure 11 shows the *in vitro* life span of cells following exposure to nuclear reactor radiation. The percentage of the remaining life span of irradiated cells against that of nonirradiated cells is plotted according to dose. We irradiated cells that had a very high proliferating potential and were at a phase equivalent to the so-called phase II of Hayflick's aging model (Hayflick and Moorhead, 1961). As in the case of X irradiation (broken line), a linear relationship without a shoulder was obtained. The value of D_0 was 260 rads. Thus, the percentage of life span shortening induced per rad is definitely greater for nuclear reactor radiation than for X rays.

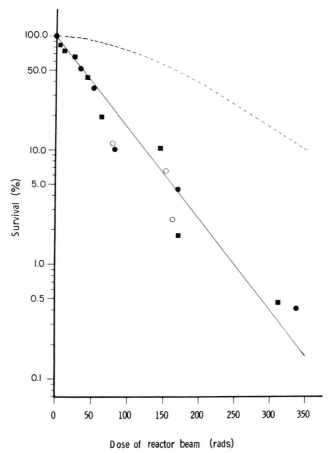

Fig. 10. Dose–survival response of normal human diploid cells after exposure to various doses of a reactor radiation beam. The radiation, which was delivered from the D_2O facility of the 5000-kW KUR reactor, was mainly thermal neutrons, which raised the secondary γ rays. The reactor beam is mixed radiation; the γ : neutron ratio was calculated to be 0.55. The survival curve was evaluated by the colony-forming ability. Cell lines: (●) SK-LU 4, at 30 PDN, (○) SK-LU 4 at 45 PDN, (■) SK-LU 13 at 11 PDN. Broken line indicates the dose–survival response after X irradiation.

Figure 12 compares the relative biological effectiveness (RBE) of nu-clear reactor radiation to X rays, in both acute and late effects. The percentage responses on the horizontal axis are percentage survival as an acute effect and percentage of life span shortening as a late effect. The broken line indicates RBE values obtained from actual results of tests, when the reactor radiation beam containing secondary γ rays was irradi-ated. The solid line indicates the calculated RBE value of the thermal

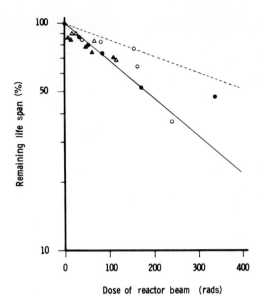

Fig. 11. Dose–response of normal human diploid cells to nuclear reactor radiation in terms of shortening of the remaining life span of the surviving cell population (solid line). The broken line shows the dose–life span response of SK-LU 13 cells after X irradiation. Cell lines: (●) SK-LU 4, at 30 PDN, (○) SK-LU 4, at 45 PDN, (△) SK-LU 13, at 14 PDN, (▲) SK-LU 13, at 31 PDN.

neutrons. The curve depicts RBE for acute effects, and the straight line, RBE for the late effects. The RBE for acute effects is dose dependent and decreases with increases in the dose. The RBE for the late effect is not dose dependent. The RBE of high-LET radiation containing β rays (nuclear reactor radiation) was 2.3 and that of thermal neutrons, 3.0.

There are no reports of studies of the late effect of ionizing radiation on normal human diploid cells other than those of our group and those of Macieira-Coelho *et al.* (1976, 1977, 1978). The radiation exposure factors were altogether different; the ^{60}Co-γ dose rate used by Macieira-Coelho was 0.28 rads/min, and the X-ray dose rate we used was 60 R/min. Therefore, the results reported by the two groups are not necessarily the same. Ours is the only report of life span shortening (late effect) due to high-LET radiation, using normal human diploid cells.

Curtis and Gebhard (1958) and Delihas and Curtis (1958) irradiated mice with fast neutrons or X rays and studied 30-day percentage survival (acute effect) and life span shortening (late effect). In this case, the RBE for acute effect was 2.2–1.7 and that for late effect, 1.7. It is impossible to compare our results to theirs, because the quality of fast neutrons differs from that of the reactor radiation beam. However, the RBE values of the

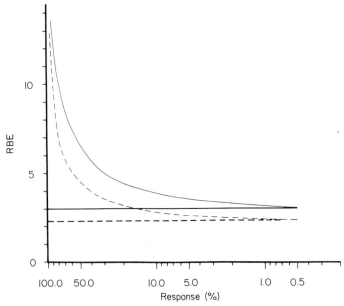

Fig. 12. Relative biological effectiveness (RBE) values of reactor radiation beams for acute (thin lines) and late (thick lines) effects in cultured human diploid cells. Percentage response implies percentage survival and percentage remaining life span for acute and late effects, respectively. The RBE values of reactor beams relative to X rays were calculated from the data in Figs. 10 and 11 (broken lines). Supposing the RBE of secondary γ rays relative to X rays was equal to 1, the RBE of high-LET particles was calculated as shown with solid lines.

reactor radiation beam for both acute and late effects were rather high, because the radiation we used was mainly thermal neutrons, and both acute and late effects were caused by a nuclear reaction that raised the secondary γ: neutron ratio to 0.55 in the absorbed dose.

The appropriateness of exploring the cause of radiation-induced life span shortening using experimental animals is still a matter of controversy (Warburg, 1975). Radiation consistently induces cancer in humans and animals, so that it is extremely difficult to evaluate the nonspecific life span-shortening effect of radiation (Lindop and Rotblat, 1961; Jablon and Kato, 1972; Kato *et al.*, 1982). The nonspecific life span shortening considered here involves a shortening of life even when such is not due to specific diseases such as carcinoma, which is, in a sense, an acceleration of aging. There are reports from studies on humans (Matanoski *et al.*, 1975) and laboratory animals (Storer, 1965) that shortening of life span was observed when deaths from tumors were excluded, but the life span-shortening effect appearing after irradiation would be obscured if the rate of carcinogenesis in irradiated animals is high. It is difficult to induce normal human diploid cells to undergo neoplastic change, using physical or chemical factors (Igel *et al.*, 1975). We found no incidence of transformed or abnormally growing cell strains resulting from X-ray or nuclear reactor radiation exposure. In other words, the cultured normal human diploid cell may serve as a useful model for evaluating the life span-shortening effect of radiation, other than carcinogenesis.

V. Repairability of Radiation-Induced Damage and Aging

In young cultured cells from individuals with Werner's syndrome, G6PD (Holliday *et al.*, 1974; Goldstein and Singel, 1974), 6PGD (Goldstein and Moerman, 1975), and HGPRT (Goldstein and Moerman, 1975) activity is more susceptible to heat inactivation than in normal cultured cells. Accumulation of these abnormal proteins is also observed in aged normal human cells (Holliday and Tarrant, 1972; Lewis and Tarrant, 1972; Holliday *et al.*, 1974; Goldstein and Moerman, 1975). These findings strongly support the "error catastrophe theory" advanced by Orgel (1963), according to which abnormal proteins appear following DNA or mRNA injury, or errors in transcription and translation lead to accelerated aging and eventually cause death.

Let us assume, according to the error catastrophe theory, that abnormalities occur in some enzymes (group) involved in the DNA repair process. Damage to DNA would accumulate in cells with sustained DNA damage due to decreased functions of the DNA repair mechanism. In other words, erroneous repair would be brought about by abnormal repair enzymes, and the damage would ultimately increase. Related to this is the question of whether or not the ability to repair DNA damage declines with age, or if the decreased ability to repair or the accumulation of damage may in turn lead to aging and death of cells and possibly to carcinogenesis.

Price *et al.* (1971) studied the incorporation of [³H]TTP in the presence of DNA polymerase, using sections of brain, liver, and myocardium of young and old mice. They observed, particularly with the brain, that incorporation was greater for the old mice, and speculated on the possibility of breakage of DNA in nondividing cells. Further, incorporation of [³H]TTP in the brain increases with X irradiation, and Modak and Price (1971) demonstrated that the number of DNA breakages in the brains of mice is equivalent to the number formed when X ray of 10 krads is given. Wheeler and Lett (1974) observed that the size of DNA of nerve cells (nondividing) derived from the cerebellum of the Beagle dog decreases with age, and "accumulation of DNA damage" has been demonstrated in nondividing cell systems.

Epstein *et al.* (1973) found that the rejoining capacity of DNA single-strand breakages induced by γ irradiation in progeria cells was much lower than in cells derived from normal human skin and established human liver cells.

However, Regan and Setlow (1974) reported that in the same progeria cells, the rejoining capacity of single-strand breakages depends on the conditions under which the cells were treated (in particular, trypsin treatment made for exfoliation of cells) or cultured, and that under appropriate conditions, repair is made fairly normal. Epstein *et al.* (1974) immediately produced counterevidence that the rejoining capacity of single-strand breakages declined even when progeria cells untreated with trypsin were used, thus emphasizing the difficulty of studies in this area.

Brown *et al.* (1976) reported deficient or decreased rejoining capacity of single-strand breakages in progeria cells. When these cells were cocultured together with normal human-derived young diploid cells or established hamster cells for 24 h in advance, rejoining of γ-ray-induced DNA single-strand breakages in progeria cells progressed normally. However, when the progeria cells were cultured together with normal human diploid cells on the verge of death, rejoining of single-strand breakages did not occur in either type of cell, suggesting that in old normal diploid cells there is a decreased repairability of the damaged DNA. Brown *et al.* (1976) cocultured two types of progeria cells obtained from different patients, and the cells recovered the capacity for rejoining single-strand breakages. This interesting finding shows that progeria cells can be classified genetically into at least two types with respect to their system for repair of DNA damage.

Clarkson and Painter (1974) and Painter *et al.* (1973) investigated the rejoining capacity of DNA single-strand breakages following X irradiation and unscheduled DNA synthesis associated with removal of dimers following UV irradiation in young and old normal human diploid cells (WI-38). They found no significant difference in DNA damage repairability between old and young cells and concluded that the decreased repairability of DNA damage is not the cause of aging of normal diploid cells.

Mattern and Cerutti (1975) induced impaired thymine derivatives [5,6-dihydroxydihydrothymine type (t')] by irradiating *Pseudomonas* phage PM 2 with γ rays. The ability to excise this thymine derivative was examined in each nucleus of old and young WI-38 cells. Cells up to the thirty-ninth generation had excision activity and showed no significant alteration due to cellular aging. However, excision was not detected in nuclei of the old cells, that is, cells after the forty-third generation. This repair deficiency occurs very rapidly compared with the decrease of DNA synthesis ability with aging (Cristofalo and Sharp, 1973). Because cells deficient in excision activity survive for several generations, the repair deficiency of DNA damage may not be a direct cause of cellular aging.

Hart and Setlow (1976) examined unscheduled DNA synthesis by [^{3}H]thymidine uptake in WI-38 cells from the eighteenth to sixtieth generations treated by UV, N-acetoxy-AFF (a chemical carcinogen), and γ rays. Decreased repairability with cellular aging was observed in each cell. However, this decrease almost parallels the decrease in capacity of DNA synthesis seen in the aging of untreated WI-38 cells. Thus it may be concluded that the decreased ability to repair DNA is one phenomena due to cellular aging.

Suzuki *et al.* (1980), using the alkaline elution method developed by Kohn *et al.* (1974), attempted to determine whether or not the rejoining capacity of DNA single-strand breakages induced by X-ray irradiation alters with aging *in vitro*. The purpose of their study was to quantitate breakage and repair of DNA single strands induced by low radiation doses rather than to use previously reported methods for DNA single-strand breakages (density gradient centrifugation). The cells used were normal human diploid cells established in our laboratory (Bau *et al.*, 1980a). They concluded that the rejoining capacity of DNA single strands broken subsequent to irradiation by 800 rads of X rays remains unchanged even with aging, *in vitro*.

Nikaido *et al.* (1980), using the host reactivation method, studied the association of aging and radiation sensitivity in cells derived from patients with hereditary diseases. First, herpes simplex virus (HSV) exposed to various doses of UV was inoculated into target cells. The HSV whose DNA damages were repaired by repair mechanisms in the target cells eliminated the infected cells and formed plaques. The number of plaques was counted to obtain the survival rate of the HSV. Using the survival rate of HSV, the magnitude of UV-damaged repairability was determined for the target cells. There was no difference in repairability among cells derived from human fetus and healthy young and old persons. Although ataxia telangiectasia (AT) cells are highly sensitive to ionizing radiation, their UV damage repairability was found to be normal. However, when xeroderma pigmentosum (XP) cells, highly sensitive to UV, were selected as target cells, the plaque formation rate of HSV exposed to UV was markedly decreased. The repairability of cells obtained from patients with Werner's syndrome also fell within the normal level. Furthermore, the repairability in all of these cells was consistent over the entire aging period.

Next, consideration will be given to cellular aging of cells genetically deficient in DNA damage repairability. Xeroderma pigmentosum cells have a particularly higher UV sensitivity compared with normal human-derived cells. This is because of the deficiency of endonuclease, an enzyme involved in the excision repair process of pyrimidine dimers, induced by UV (Cleaver, 1968, 1973; Setlow et al., 1969). However, the life span of cultured XP cells was found to be identical with that of normal human diploid cells (Goldstein, 1971; Nikaido et al., 1980). Ataxia telangiectasia cells are highly sensitive to ionizing radiation compared with normal human diploid cells (Taylor et al., 1975; Vincent et al., 1975). Paterson et al. (1976) reported a significant decrease in removability of impaired bases in DNA induced in AT cells by γ rays. As the AT cells used were fourteenth to fifty-fourth generation, it cannot be said that the life span was short in this culture system.

Is there any association between aging of cells in the body and DNA repairability? Wheeler and Lett (1974) irradiated the cerebella of Beagles aged 7 weeks to 13 years with γ rays of 4700 rads. Nerve cell DNA was extracted at an appropriate time to examine the rejoining capacity of single-strand breakages, but no difference could be found in the repairability attributable to aging.

Thus, it is most difficult to detect an association between cellular aging and repairability of radiation-induced DNA damage.

VI. Discussion

To elucidate the mechanism of radiation-induced late effects on cells, it seems necessary to investigate the relationship between cellular proliferation and aging. As the aging of human fibroblasts in culture system progresses there is a decrease in proliferation capacity and enlargement of cellular volume. Mitsui and Schneider (1976a,b) found, in a detailed examination of this relationship, that cessation of cellular proliferation occurred at random during subculture, and that when proliferation ceased, cellular volume and nuclear size increased. Among their data, the finding that cells with a smaller volume and active proliferation capacity exist even toward the end of subculture is deemed important. This demonstrates that individual doubling capacity is markedly heterogeneous in a cell population. That cells lose proliferative ability in the early period of subculture was confirmed by an autoradiographic method examining [^{3}H]thymidine uptake (Cristofalo and Huang, 1976) and by cinemicrophotographic studies (Absher et al., 1975).

Bell et al. (1978) suggested that cellular aging might be one model representing cellular differentiation. They noted that each cell in a population has a fixed life span and that there was a marked heterogeneity of life span among the cells. Furthermore, because the heterogeneity of cellular life span is omnipresent, the life span of a cell population, though being a mean, remains quite stable. This phenomenon is considered to be an important feature for the pattern of cellular differentiation.

We (Ban *et al.*, 1980b) made an attempt to isolate a subpopulation of cells having the longest life span. To remove nondividing cells and cells with a lower doubling potential selectively, colony formation was performed successively to sort out lineages with doubling potentials greater than those of the original population. A representative method is shown in Fig. 13. Cellular life spans obtained from several colony formations are always longer than the life span of the parental population. Accordingly, if colony formation is repeated many times, a subpopulation with a longer life span can be isolated. Using this method, we studied the modification

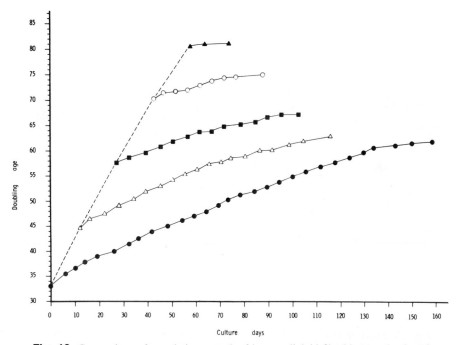

Fig. 13. Comparison of population growth of human diploid fibroblasts and substrains that were cloned by the successive colony-forming method. First cloning was started at age 33 PDN of parental strain (●). These colonial cells were designated as substrain I (△) and used for mass cultivation or colony formation. Next, substrains were obtained from the second cloning, and designated substrain II (■). The cells of substrain II passed two colony formations and produced substrain III (○) and substrain IV (▲), in that order.

of the maximum doubling potential obtained by successive colony formation in a human diploid cell strain exposed to X rays (Fig. 14). As colony formation rate decreased rapidly along with cellular aging, the fourth colony formation could not be performed for the 100- and 400-rad–exposed groups. However, the longest life span for the 200- and 600-rad–exposed groups was identical with that for the nonexposed group. Thus it may be concluded that X rays shorten the life span of a cell population (Figs. 3–9, Table IIIA, B, C) but do not modify the longest life span.

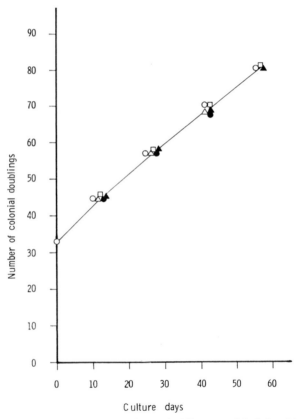

Fig. 14. Effect of X irradiation on maximum doubling potential. Cells with the ability to multiply into colonies after irradiation recovered and underwent successive colony formation, as shown in Fig. 13. The number of colonial doublings was calculated as the mean doubling for each colony formation step. Cells that survived after exposure to 100 (△) or 400 R (●) underwent three successive colony formations, whereas cells that survived 0 (○), 200 (□), or 600 R (▲) underwent four colonial formations. Growth rates of all groups were the same throughout all steps.

TABLE IIIA

Distribution of Chromosome Numbers in Cells Derived from the Lung, Skin, and Kidney

Cell origin	Number of metaphases scored	Chromosome counts				
		44	45	46	47	70+
Lung	50	1	1	45	1	2
Skin	50	0	0	48	0	2
Kidney	50	0	6	37	0	7

TABLE IIIB

Chromosome Aberrations in Cells with 44 to 47 Chromosomes

Cell origin	Number of metaphases	Number of aberrant cells			Isochromatid
		Single chromatid			
		Gaps	Breaks	Deletions	Breaks
Lung	48	1 (Bq)[a]	0	0	0
Skin	48	1 (Bq)	1 (Cp)	1	1
Kidney	43	8	0	0	6

[a] Parentheses show the position of aberration.

TABLE IIIC

In Vitro Life Span of Fibroblasts (Fibroblast-like Cells) Proliferating from Various Tissues

Cell origin	PDN[a]	Culture term[b] (months)
Lung	62.0	9.0
Breast skin	18.9	2.3
Femoral bone marrow	9.0	1.3
Kidney	7.8	1.0
Liver	13.1	3.0

[a] PDN, population doubling number of cell population before cells cease to proliferate.

[b] Culture term shows the period during which subculture is feasible. There are cells surviving for more than several months even after they cease to divide, if the culture medium is regularly changed.

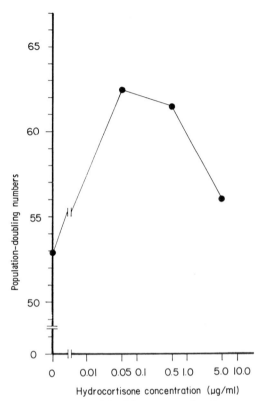

Fig. 15. Population-doubling potentials of SK-LU 13 cells subcultured in hydrocortisone-containing medium.

Hydrocortisone is well known for its potential to extend cell life span *in vitro*, under certain conditions (Macieira-Coelho, 1966; Cristofalo, 1975). Figure 15 shows the life spans of cell populations that were subcultured in culture media containing hydrocortisone of various concentrations (Ban *et al.*, 1980b). This experiment was done using cells that had already undergone 12 population doublings in a medium without hydrocortisone. The life span extension effect of hydrocortisone was most effective at a concentration of 0.5 μg/ml, when extended life span was observed in approximately 24% of the cells. However, this effect decreased as the concentration was increased. As shown in Fig. 16, successive colony formation was attempted with younger cells (12 PDN) in the medium containing hydrocortisone of the same concentration, and alteration in the longest life span was examined.

Life spans for hydrocortisone-treated and nontreated groups were all

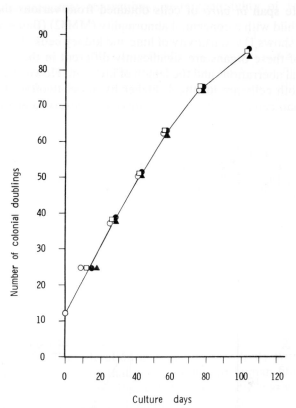

Fig. 16. Effect of hydrocortisone on maximum doubling potential. Cells multiplying into colonies recovered and underwent the successive colony formations shown in Fig. 14. Colony-forming cells underwent successive colony formation five times in growth medium (○) and six times in medium containing 0.05 (□), 0.50 (●), or 5.0 μg/ml (▲) of hydrocortisone. Growth speeds of all groups were the same through all steps.

but identical. Therefore, hydrocortisone does not seem to bring about significant extension in the longest life span. X rays and hydrocortisone do not greatly affect the longest life span, but they are related, to a great extent, to the shortening and extension of life spans of cell populations. It is not yet clear what implication this has in the modification system of the cellular life span. A current hypothesis is that cells that have doubling potential progress to an irreversible nondividing state. Such a progression may be modified by X rays or hydrocortisone.

A search for the aging process in cells with chromosomal abnormalities is a new approach for studying the mechanism of cellular aging, but such reports are few. Table III shows the frequency of chromosomal aberra-

Ban, S., Nikaido, O., and Sugahara, T. (1980b). Modifications of doubling potential of cultured human diploid cells by ionizing radiation and hydrocortisone. *Exp. Gerontol.* **15**, 539–549.

Ban, S., Ikushima, T., and Sugahara, T. (1981). Reduction in proliferative life span of human diploid cells after exposure to a reactor radiation beam. *Radiat. Res.* **87**, 1–9.

Ban, S., Iida, S., Chin, N., and Awa, A. A. (1982). *In vitro* life span and UV sensitivity in cells obtained from a multimalformed premature human fetus. *J. Radiat. Res.* **23**, 88–98.

Beebe, G. W., Kato, H., and Land, C. E. (1975). Studies of the mortality of A-bomb survivors. VI. Mortality and radiation dose, 1950–1974. *Radiat. Res.* **75**, 138–201.

Bell, E., Marek, L. F., Levinstone, D. S., Merril, C., Sher, S., Young, I. R., and Eden, M. (1978). Loss of division potential *in vitro:* aging or differentiation? *Science (Washington, D.C.)* **202**, 1158–1163.

Brown, T., Epstein, J., and Little, J. B. (1976). Progeria cells are stimulated on repair DNA by co-cultivation with normal cells. *Exp. Cell Res.* **97**, 291–296.

Clarkson, J. M., and Painter, R. B. (1974). Repair of X-ray damage in aging WI-38 cells. *Mutat. Res.* **23**, 107–112.

Cleaver, J. E. (1968). Defective repair replication of DNA in xeroderma pigmentosum. *Nature (London)* **218**, 652–656.

Cleaver, J. E. (1973). DNA repair with purines and pyrimidines in radiation and carcinogen-damaged normal and xeroderma pigmentosum human cells. *Cancer Res.* **33**, 362–369.

Court-Brown, W. M., and Doll, R. (1958). Expectation of life and longevity of physicians. *Br. Med. J.* **ii**, 181–187.

Cristofalo, R. A. V., Jr., and Huang, P. C. (1976). The proportion of cells labeled with tritiated thymidine as a function of population doubling level in cultures of fetal, adult, mutant, and tumor origin. *Exp. Cell Res.* **102**, 31–42.

Cristofalo, V. J. (1975). The effect of hydrocortisone on DNA synthesis and cell division during aging *in vitro*. *Adv. Exp. Med. Biol.* **53**, 7–22.

Cristofalo, V. J., and Sharf, B. B. (1973). Cellular senescence and DNA synthesis. *Exp. Cell Res.* **76**, 419–427.

Curtis, H. J., and Gebhard, K. (1958). The relative biological effectiveness of fast neutrons and X-rays for life shortening in mice. *Radiat. Res.* **9**, 278–284.

Danes, B. S. (1971). Progeria: a cell culture study on aging. *J. Clin. Invest.* **50**, 2000–2003.

Delihas, N., and Curtis, H. J. (1958). The relative biological effectiveness of fission neutrons for the production of acute mortality in mice. *Radiat. Res.* **8**, 166–180.

Epstein, J., Williams, J. R., and Little, J. B. (1973). Deficient DNA repair in human progeroid cells. *Proc. Natl. Acad. Sci. USA* **70**, 977–981.

Epstein, J., Williams, J. R., and Little, J. B. (1974). Rate of DNA repair in progeria and normal human fibroblasts. *Biochem. Biophys. Res. Commun.* **59**, 850–857.

Gey, G. O., Coffman, W. D., and Kubicek, M. T. (1952). Tissue culture studies of the proliferative capacity of cervical carcinoma and normal epithelium. *Cancer Res.* **12**, 264–265.

Goldstein, S. (1969). Life span of cultured cells in progeria. *Lancet* **i**, 424.

Goldstein, S. (1971). The role of DNA repair in aging of cultured fibroblasts from xeroderma pigmentosum and normals. *Proc. Soc. Exp. Biol. Med.* **137**, 730–734.

Goldstein, S., and Moerman, E. J. (1975). Heat-labile enzymes in Werner's syndrome fibroblasts. *Nature (London)* **255**, 159.

Goldstein, S., and Singal, D. P. (1974). Alteration of fibroblast gene products *in vitro* from a subject with Werner's syndrome. *Nature (London)* **251**, 719–721.

Guilly, Y. L., Simon, M., Lenoir, P., and Bourel, M. (1973). Long-term culture of human adult liver cells: morphological changes related to *in vitro* senescence and effect of donor's are on growth potential. *Gerontologia (Basel)* **19**, 303–313.

Hart, R. W., and Setlow, R. B. (1976). DNA repair in late-passage human cells. *Mech. Ageing Dev.* **5**, 67–77.

Hayflick, L. (1965). The limited *in vitro* lifetime of human diploid cell strains. *Exp. Cell Res.* **37**, 614–636.

Hayflick, L. (1974). The longevity of cultured human cells. *J. Am. Geriatr. Soc.* **22**, 1–12.

Hayflick, L., and Moorhead, P. S. (1961). The serial cultivation of human diploid cell strains. *Exp. Cell Res.* **25**, 585–621.

Holliday, R., and Tarrant, G. M. (1972). Altered enzymes in aging human fibroblasts. *Nature (London)* **238**, 26–30.

Holliday, R., Porterfield, J. S., and Gibbs, D. D. (1974). Premature aging and occurrence of altered enzyme in Werner's syndrome fibroblasts. *Nature (London)* **248**, 762–763.

Igel, H. J., Freeman, A. E., Spiewak, J. E., and Kleinfeld, K. L. (1975). Carcinogenesis *in vitro*. II. Chemical transformation of diploid human cell cultures: a rare event. *In Vitro* **2**, 117–129.

Jablon, S., and Kato, H. (1972). Studies of the mortality of A-bomb survivors. V. Radiation dose and mortality, 1950–1970. *Radiat. Res.* **50**, 649–698.

Kato, H., Brown, C. C., Hoel, D. G., and Schull, W. J. (1982). Life span study report 9. Part 2. Mortality from causes other than cancer among atomic bomb survivors, 1950–1978. *Radiat. Eff. Res. Found. Tech. Rep.* No. 05-81.

Kohn, K. W., Friedman, C. A., Ewig, R. A. G., and Iqbal, Z. M. (1974). DNA chain growth during replication of asynchronous L1210 cells. Alkaline elution of large DNA segments from cells lysed in filters. *Biochemistry* **13**, 4134–4139.

Kohn, K. W., Ewig, R. A. G., Erickson, L. C., and Zwelling, L. A. (1981). Measurement of strand breaks and cross-links by alkaline elution. *In* "DNA Repair: A Laboratory Manual of Research Procedures" (E. C. Friedberg and P. C. Hanawalt, eds.), pp. 379–401. Dekker, New York.

Lavin, M. F., Chen, P. C., and Kidson, C. (1978). Ataxia telangiectasia: characterization of heterozygotes. *In* "DNA Repair Mechanisms" (P. C. Hanawalt, E. C. Friedberg, and C. F. Fox, eds.), pp. 651–654. Academic Press, New York.

Lewis, C. M., and Tarrant, G. M. (1972). Error theory and aging in human diploid fibroblasts. *Nature (London)* **239**, 316–318.

Lindop, P. J., and Rotblat, J. (1961). Long-term effects of a single whole-body exposure of mice to ionizing radiations. II. Causes of death. *Proc. R. Soc. London Ser. B* **154**, 350–368.

Lindop, P. J., and Rotblat, J. (1962). The age factor in the susceptibility of man and animals to radiation. *Br. J. Radiol.* **35**, 23–31.

Macieira-Coelho, A. (1966). Action of cortisone on human fibroblasts *in vitro*. *Experientia* **22**, 390–391.

Macieira-Coelho, A., Diatloff, C., and Malaise, E. (1976). Doubling potential of fibroblasts from different species after ionizing radiation. *Nature (London)* **261**, 586–588.

Macieira-Coelho, A., Diatloff, C., Billarden, C., Bourgeois, C. A., and Malaise, E. (1977). Effect of low dose rate ionizing radiation on the division potential of cells *in vitro*. III. Human lung fibroblasts. *Exp. Cell Res.* **104**, 215–221.

Macieira-Coelho, A., Diatloff, C., Billard, M., Fertil, B., Malaise, E., and Fries, D. (1978). Effect of low dose rate irradiation on the division potential of cells *in vitro*. IV. Embryonic and adult human lung fibroblast-like cells. *J. Cell. Physiol.* **95**, 235–238.

Martin, G. M., Gartler, S. M., Epstein, C. J., and Motulsky, A. G. (1965). Diminished lifespan of cultured cells in Werner's syndrome. *Fed. Proc., Fed. Am. Soc. Exp. Biol.* **24**, 678.

Martin, G. M., Sprague, C. A., and Epstein, C. J. (1970). Replicative life-span of cultivated human cells. Effects of donor's age, tissue, and genotype. *Lab. Invest.* **23**, 86–92.

Matanoski, G. M., Seltser, R., Sartwell, P. E., Diamond, E. L., and Elliot, E. A. (1975). The current mortality rates of radiologists and other physician specialists: deaths from all causes and from cancer. *Am. J. Epidemiol.* **101,** 188–198.

Mattern, M. R., and Cerutti, P. A. (1975). Age-dependent excision repair of damaged thymine from γ-irradiated DNA by isolated nuclei from human fibroblasts. *Nature (London)* **254,** 450–452.

McGrath, R. A., and Williams, R. W. (1966). Reconstruction *in vivo* of irradiated *Escherichia coli* deoxyribonucleic acids; the rejoining of broken pieces. *Nature (London)* **212,** 534–535.

Mitsui, Y., and Schneider, E. L. (1976a). Relationship between cell replication and volume in senescent human diploid fibroblasts. *Mech. Ageing Dev.* **5,** 45–56.

Mitsui, Y., and Schneider, E. L. (1976b). Increased nuclear sizes in senescent human diploid fibroblast culture. *Exp. Cell Res.* **100,** 147–152.

Modak, S. P., and Price, G. B. (1971). Exogenous DNA polymerase-catalysed incorporation of deoxyribonucleotide monophosphates in nuclei of fixed mouse-brain cells. Changes associated with age and X-irradiation. *Exp. Cell Res.* **65,** 289–296.

Mori, T., Horikawa, M., Nikaido, O., and Sugahara, T. (1978). Comparative studies on protective effect of various sulfhydryl compounds against cell death and DNA strand breaks induced by X-rays in cultured mouse L cells. *J. Radiat. Res.* **19,** 319–335.

Nikaido, O., Ban, S., and Sugahara, T. (1980). Population doubling numbers in cells with genetic disorders. *Adv. Exp. Med. Biol.* **129,** 303–311.

Orgel, L. E. (1963). The maintenance of the accuracy of protein synthesis and its relevance to aging. *Biochemistry* **49,** 517–521.

Painter, R. B., Clarkson, J. M., and Young, B. R. (1973). Ultraviolet-induced repair replication in aging diploid human cells (WI-38). *Radiat. Res.* **56,** 560–564.

Paterson, M. C., Smith, B. P., Lohman, P. H. M., Anderson, A. K., and Fishman, L. (1976). Defective excision repair of γ-ray-damaged DNA in human (ataxia telangiectasia) fibroblasts. *Nature (London)* **260,** 444–446.

Price, G. B., Modak, S. P., and Makinodan, T. (1971). Age-associated changes in the DNA of mouse tissue. *Science (Washington, D.C.)* **171,** 917–920.

Puck, T. T., and Marcus, P. I. (1955). A rapid method for viable cell titration and clone production with HeLa cells in tissue culture: the use of X-irradiated cells to supply conditioning factors. *Proc. Natl. Acad. Sci. USA* **41,** 432–437.

Puck, T. T., and Marcus, P. I. (1956). Action of X-rays on mammalian cells. *J. Exp. Med.* **103,** 653–666.

Regan, J. D., and Setlow, R. B. (1974). DNA repair in human progeroid cells. *Biochem. Biophys. Res. Commun.* **59,** 858–864.

Seltser, R., and Sartwell, P. E. (1965). The influence of occupational exposure to radiation on the mortality of American radiologists and other medical specialists. *Am. J. Epidemiol.* **81,** 2–22.

Setlow, R. B., Regan, J. D., German, J., and Carrier, W. L. (1969). Evidence that xeroderma pigmentosum cells do not perform the first step in the repair of ultraviolet damage to their DNA. *Proc. Natl. Acad. Sci. USA* **64,** 1035–1041.

Stanley, J. F., Pye, D., and MacGregor, A. (1975). Comparison of doubling numbers attained by cultured animal cells with life span of species. *Nature (London)* **255,** 158–159.

Storer, J. B. (1965). Radiation resistance with age in normal and irradiated populations of mice. *Radiat. Res.* **25,** 435–459.

Suzuki, F., Watanabe, E., and Horikawa, M. (1980). Repair of X-ray-induced DNA damage in aging human diploid cells. *Exp. Cell Res.* **127,** 229–307.

Taylor, A. M. R. (1978). Unrepaired DNA strand breaks in irradiated ataxia telangiectasia lymphocytes suggested from cytogenetic observations. *Mutat. Res.* **50,** 407–418.

Taylor, A. M. R., Harnden, D. G., Arlett, C. F., Harcourt, S. A., Lehmann, A. R., Stevens, S., and Bridges, B. A. (1975). Ataxia telangiectasia: a human mutation with abnormal radiation sensitivity. *Nature (London)* **258,** 427–429.

Till, J. E., and McCulloch, E. A. (1961). A direct measurement of the radiation sensitivity of normal mouse bone marrow cells. *Radiat. Res.* **14,** 213–222.

Vincent, R. A., Jr., Sheridan, R. B., III, and Huang, P. C. (1975). DNA strand breakage repair in ataxia telangiectasia fibroblast-like cells. *Mutat. Res.* **33,** 357–366.

Warburg, H. E., Jr. (1975). Radiation-induced life-shortening and premature aging. *Adv. Radiat. Biol.* **5,** 145–179.

Warren, S. (1956). Longevity and causes of death from irradiation in physicians. *JAMA J. Am. Med. Assoc.* **126,** 464–468.

Wheeler, K. T., and Lett, J. T. (1974). On the possibility that DNA repair is related to age in non-dividing cells. *Proc. Natl. Acad. Sci. USA* **71,** 1862–1865.

27 Rapid Assay for Measurement of Chemosensitivity of Human Tumors in Vitro

Li-Hui Wei

Department of Gynecology and Obstetrics
People's Hospital of Peking Medical College
Peking, China

Ohtsura Niwa

Department of Experimental Radiology
Faculty of Medicine, Kyoto University,
Kyoto 606, Japan

I. Introduction

Biochemical and cell biological analyses of human cancer have been greatly facilitated by the introduction of tissue culture techniques for the cultivation of human cancer cells as well as xenograft techniques using athymic *nude* mice as recipients of human cancer. The first report of a successful establishment of a human cancer cell line, HeLa cells from cervical carcinoma, was made as early as 1952 (Gay *et al.*). This was soon followed by the pioneering work of Puck and Marcus (1956), who determined the radiosensitivity of HeLa cells by assaying colony-forming abil-

Modification of Radiosensitivity in Cancer Treatment
Copyright © 1984 by Academic Press Japan, Inc.
All rights of reproduction in any form reserved.
ISBN 0-12-676020-9

ity of the cells *in vitro*. Their work demonstrated for the first time that the sensitivity of human cancer cells to anticancer drugs could be assayed *in vitro*, using tissue culture techniques. The development of soft agar assay now enables prediction of the sensitivity to therapeutic agents of tumor cells derived directly from human cancer tissues (Hamberger and Salmon, 1977a).

Nude mice lack a thymus gland and as a result also lack functional cellular immunity (Pantelouris, 1968). Malignant tissues from patients were successfully transplanted into *nude* mice (Rygaard and Povisen, 1969; Giovanella *et al.*, 1972). Attempts were made to use xenograft of human tumors in *nude* mice as an *in vivo* model system for analysis of the response of the tumors to therapeutic agents (Tokita *et al.*, 1980; Giuliani *et al.*, 1981).

Understanding of cellular responses of cancer cells to a variety of anti-cancer agents, as determined by *in vitro* tissue culture systems or by *in vivo* xenograft system using *nude* mice, can aid in prediction of clinical responses of such tumors to chemotherapeutic agents. However, these *in vitro* and *in vivo* systems require long periods of time and a large number of tissue culture materials and mice. We developed the well method, a rapid and a convenient method of assaying the chemosensitivity of human cancer cells. Using multiwell dishes, this method allows for prediction of the response of cells to specific agents in only 3 days. The results obtained are comparable to these seen with conventional colony assays.

II. Materials and Methods

A. Cells and Cell Culture

Three strains of normal and malignant cells, normal human diploid cells and cells derived from carcinoma of the gallbladder and from carcinoma of the colon, and one malignant human cell line, HeLa cells, were used.

Normal human diploid cells derived from skin biopsy of a healthy adult donor were kindly provided by Dr. T. Yagi of the Radiation Biology Center, Kyoto University.

Tumorous tissues, which were determined to be carcinomas of the gallbladder and of the colon, were obtained from Kyoto National Hospital and Kyoto University Hospital. After washing in Eagle's MEM supplemented with 200 units/ml penicillin, 100 μg/ml streptomycin, and 10% heat-inactivated calf serum, tissues were minced into pieces 1–2 mm in diameter. The tissue fragments were placed in 6-cm diameter plastic dishes with 2 ml of α MEM supplemented with antibiotics and 10% heat-inactivated calf serum. Within 4 days tissue fragments were firmly attached to the dish surface and the cells began to migrate out of the fragments, eventually forming a monolayer around the fragments. When the cells were trypsinized and subcultured, the tumor cells and fibroblasts showed different sensitivities to trypsinization. Tumor cells derived from colon cancer showed typical epithelial morphology and adhered to the dish surface more firmly than did the fibroblasts. As a consequence, fibroblasts could be selectively eliminated through trypsinization. Tumor cells derived from patients with gallbladder cancer had a round and refractile morphology. On trypsinization, these cells were quickly recovered in the medium while fibroblasts remained in the monolayer. Therefore, the differential sensitivity to trypsinization of tumor cells and fibroblasts was exploited to obtain a homogeneous population of cells consisting entirely of tumor cells. After several passages of the culture with a particular trypsinization condition, fibroblasts were completely eliminated from the culture.

HeLa cells were obtained from Flow Laboratory, Stanmore, N.S.W., Australia.

Cells used in the present study are listed in Table I.

B. Drug Sensitivity of the Cells

Sensitivity of the cells to eight anticancer drugs (5-fluorouracil, vincristine, bleomycin, actinomycin D, cis-dichlorodiamineplatinum, adriamycin, mitomycin C, and daunomycin) was tested either by the colony method or by the well method we developed.

For the colony method, 2×10^5 cells were seeded onto a plastic dish (6 cm diameter). After an overnight incubation, cultures were treated with anticancer drugs dissolved in medium for 3 h at 37°C. Dishes were washed

TABLE I

Types of Cells Examined

Cell type	Passage	Colony formation	Plating efficiency (%)	Doubling time (h)	Saturation (cell no./ 6-cm dish)
Human diploid	*in vitro*	+	10–30	24	5×10^6
HeLa	*in vitro*	+	100	24	2×10^6
Gall bladder carcinoma no. 1	*in vitro* *in vivo*	+	10–30	59	8×10^5
Colon carcinoma	*in vitro*	+	10–30	45	2×10^6

twice with fresh medium, and cells were collected by trypsinization. Appropriate numbers of the cells were seeded onto plastic dishes, and the colonies formed within 2 weeks were fixed, stained, and scored.

For the well assay, 5×10^3 cells were seeded into each well of 96 multiwell dishes (Falcon). From 3 h to an overnight incubation at 37°C, twofold dilution of anticancer drugs dissolved in medium was added to each well. Cultures were incubated for 3 h at 37°C, washed twice, and fresh medium added. Each well was observed daily under a low-magnification microscope after staining with 0.003% neutral red. A well was scored as + when it had healthy cells with a morphology identical to control cells. A ± score was given to the well in which cells showed differences in morphology; a − score was assigned to the wells in which the cells had all died. The well that was scored as + on the third day after

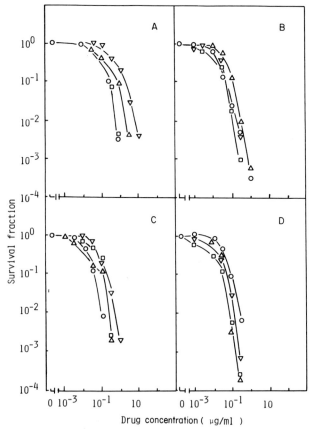

Fig. 1. Chemosensitivity of normal and malignant human cells assayed by the colony method: (○) Normal human diploid cells, (□) HeLa cells, (△) gallbladder carcinoma cells, (▽) colon cancer cells. (A) 5-fluorouracil, (B) vincristine, (C) bleomycin, (D) actinomycin D.

the drug treatment remained + for the subsequent observations. Thus experiments were usually terminated on the third day.

III.   Results

A.   Drug Sensitivity of the Cells Assayed by the Colony Method

Human diploid cells, HeLa cells, gallbladder cancer cells, and colon cancer cells were tested for their sensitivity to eight anticancer drugs, using the colony method (Figs. 1 and 2).

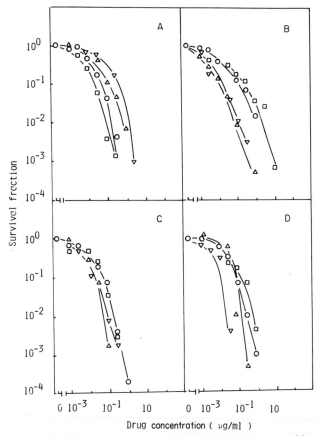

Fig. 2. Chemosensitivity of normal and malignant human cells assayed by the colony method. Symbols are as in Fig. 1. (A) *cis*-Dichlorodiamineplatinum, (B) adriamycin, (C) mitomycin C, (D) daunomycin.

Among the four types of human cells studied, colon cancer cells were the most resistant to 5-fluorouracil and to *cis*-dichlorodiamineplatinum, whereas these cells were the most sensitive to vincristine and actinomycin D. The HeLa cells were the most sensitive to 5-fluorouracil and *cis*-dichlorodiamineplatinum, and the most resistant to vincristine and to actinomycin D.

The sensitivity to vincristine varied widely among the four types of cells. More than a 10-fold difference in D_{10} value was observed among the cells. The response to adriamycin, however, showed the smallest deviation among the cells. Less than a threefold difference in D_{10} values was noted for this drug between the most sensitive (HeLa cells, $D_{10} = 4.7 \times 10^{-2}$ μg/ml) and the most resistant (gallbladder cells, $D_{10} = 1.26 \times 10^{-1}$ μg/ml) cells.

B.   Drug Sensitivity of the Cells Assayed by the Well Method

Five thousand cells were seeded into 96 multiwell dishes. Anticancer drugs were serially diluted twofold. In the usual experiment, 12 dilutions were prepared for each drug. Each dilution was tested on duplicate wells. Multiwell dishes have 96 wells (12 × 8). Thus, four anticancer drugs could be tested in one dish.

Results obtained for mitomycin C were plotted in parallel with the results obtained by the colony method (Fig. 3). As is clear from the figure, cytotoxicity was evident at a lower concentration when observations were made on a later day. Time course of a + well becoming − differed for each type of cell tested. For example, the highest concentration that showed no effect (scored as +) gradually decreased when human diploid cells were tested, whereas the highest concentration of the drug with no effect suddenly decreased on the third day when colon cancer cells were assayed. However, the highest concentration of mitomycin C without any morphological change of the cells in the well on the third day was unchanged with further observations of all four cell types examined (data not shown). The same held for seven other anticancer agents tested. Thus the data on the third day were taken as the end point.

Detailed analysis of the results by the well method obtained for eight therapeutic agents indicated that the highest concentrations of the drugs without effect fell on the same range as D_{10} values assayed by the colony method. Similarly, the highest concentrations of the drugs that gave ± results corresponded approximately to doses that reduced the survival of the cells to 1% level.

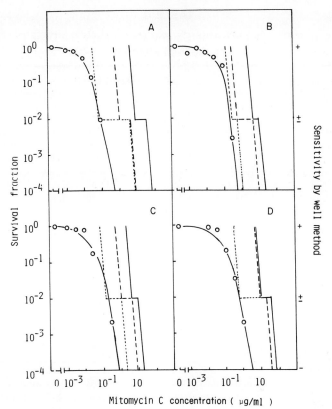

Fig. 3. Comparison of the well and colony methods. Observation made on the first day after the drug treatment (————); observation made on the second day (— — — —); observation made on the third day (----).

C.   Comparison of Findings with the Colony and the Well Methods

The D_{10} values of human diploid cells, HeLa cells, gallbladder cancer cells, and colon cancer cells for eight anticancer drugs, and the highest dose that gave a + result in the well assay are given in Table II. The values determined by these two methods are in good agreement. The one exception was the sensitivity of colon cancer cells to actinomycin D. The dose determined by the well method was four times higher than the D_{10} value seen with the colony method. All other values are within threefold deviation.

TABLE II

Comparison of D_{10} Values by the Colony Method and the Dose Determined by the Well Method[a]

	D_{10} and Dose (μg/ml)							
	Human dip-loid		HeLa		Gall-1		Colon	
Drug and concentration (μg/ml)	Colony D_{10}	Well	Colony D_{10}	Well	Colony D_{10}	Well	Colony D_{10}	Well
5-FU	6.02	4.68	2.24	2.34	11.4	37.5	4.47	9.37
VCR ($\times 10^{-1}$)	12.6	11.7	23.4	11.7	1.10	1.46	1.17	0.73
BLM	5.62	2.34	5.76	9.37	2.51	1.17	1.99	2.34
Act-D ($\times 10^{-1}$)	7.94	5.86	10.1	5.86	8.32	2.92	1.26	5.86
CisPt ($\times 10^{-1}$)	3.55	5.86	2.81	5.86	6.31	2.92	17.8	46.8
ADM ($\times 10^{-2}$)	6.31	3.66	4.17	3.66	12.6	7.32	11.2	14.6
MMC ($\times 10^{-2}$)	3.55	3.66	18.5	14.6	7.94	7.32	19.5	29.3
DAM ($\times 10^{-2}$)	15.8	14.6	3.24	1.83	4.47	1.83	6.03	7.32

[a] Abbreviations: 5-FU, 5-fluorouracil; VCR, vincristine; BLM, bleomycin; Act-D, actinomycin D; CisPt, *cis*-dichlorodiamineplatinum; ADM, adriamycin; MMC, mitomycin C; DAM, daunomycin. Gall-1, gallbladder carcinoma cell no. 1.

IV. Discussion

Colony formation assay provides precise and quantitative data on the response of cells to anticancer agents. The soft agar clonogenic assay aids in predicting which agent to prescribe for treatment of a particular cancer (Hamberger and Salmon, 1977a,b; Salmon *et al.*, 1978; Pavelic *et al.*, 1980). However, these assays are not only time consuming but also require a large number of dishes for accurate measurement of the cellular responses. Rapid methods have been developed using incorporation of [^{3}H]thymidine into acid-insoluble fraction of cells treated with therapeutic agents (Murphy *et al.*, 1975; Bech-Hansen *et al.*, 1977; Raich, 1978; Tanigawa *et al.*, 1982).

Another rapid test, the tissue culture microtest, is similar to the one we developed here and is useful for the prediction of the clinical response of human cancer (Holmes and Little, 1974). In this test, biopsied tumor tissues are seeded directly onto microwell dishes. The cell number in each well is counted 3 days after treating the cells with drugs, and this number serves as a measure of the cellular response to the drugs. Of 13 microtests, only one differed from the clinical result.

In the present study, the well and colony methods were compared. Results were obtained for a combination of four types of cells and eight anticancer agents. To our knowledge, this is the first attempt to compare the well and colony methods. In most cases, the effective drug concentration estimated by both methods fell within the same dose range. Although the results obtained by the well method are qualitative, the short period of time and small amount of materials required shows the usefulness of this approach. Using only one multiwell dish, we were able to screen four different anticancer drugs. Because large amounts of experimental data should eventually lead to a better prognosis for cancer patients, the convenience of the well method permits a large-scale study of chemosensitivity of cancer tissues obtained clinically.

Acknowledgments

We thank Drs. N. Tanigawa and Y. Mizuno for pertinent advice during the experiments.

References

Bech-Hansen, N. T., Sarangi, F., Sutherland, D. J. A., and Ling, V. (1977). Rapid assays for evaluating the drug sensitivity of tumor cells. *J. Natl. Cancer Inst. (US)* **59**, 21–27.

Gay, G., Coffman, W., and Kubiceck, M. (1952). Tissue culture studies of the proliferative capacity of cervical carcinoma and normal epithelium. *Cancer Res.* **12**, 264–265.

Giovanella, B. C., Sterlin, J. S., and Williams, L. J. (1972). Development of invasive tumors in the *nude* mouse after injection of cultured human melanoma cells. *J. Natl. Cancer Inst. (US)* **48**, 1531–1533.

Giuliani, F. C., Zirvi, K. A., and Kaplan, N. O. (1981). Therapeutic response of human tumor xenografts in athymic mice to doxorubicin. *Cancer Res.* **41**, 325–335.

Hamberger, A. W., and Salmon, S. E. (1977a). Primary bioassay of human tumor stem cells. *Science (Washington, D.C.)* **197**, 461–463.

Hamberger, A. W., and Salmon, S. E. (1977b). Primary bioassay of human myeloma stem cells. *J. Clin. Invest.* **60**, 846–854.

Holmes, H. L., and Little, L. M. (1974). Tissue-culture microtest for predicting response of human cancer to chemotherapy. *Lancet* **2**, 985–987.

Murphy, W. K., Livingston, R. B., Ruiz, V. G., Gercovich, F. G., George, S. L., Hart, J. S., and Freireich, E. J. (1975). Serial labeling index determination as a predictor of response in human solid tumors. *Cancer Res.* **35**, 1438–1444.

Pantelouris, E. M. (1968). Absence of thymus in a mouse mutant. *Nature (London)* **217**, 370–371.

Pavelic, Z. P., Slocom, H. K., Rustum, Y. M., Creaven, P. J., Nowak, N. J., Karakousis, C., Takita, H., and Mittelman, A. (1980). Growth of cell colonies in soft agar from biopsies of different human solid tumors. *Cancer Res.* **40,** 4151–4158.

Puck, T. T., and Marcus, P. I. (1956). Action of X-rays on mammalian cells. *J. Exp. Med.* **103,** 653–666.

Raich, P. C. (1978). Prediction of therapeutic response in acute leukemia. *Lancet* **1,** 74–76.

Rygaard, J., and Povison, C. O. (1969). Heterotransplantation of a human malignant tumor to *nude* mice. *Acta Pathol. Microbiol. Scand.* **77,** 758–760.

Salmon, S. E., Hamberger, A. W., Soehnlen, B., Durie, B. G. M., Albert, D. S., and Moon, T. E. (1978). Quantitation of differential sensitivity of human tumor cells to anticancer drugs. *N. Engl. J. Med.* **298,** 1321–1327.

Tanigawa, N., Kern, D. H., Hikasa, Y., and Morton, D. L. (1982). Rapid assay for evaluating the chemosensitivity of human tumors in soft agar culture. *Cancer Res.* **42,** 2159–2164.

Tokita, H., Tanaka, N., Sekimoto, K., Ueno, T., Okamoto, K., and Fujimura, S. (1980). Experimental model for combination chemotherapy with metronidazole using human uterine cervical carcinoma transplanted into *nude* mice. *Cancer Res.* **40,** 4278–4294.

Index

A

Absorbed power, measurement of, hyperthermia and, 315–317
Actinomycin D
  assay of tumor cell sensitivity to, 525–526, 528, 529, 530
  SLD and PLD repair and, 229, 237
Adenocarcinoma, spontaneous, chlorpromazine and, 303
Adenosine triphosphate, chlorpromazine and, 300
Adenylate cyclase, activation of, 267
Adrenochrome derivatives, radiation protection by, 32–34, 49
  combination with other drugs, 64
  in mice and humans, 67
Adrenochrome monoguanylhydrazone methane-sulfonate, clinical trials of, 64–68
Adriamycin
  assay of tumor cell sensitivity to, 525, 527, 528, 530
  DNA and, 236
Aging, repairability of radiation-induced damage and, 507–510
Alcohols, radioprotection and, 51
Alkylating agents
  and nucleoside analogs, experimental cancer therapy and, 241–242
  PLD repair and, 230
  therapeutic gain and, 159–161
DL-5-Alkylthiomethyl-5-methylhydantoin, radioprotection and, 50
S-(2-Aminoethyl)isothiouronim (AET), radioprotection by, 37–39, 47
  combination with other drugs and, 53
Aminomisonidazole, toxicity of, 157
S-2-(5-Aminopentylamino)ethylphosphorothioic acid, radio protection and, 49, 50

p-Aminopropiophenone, radioprotection and, 48
  combination with other drugs, 53
2-(3-Aminopropylamino)ethylmercaptan, radioprotection and, 51
S-2-(3-Aminopropylamino)ethylphosphothioic acid, see WR-2721
Anesthetics, local, cell killing by bleomycin and, 239
Animals, species, *in vitro* lifespan of cells and, 497
Anoxic chamber system, principle of, 131–132
Aphidicolin, PLD repair and, 231
Aqueous solutions
  deoxygenated, products of irradiation, 87–88
  oxygen containing, products of irradiation, 88–89
1-β-D-Arabinofuranosyladenine, experimental cancer therapy and, 240, 241, 242
Arrhenius plot
  Chinese hamster V-79 thermal survival and, 445–447
  for thermal cell killing, 339, 340
  of thermal killing of GHE cells, 355, 356
Ascites tumor cells, chlorpromazine and, 303
Ataxia telangiectasia cells
  characterization of repair deficiency in, 254–256
  dose–survival curves of, 489, 491
  radiosensitivity, DNA repair and DNA replication in, 489
  assay of radiosensitivity, 467
  cell labeling and alkaline elution method, 466–467
  colony-forming method, 465
  discussion, 473–474
  establishment of cell strains and culture medium, 464–465

533